W.B. SAUNDERS COMPANY
PHILADELPHIA LONDON TORONTO
MEXICO CITY RIO DE JANEIRO
SYDNEY TOKYO HONG KONG

1986

LABORATORY IMMUNOLOGY AND SEROLOGY

SECOND EDITION

Neville J. Bryant, ART, FACBS

Technical Director, Serological Services, Ltd., Toronto
President, Serological Serums, Ltd.
Toronto, Ontario, Canada

W. B. Saunders Company: West Washington Square
                          Philadelphia, PA   19105

Library of Congress Cataloging in Publication Data

Bryant, Neville J.
   Laboratory immunology and serology.

   Includes bibliographies and index.
1. Serology—Technique.   2. Immunodiagnosis.
   I. Title. [DNLM: 1. Allergy and immunology—laboratory
manuals.   2. Serology—laboratory manuals. QW 525
B915L]

RB46.5.B79 1986   616.07′561   85-11871

ISBN 0-7216-1059-5

Editor: Baxter Venable
Designer: Bill Donnelly
Production Manager: Laura Tarves
Illustration Coordinator: Peg Shaw

Laboratory Immunology and Serology   ISBN   0-7216-1059-5

Last digit is the print number: 9   8   7   6   5   4   3   2   1

PREFACE

This book is designed for students of medical technology studying the sciences of serology and immunology as a separate entity, or as part of a microbiology course. The material provides the theory and practical procedures necessary for a basic yet thorough understanding of serological principles.

In response to readers' requests, the immunology section of the book in this, the second edition, has been greatly enlarged. The material presented, however, remains at an introduction level, unencumbered by the research information which is of little use to the student.

Again, each chapter is preceded by a set of learning objectives and each contains a set of review questions with answers given at the end of the book. General references are given after each chapter that will direct the student to other texts containing specific information about the subject under discussion.

The book attempts to say nothing startling or new; its purpose is to introduce the student to the fascinating science of serology and immunology and, perhaps, to whet the student's appetite for further, more advanced study.

Many people have contributed in one way or another to the preparation of the second edition, and I wish to express my gratitude to them. Most especially, my thanks go to Nancy Harrison, who performed many of the tasks necessary to achieve the completion of the text with diligence and cheerfulness.

Appreciation is also due to the people at W. B. Saunders Company, who are always supportive and patient—most especially Baxter Venable, my editor, whose interest in this project is always there, and who has shown patience, support and inspiration during the lengthy preparation of this second edition.

NEVILLE J. BRYANT

CONTENTS

ONE

INTRODUCTION: NONSPECIFIC (NATURAL, INNATE) IMMUNITY

OBJECTIVES

The student shall know, understand, and be prepared to explain:

1. A brief history of immunology
2. Types of nonspecific immunity
3. The concepts of susceptibility and nonsusceptibility
4. The role of the epithelial barriers in nonspecific immunity
5. Inflammation, with special emphasis on the vascular and cellular response
6. Phagocytosis, encompassing the contributing mechanisms: chemotaxis, opsonization, ingestion, and degranulation
7. The concepts of nonspecific humoral immunity with respect to:
   a. "Natural antibody"
   b. Lysozyme
   c. Properdin
   d. Betalysin
   e. Interferon
   f. Complement

The science of immunology represents that area of biology that is concerned with the processes by which all living organisms (including human beings) defend themselves against infection (*i.e.,* the study of immunity).

The term *immunity* can be used to imply "resistance" in its broadest sense, including resistance to infectious agents, foreign particles, toxins (poisonous substances), living cells, and cancer.

The principles of immunology stem almost from the earliest written observations of humankind, in which it was noted that individuals who recovered from a certain disease rarely contracted the same disease again. This observation prompted deliberate attempts to induce immunity: In A.D. 1500, the Chinese developed a custom of inhaling crusts from smallpox lesions to prevent the development of smallpox in later life. The procedure was, at best, hazardous. By 1718, the practice of injecting material from crusts or fluids from smallpox blisters (known as "variolation") was used extensively throughout the Eastern world and was introduced into Western medicine by Lady Montagu, the wife of the British ambassador to Turkey, who had her children so treated. By the time that the American colonies developed into an independent nation, variolation was a reasonably common practice, and clear evidence had been obtained that it was effective in most cases. The problem that could not be overcome, however, was that the virus used could be transmitted; therefore, protection by variolation was hazardous to the community at large.

In 1798, an English physician, Jenner, published his monumental work on vaccination, describing a related, yet safe, procedure. Realizing that individuals who had had cowpox were spared in smallpox epidemics, he inoculated a boy with pus from an individual who had cowpox and subsequently reinoculated the same boy with infectious pus from a patient in the active state of smallpox. No disease state followed these inoculations, and the experiment was repeated several times with great success. The term *vaccination* (L. *vacca* = cow) was applied to the procedure and referred specifically to the injection of smallpox "vaccine." The term has now come to mean any immunizing procedure in which vaccine is injected.

Jenner's discovery provided the first clear evidence that active immunization could be used safely to prevent an infectious disease, that attenuated (thinned, weakened) viruses could be used for effective active immunization, and that resistance to infection might be related to the speed and intensity of inflammatory reactions. The concept of interference of one virus infection by another was also suggested in Jenner's work.

Almost 70 years later, these discoveries were extended by Pasteur, who showed that heat could kill bacteria, and, from this observation, the term *pasteurization,* came into use. In addition, Pasteur recognized and exploited the general principles underlying vaccination through the observation that the inoculation of the causative agents of chicken cholera and anthrax in animals induced immunity against these diseases. Later, he also made the outstanding contribution of vaccination against rabies.

In the two decades before 1900, Elie Metchnikoff, a Russian biologist, who was one of the major pioneers of immunology, elucidated the role of phagocytosis and cellular immunity. Within the same period of time, killed vaccines were introduced, complement (alexin) was described, and the comparative roles of complement and cell lysis were elucidated.

Discoveries in the field of immunology during the twentieth century have been numerous and have profoundly influenced the development of every branch of medicine and surgery. In 1903, Write and Douglas demonstrated that acquired immunity resulted from both humoral and cellular elements and described opsonization. As a result of these observations and discoveries, the term *antigen* (antibody + Gr. *gennan* = to produce) came into regular use to describe the agent that conferred immunity on the host by the production of specific antibody.

In 1902, Richet and Portier provided evidence that the immune reaction could be damaging as well as beneficial by showing anaphylaxis to be an immunologic reaction. The following year, the Arthus reaction was described, and, at about the same time, von Pirquet and Schick showed as part of their studies of serum sickness that diseases of the skin, heart, joints, blood vessels, and kidneys, as well as fever, could be caused by the body's immunologic reaction to foreign protein. By 1920, the immunologic basis of certain kinds of allergy had also been reported by Prausnitz and Kustner.

In another direction of inquiry, Paul Ehrlich was the first to use quantitative measurements of immune reactions. Then, in 1928, Alexander Fleming discovered penicillin, and, in 1932, Gerhard Domagk developed prontosil, which was found to be an effective antibacterial agent against streptococcus. Later, the active ingredient was found to be sulfanilamide, which proved to be active against a wide variety of organisms.

The understanding of immune reactions has been enhanced by the techniques for analysis of these processes, including the precise chemical methods for measurement of antigens and antibodies through precipitin analysis (introduced by Heidelberger, 1924-1926), immunoelectrophoresis (Grabar and Williams, 1953), and so forth.

Studies of immunodeficiency and structure-function relationships in the lymphoid system were initiated as a result of the discovery of hypogammaglobulinemia (Burton, 1952), which eventually led to the dissection of the immune system into two separate areas, known as the T- and B-cell systems.

In addition, the studies of Medawar *et al.* (1944, 1945) initiated interest in transplantation and showed that the immunologic processes are clearly involved in allograft rejection of normal organs.

At the present time, it is safe to say that immunology has an impact on all medical disciplines. Many patients are recognized who have immunologic deficiencies or abnormal immune responses as the sole basis for their disease. It is therefore clear that no other body of knowledge is as important for medical personnel to study and understand as are the fundamentals of the immune process.

NONSPECIFIC IMMUNITY

Two types of immunity are recognized: (1) that which is present at the time of birth or that develops during maturation ("natural"), and (2) that which is acquired as a result of prior experience with a foreign substance.

Nonspecific ("natural" or "innate") immunity, therefore, is the process by which all animals (including humans) resist the invasion of foreign or potentially harmful microorganisms by natural means (*i.e.,* without the production of protective antibodies). This includes the concepts of susceptibility and nonsusceptibility, epithelial barriers, antibacterial agents, inflammation, complement, phagocytosis, acid pH of stomach, normal intestinal flora, and so forth.

Susceptibility and Nonsusceptibility

Certain animal species are resistant to particular disease states, whereas other species are highly susceptible to them. This phenomenon is not clearly understood, although there is growing evidence that it is controlled to some extent by hereditary or genetic influences. An example of this would be the Fy^a and Fy^b (Duffy) receptors on the erythrocyte membrane, which are believed to be associated with susceptibility to malaria. Studies by Miller and colleagues (1975, 1976) showed that the red cells of individuals who had not inherited the Fy^a or Fy^b receptors (*i.e.*, individuals of Duffy phenotype Fy[a − b −]) were resistant to invasion *in vitro* with *Plasmodium knowlesi*. Of 17 volunteers exposed to the bites of *Plasmodium vivax*–infected mosquitoes, only those with the red cell phenotype Fy(a − b −) were resistant to erythrocyte infection.

The concepts of susceptibility and nonsusceptibility are not confined to species differences; they are evident among different races of humans and can be affected by age and the influence of hormones.

The Epithelial Barriers

The skin and mucous membranes provide the body with a physical barrier against invasion and, in addition, possess certain active mechanisms for the killing of bacteria and other organisms. This protection is in many ways remarkable, because many epithelial surfaces consist of only a single layer and are exposed to large numbers of bacteria. Complete sterilization of these surfaces by artificial means is impossible except, perhaps, for brief periods of time.

The self-sterilizing power of the skin is achieved by desiccation (drying), epithelial desquamation (shedding), pH, and, most important, the secretion of fatty acids that have antibacterial properties.

Mucosal surfaces, by contrast, are protected by a so-called slime layer, which has been shown to possess antibodies of the IgA class (see page 15) and other antimicrobial and antiviral substances. The bacterial enzyme *lysozyme* is present in abundance in such secretions (*e.g.*, saliva, tears), as well as in the granules of polymorphs and macrophages, and is widely distributed throughout the body fluids. This enzyme is especially effective in lysing certain bacteria (*e.g.*, *Micrococcus lysodeikticus*).

In addition to this, a nonspecific antiviral agent known as *interferon*, which inhibits intracellular viral replication, is itself synthesized by cells in response to viral infection. It is evident that interferon is a major factor in the recovery from (as distinct from the prevention of) viral infections.

Inflammation

Inflammation is the term used to describe the condition into which tissues enter as a reaction to injury—the classic signs of which are pain, heat, redness, and swelling, and sometimes a loss of function. The inflammatory process involves the *cellular defenses* of the body, which are among the most efficient and adaptive of all mechanisms available for the resistance to invasion by parasitic microorganisms. In addition, the *vascular response* aids in preventing the invasion of bacterial agents beyond the periphery of the body.

In brief, the inflammatory process is characterized by the vascular response and the cellular responses.

The Vascular Response. The primary response in acute inflammation is the dilation of the artery so that more blood passes to the area of injury. This increased content of blood is termed *hyperemia* and is the reason why the inflamed area appears red. As a result of this, plasma leaks from the vessels, making the blood more viscoid; the lubricating action of the plasmatic zone is impaired; and the stream of blood slows down (referred to as *stasis*). At the same time, the endothelial cells become swollen, and the spaces between adjacent cells become widened, thereby permitting plasma and cells to pass between them.

The most characteristic feature of acute inflammation is the formation of an exudate that has both a fluid and a cellular component. The fluid exudate is formed as a result of increased vascular permeability, which allows the plasma proteins to leak through the vessel wall, causing the osmotic pressure effect of the plasma proteins to be lost. In addition, there is an alteration in the "ground substance," which becomes more fluid, thus allowing the exudate to diffuse into the surrounding tissues more readily, preventing an immediate rise in tissue tension. Although it is normal for the tissues to drive fluid back into the venules, tissue tension does eventually increase, thus limiting the amount of exudate formed and causing pain.

The fluid exudate has almost the same composition as plasma, and it contains antibacterial substances (*e.g.*, complement) as well as specific antibodies. Drugs and antibiotics, if present in the plasma, also appear in the exudate.

In addition to these effects, the fluid exudate serves to dilute any irritating chemicals and bacterial toxins that might be present. In addition, the fibrinogen that is in the exudate is converted to fibrin by the action of tissue thromboplastins, and a fibrin clot forms. This fibrin forms a fine network of fibers, which provides a union between severed tissues, acts as a barrier against bacterial invasion, and aids phagocytosis (discussed later in this chapter).

The Cellular Response. The cellular response begins when white cells move into the plasmatic zone at the site of injury and stick to the altered vessel wall. At first, this adhesion is brief, after which the cells either roll gently along the endothelial lining or get swept back into the blood stream. Later, however, the cells adhere more firmly and line the endothelium, forming masses that may even block the lumen (known as *pavementation of the endothelium*). These adhering white cells will eventually push pseudopodia between adjacent endothelial cells, penetrate the basement membrane, and emerge on the external surface of the vessel (known as *emigration of the white cells*). The gap that is left by the emigrating white cells soon closes behind it, although sometimes a few red cells escape at the same time.

A characteristic feature of the cellular exudate is that in the initial stages of development, neutrophil polymorphonuclear leukocytes (polymorphs) predominate, but, as time goes by, these are replaced by monocytes (probably due to the faster migration and limited life span of polymorphs, which die off, leaving the long-lived mononuclear cells to replace them). Lymphocytes are also found in areas of inflammation, particularly during the healing process, although in certain instances (*e.g.,* viral infections, acute dermatitis), they are the predominant cell in the early stages of inflammation.

The function of the cellular exudate is to enact the process known as *phagocytosis.*

Phagocytosis

The action of the phagocytes is one of the most remarkable and fascinating of all body defense mechanisms. Early descriptions of the phenomenon known as phagocytosis are attributed to Elie Metchnikoff (1907), a Russian-born biologist, who recognized that specialized phagocytic (eating) cells provide a defense mechanism against invasion by engulfing foreign particulate matter, which they then attempt to destroy enzymatically. Metchnikoff observed that the process is a very general one and can be observed in animals of all stages of evolution.

The mechanisms contributing to phagocytosis include *chemotaxis, opsonization, ingestion,* and *degranulation.*

Chemotaxis. Chemotaxis is a process in which cells tend to move in a certain direction under the stimulation of chemical substances. This stimulation can cause two effects: (1) the cells may move

toward the stimulating substance (known as *positive* chemotaxis), or (2) the cells may move *away* from the stimulating substance (known as *negative* chemotaxis). Without the influence of these chemotactic substances, cell motion is random.

Leukocytes have never been shown to display negative chemotaxis; they are always drawn *toward* the substance and, therefore, to the site of injury. This is a critical early step in phagocytosis.

A considerable amount of research has been devoted to the identification of the chemicals responsible for chemotaxis in acute inflammation in humans. Agents such as starch and certain bacteria have been shown to attract both polymorphs and monocytes *in vitro.* Other chemotactic agents are antigen-antibody complexes and dead tissue, although these function only if complement is present and activated (C567 and the anaphylatoxins C3a and C5a being the chemotactic agents).

Opsonization. Of great importance in the phagocytic process is a group of antibodies known as serum opsonins (*i.e.,* antibodies and complement components). These antibodies interact with the surface of bacteria, rendering it acceptable to the phagocyte. Antibodies are able to opsonize by themselves, or they can cause the complement system (see page 24) to generate C3 (C1423), which coats the bacterium. Phagocytes apparently possess surface Fc receptors for Ig and C3 receptors that recognize and interact with antibodies and activated C3. Because time is required for these antibodies to develop, they are of greater significance in the later stages of inflammation than in the earlier stages.

Ingestion. Once the phagocyte has recognized that a particle is foreign, engulfment occurs by active ameboid motion (*i.e.,* resembling an ameba in movement). The phagocyte extends its cytoplasmic membrane around the invading organism, which is eventually surrounded and completely enclosed. This final structure containing the phagocytosed particle is known as the phagocytic "vacuole" or "phagosome" (Fig. 1–1).

Degranulation. When ingestion of the foreign particle is complete, cytoplasmic lysosomes (minute cell particles), which contain certain hydrolytic enzymes and peroxidase, approach the phagosome (vacuole), fuse with it, rupture, and discharge their contents into it. The mechanisms by which this phenomenon occurs are unknown. The cell then becomes degranulated as foreign materials (with the exception of inert materials) are digested. Bacteria are not always destroyed by hydrolytic enzymes. Some may survive and eventually break out of the cell again.

Nonspecific Immunity of Body Fluids

Body fluids and secretions have long been known to possess antibacterial properties. In many in

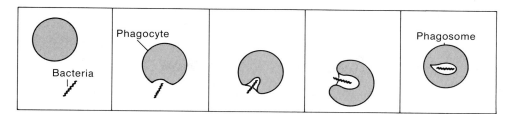

Figure 1–1. Phagocytosis (ingestion of foreign matter).

stances, the action of specific antibody and complement accounts for these properties; however, additional substances that play a significant role in nonspecific defense may be present.

"Natural" Antibody. An antibody that is present in a host and reacts with substances with which the host has had no known contact is referred to as "natural" antibody. Three possible mechanisms have been proposed to explain their formation:

1. *Genetic.* It is possible that natural antibody production is under genetic control and, therefore, that no antigenic stimulation of any kind is required for this production.
2. *Cross-reaction.* It has also been proposed that natural antibodies may be produced as a result of stimulation by specific antigens that have similar (but not identical) antigenic determinant groups that cross-react with the particular antigen by virtue of these chance similarities.
3. *Antigenic stimulation.* It is also possible that "natural" antibodies arise as the result of direct, specific antigenic stimulation—the antigens gaining access to the host by natural means. This possibility is the one that has achieved the widest general acceptance.

Lysozyme. Lysozyme is an enzyme found in many types of cells, which has been shown to have antibacterial activity. The enzyme functions by virtue of mucolytic properties that cleave acetyla-mino-sugars, the backbone of both gram-positive and gram-negative bacteria. Certain basic polypeptides (with large amounts of lysine) have been shown to kill anthrax. A synergistic action of the effect of lysozyme and complement has been observed in *in vitro* studies.

Properdin. Properdin is a serum protein that exerts bactericidal and viricidal effects in the presence of the third component of complement (C3) and magnesium ions. Originally described as a naturally occurring euglobulin with a broad spectrum of activity against bacteria, evidence now suggests that the presence of minute amounts of "natural" antibody accounts for the properdin effect. Properdin, however, is indistinguishable from these antibodies by virtue of the fact that they are capable of combining with certain monomolecular antigens to activate the complement sequence at the level of the third component (see Complement Activation—The Alternative Pathway, page 32).

Betalysin. The serum from many animal species contains a heat-stable substance with antibacterial activity. This substance (which is not present in plasma from the same animal) is known as betalysin. The substance is released during coagulation and probably functions through an enzymatic alteration of the cell surfaces of susceptible bacteria.

Interferon. Interferon is a nonspecific inhibitor of viral replication, its action being at the cellular level. It is a substance that has a molecular weight of about 25,000, which is released from infected cells following viral infection. It is also released from sensitized lymphocytes upon interaction with specific antigens and nonspecific stimulators (*e.g.,* phytohemagglutinins, PHA). Interferon is known to be significant in the recovery mechanism of viral infections, being particularly well suited to cell-mediated responses involving interactions *in vivo*.

Complement. Complement may be regarded as a group of nonspecific serum components, which, when activated by the interaction of antigen and antibody, combine in a fixed sequence and thereby enhance the effect of antibody (see Chapter 3).

The following is a brief summary of the biologic functions of complement in immune defense:

1. *Cytolysis.* A few species of bacteria are lysed by complement—primarily the gram-negative organisms, such as *Escherichia coli*. This is achieved through the full activation of the complement system, which allows lysozyme to reach the plasma membrane, where it destroys the mucopeptide layer.
2. *Immune Adherence* (C3b). This leads to the phagocytosis of microorganisms after coating with opsonizing antibody and complement or after complement activation via the alternative pathway (see page 32). Because many C3 molecules are bound to the surface membrane at each complement activation site, adherence to macrophages and polymorphs will occur more frequently through C3 than through IgG binding.
3. *Immunoconglutinin.* This may play a role in defense by agglutinating relatively small complexes containing bound C3, thereby making them more susceptible to phagocytosis.
4. *Inflammation.* The split fragments from complement components during consumption stimulate two helpful features of acute inflammation:

a. *Chemotactic factors.* By chemotaxis, phagocytic neutrophil polymorphs are attracted to the site of complement activation.

b. *Anaphylatoxin.* Anaphylatoxin, through histamine release, increases vascular permeability and hence the flow of serum antibody and complement to the infected area.

5. *Others.* Complement is also implicated in disease processes involving cytotoxic and immune complex–mediated hypersensitivities:

a. *Cytotoxic reactions.* These are not uncommon findings in nephrotoxic nephritis and autoimmune hemolytic anemia.

b. *Immune complexes.* These are formed in antibody excess, giving rise to immune vasculitis of the Arthus type. Soluble complexes formed in antibody excess give "serum-sickness"–type reactions.

In paroxysmal nocturnal hemoglobinuria (PNH), red cells are particularly sensitive to complement lysis due to an ability to fix the activated trimolecular complex C$\overline{567}$ at night when the pH of the plasma decreases. It should be noted that this is an erythrocyte membrane defect and is not due to an abnormality in the complement system.

Other Nonspecific Factors. Plant extracts, the sera of invertebrates, and other body fluids of animals have been shown to have antibacterial activity. Although the properties of most of these substances have not been extensively studied, it is apparent that these antibacterial properties have arisen as a result of evolutionary selection rather than as a result of exposure to specific microorganisms or antigenic determinants. Several non–antibody serum proteins can also be included among these.

Accumulation of metabolic intermediaries at sites of inflammation is associated with a lowering of the pH, which has an antibacterial effect, as have basic peptides and histones, which are released at the sites of inflammation by dead or dying cells.

Other Aspects of Nonspecific Immunity

Nonspecific immunity is controlled by genetic factors (as evidenced by interspecies differences in susceptibility and nonsusceptibility, racial and individual differences, and certain immunologic deficiency diseases, which are known to be genetically determined) and by the endocrine system (as evidenced by observations of susceptibility and nonsusceptibility influenced by hormones, adrenal hormones, thyroid hormones, sex hormones, and pineal hormones).

In addition, nonspecific immunity has been shown to be influenced by nutritional factors, age, and environmental and therapeutic factors such as exercise and exposure, irradiation, local wound care, drugs, and anesthesia.

Certain selected diseases have been shown to affect nonspecific immunity, either through an increase or decrease in the capacity for phagocytosis and/or a diminished or increased capacity for intracellular killing of bacteria. These include diabetes mellitus, cancer, and uremia. Prematurity and burn injury may also affect nonspecific immunity in this way, as can shock, infection, and alcohol intoxication.

Nonspecific immunity can be stimulated by drugs such as endotoxin (in small doses) tuberculin, zymosan, and restim. An increase in body temperature is also associated with an increase in metabolic function, which has a beneficial effect on nonspecific immunity. In addition, the transfusion of viable leukocytes from both normal donors and patients with chronic myelogenous leukemia is often effective in temporarily elevating the leukocyte count and thereby exerting a favorable effect on nonspecific immunity.

REVIEW QUESTIONS

MULTIPLE CHOICE

Choose the phrase, sentence, or symbol that completes the statement or answers the question. More than one answer may be correct in each case. Answers are given at the end of this book.

1. The process by which an animal resists the invasion of foreign or potentially harmful microorganisms by natural means (*i.e.,* without the production of protective antibodies) is known as:
   (a) humoral immunity
   (b) innate immunity
   (c) epithelial immunity
   (d) none of the above
   (*Introduction*)

2. The self-sterilizing power of the skin is achieved by:
   (a) desiccation
   (b) epithelial desquamation
   (c) pH
   (d) the secretion of fatty acids that have antibacterial properties
   (*The Epithelial Barriers*)

3. The mucosal surfaces of the body are protected by a so-called slime layer, which has been shown to possess antibodies of the:
   (a) IgM class
   (b) IgG glass
   (c) IgA class
   (d) IgE class
   (*The Epithelial Barriers*)

4. The classic signs of inflammation are:
   (a) pain
   (b) heat
   (c) redness
   (d) swelling
   (*Inflammation*)

5. The "slowing" of the blood stream is referred to as:
   (a) hyperemia
   (b) stasis
   (c) the vascular response
   (d) none of the above
   (*Inflammation: The Vascular Response*)

6. The fluid exudate in acute inflammation:
   (a) is formed as a result of decreased vascular permeability
   (b) has almost the same composition as plasma
   (c) contains drugs and antibiotics if these are present in the plasma
   (d) contains specific antibodies
   (*Inflammation: The Vascular Response*)

7. The cellular exudate in acute inflammation:
   (a) contains neutrophil polymorphonuclear leukocytes
   (b) has almost the same composition as plasma
   (c) enacts the process of phagocytosis
   (d) contains lymphocytes only
   (*Inflammation: The Cellular Response*)

8. The mechanisms contributing to phagocytosis include:
   (a) chemotaxis
   (b) opsonization
   (c) ingestion
   (d) degranulation
   (*Phagocytosis*)

9. An antibody that is present in a host and reacts with substances with which the host has had no known contact is referred to as:
   (a) innate antibody
   (b) humoral antibody
   (c) natural antibody
   (d) erythrocyte antibody
   (*Nonspecific Humoral Immunity*)

10. The biologic functions of complement in immune defense include:
    (a) cytolysis
    (b) immune adherence
    (c) chemotaxis
    (d) opsonization
    (*Nonspecific Humoral Immunity: Complement*)

11. Nonspecific immunity has been shown to be influenced by:
    (a) nutritional factors
    (b) age
    (c) environmental factors
    (d) therapeutic factors
    (*Other Aspects of Nonspecific Immunity*)

12. Nonspecific immunity may be stimulated by:
    (a) zymosan
    (b) anesthesia
    (c) leukocyte transfusions
    (d) all of the above
    (*Other Aspects of Nonspecific Immunity*)

ANSWER "TRUE" OR "FALSE"

13. The Duffy receptors on the red cell membrane are believed to be associated with susceptibility to tuberculosis.
    (*Susceptibility and Nonsusceptibility*)

14. The bacterial enzyme lysozyme is present in abundance in body secretions.
    (*The Epithelial Barriers*)

15. The antiviral agent known as *interferon* is synthesized by cells in response to viral infection.
    (*The Epithelial Barriers*)

16. In the early stages of the development of the cellular exudate in acute inflammation, the predominant cells present are monocytes.
    (*Inflammation*)

17. Leukocytes always display negative chemotaxis.
    (*Chemotaxis*)

18. Serum opsonins interact with the surface of bacteria, rendering it acceptable to the phagocyte.
    (*Opsonization*)

19. *Escherichia coli* is lysed by complement activation.
    (*Complement*)

20. Properdin exerts bactericidal and viricidal effects in the presence of the trimolecular complement complex C567.
    (*Properdin*)

General References

Alexander, J. W., and Good, R. A.: Fundamentals of Clinical Immunology. Philadelphia, W. B. Saunders Company, 1977.

Barrett, J. T.: Textbook of Immunology, 4th ed. St. Louis, The C. V. Mosby Co., 1983.

Bellanti, J. A.: Immunology II. Philadelphia, W. B. Saunders Company, 1978.

Bellanti, J. A.: Immunology: Basic Processes. Philadelphia, W. B. Saunders Company, 1979.

Henry, J. B. (Ed.): Clinical Diagnosis and Management by Laboratory Methods, 17th ed. Philadelphia, W. B. Saunders Company, 1984.

Parker, C. W.: Clinical Immunology, Philadelphia, W. B. Saunders Company, 1980.

Roitt, M.: Essential Immunology, 2nd ed. Oxford, Blackwell Scientific Publications, 1974.

Walter, J. B.: An Introduction to the Principles of Disease. Philadelphia, W. B. Saunders Company, 1977.

TWO

SPECIFIC IMMUNITY

The student shall know, understand, and be prepared to explain:
1. The concepts of specific immunity
2. Antigens and antibodies
3. The structure of immunoglobulins
4. The general function of immunoglobulin
5. Immunoglobulin domains
6. Types of immunoglobulin, including:
   a. IgG
   b. IgM
   c. IgA
   d. IgE
   e. IgD
7. The function and characteristics of the above-mentioned immuno-globulins
8. Cells involved in specific immunity, including:
   a. The T-lymphocytes
   b. The B-lymphocytes
   c. Null cells
   d. NK cells

Unlike nonspecific immunity, the processes of specific (or "acquired") immunity are an adaptive response to foreign antigenic stimulus, which results in the acquisition of immunologic memory and the production of antibody, which reacts *specifically* with the antigen that caused its production.

Immunity against infectious diseases may be conferred basically in two ways: (1) by actual infections or inoculation that causes the production of specific protective antibodies (known as "active" immunity), or (2) by artificial transmission of antibodies, which afford temporary protection against invading antigen (known as "passive" immunity).

In some cases, a certain degree of "cross-immunity" is afforded when there is a relationship or similarity between causative agents. In this way, immunity against one infectious agent may contribute some immunity against other infectious agents.

Several factors are involved in the *degree* of protection produced as a response to infection or inoculation. In this connection, the size of the infecting dose, the route of administration, and the type of infective agent are contributory.

Active immunity may therefore be defined as "the state of resistance developed by an individual following effective contact with foreign microorganisms or their products." Such contact may be caused by:

1. Clinical or subclinical infection
2. The injection of live or killed microorganisms or their antigens
3. The absorption of bacterial products (*e.g.*, toxins).

The antibodies produced by the host in response to any of these events may take from a few days to a few weeks to develop, yet they usually persist for years, offering protection against reinfection. The agents used in active immunization are either live, killed, or attenuated (*i.e.*, thinned: *L. atten-uare* = to thin).

When foreign antigen gains entrance into the body, two types of immunologic reactions may occur. These are different but fundamentally similar mechanisms, known as humoral or cell-mediated immunity.

Humoral Immunity. Humoral immunity refers to the synthesis and release of free antibody (humoral antibody) into the blood and other body fluids. This antibody is then capable of direct combination with and neutralization of bacterial toxins by coating bacteria to enhance their phagocytosis, and so forth.

Cell-Mediated Immunity. Cell-mediated immunity refers to the production of "sensitized" lymphocytes, which take part in such reactions as the rejection of tissue transplants, the delayed hypersensitivity to tuberculin seen in persons immune to tubercle bacilli, destruction of cancer cells, and destruction of parasites.

ANTIGENS AND ANTIBODIES

As previously mentioned, active immunity against disease is achieved by the production of antibody (or cellular responses) in the host against a specific invading foreign antigen. An antigen is, in fact, any substance that is capable of stimulating the production of antibody. Antibody, conversely, refers to a group of plasma proteins (the immunoglobulins) that are formed as a result of exposure to antigen and that react *specifically* with that particular antigen. (Note: The outstanding characteristic of an antibody is its specificity; this implies that an antibody, once formed, is capable of reacting ONLY with the antigen that elicited its production.) Stimulation with a new antigen causes the production of a new antibody. This general rule is not absolute, as in cases of "cross-immunity"—see later in this text.

Antigens

An antigen is usually defined as any molecular structure that, when introduced parenterally into an animal, is capable of causing the production of antibodies by that animal. The antibody formed is capable of specific combination with the antigen that elicited its production. The antibodies produced are heterogenous with respect to immunoglobulin class, affinity for antigen, and specificity. At the present time, many authorities use the term *immunogen* when referring to antigen, and these terms have come to be used synonymously.

Antigenic substances of low molecular weight (*i.e.*, less than 5000) rarely stimulate the formation of antibodies and are known as *haptens*. These haptens can, however, provide antigenic specificity when coupled with a larger molecule. High molecular weight molecules of 500,000 or greater with complex protein or polypeptide-carbohydrate structures are the best antigens. The reason for this is that the entire molecule does not function as an immunoglobulin- or lymphokine-inducing structure. Instead, within each molecule, there are specific regions of limited size that function as the antigenic determinant sites, also known as *spitopes*. The number of these antigen determinant sites per molecule of antigen is referred to as the valence of the antigen. (Note: Valence, in this context, has no relationship to the ionic condition of the antigen.) It therefore follows that the larger a molecule is, the greater the number of antigenic sites, and thus the greater the variety and quantity of antibody that will be formed.

In addition to size, the foreign molecule must possess a chemical structure that is unfamiliar to the host. Again, the more diverse the chemical structure, the more antigenic the molecule becomes.

Lastly, the route of parenteral administration of the antigen is instrumental in the degree of antibody production. Generally, intravenous (into the vein) and intraperitoneal (into the peritoneal cavity) routes are effective. The intradermal (into the dermis, or skin) route offers stronger stimulus than the subcutaneous (beneath the skin) or intramuscular (into the muscle) route.

Several terms are used when describing antigens. These include autologous antigen, heterologous antigen, homologous antigen, and heterophil antigen. The meanings of these terms follow:

1. *Autologous antigen.* In simple terms, this refers to one's own antigen, which, under appropriate circumstances, would stimulate the production of autoantibody. Autologous antigen is therefore synonymous with autoantigen.
2. *Heterologous antigen.* This is merely a different antigen from that which was used in the immunization and which may or may not react with the antibody formed, depending upon the chemical similarity to the immunizing antigen.
3. *Homologous antigen.* This refers to the antigen used in the production of antibody.
4. *Heterophil antigen.* Also known as heterogenetic antigens, these are antigens that exist in unrelated plants or animals but which are either identical or so closely related that antibodies to one will cross-react with antibodies to the other.

Antibodies

Basically, antibodies may be viewed as substances produced in response to antigenic stimulation that are capable of specific interaction with the provoking antigen. It has now become common practice when referring to antibodies to use the general term *immunoglobulin* because of the heterogeneity in the types of molecules that can function as antibodies. In humans, five distinct structural types or "classes" of immunoglobulin have been isolated: immunoglobulin G (abbreviated IgG), IgM, IgA, IgD, and IgE.

Structure of Immunoglobulins

Each of the immunoglobulin classes has a basic structural similarity. The single structural unit consists of two sizes of peptide chain, termed "heavy" and "light" chains. A model for the basic immunoglobulin molecule was proposed by Porter in the 1950s, which showed a symmetrical, four-peptide unit, consisting of two heavy chains and two light chains linked by interchain disulfide bonds (Fig. 2–1). The molecule appears to be Y-shaped, the arms of the Y swinging out to an angle of 180 degrees from the horizontal.

In 1959, Porter demonstrated that treatment of IgG (which consists of a single structural unit) with the enzyme papain splits the molecule into three fragments. Two of these fragments appeared to be identical and were subsequently shown to be capable of binding specifically with antigen, although they were not capable of causing agglutination or precipitation reactions. These two fragments were called *Fab* (**f**ragment capable of **a**ntigen **b**inding); each is composed of one light chain and one half of one heavy chain. The remaining fragment (in rabbit IgG) was found to crystallize upon purification and was therefore called *Fc* (**f**ragment **c**rystalline). This Fc fragment was found to be composed of two halves of two heavy chains and was

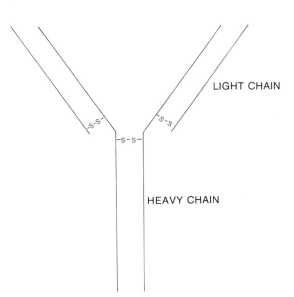

Figure 2–1. The model for the basic immunoglobulin molecule proposed by Porter.

further found to be involved in complement activation, fixation to the skin, and placental transport, although it does not have the ability to combine with antigen (Fig. 2–2).

Treatment of IgG with the enzyme pepsin results in a slightly different Fab-type fragment that not only retains the ability to bind with antigen but is also capable of causing agglutination or precipitation reactions. This fragment is known as $F(ab')_2$. It has two antigen-binding sites and is composed of two light chains and two halves of heavy chains. The remainder of the molecule is split into many small fragments by pepsin digestion (Fig. 2–3).

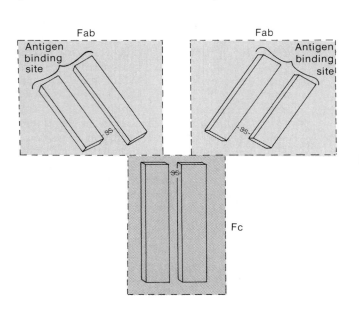

Figure 2–2. Cleavage of antibody molecule by papain.

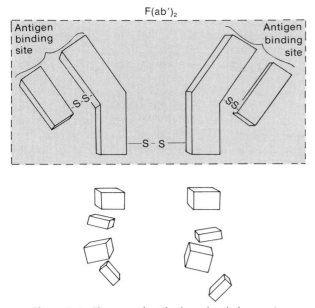

Figure 2–3. Cleavage of antibody molecule by pepsin.

glubulin—the myeloma protein, or M-protein, which appears in the serum, often in high concentrations. Purification of the myeloma protein renders a preparation of an immunoglobulin with a unique structure.)

Analysis of a number of purified myeloma proteins has revealed that the amino acid sequence of the heavy and light chains contains a "constant" region, where the amino acid sequence is identical for the type and subtype, and a "variable" region, consisting of the first 110 to 120 amino acids, which vary widely between type and subtype. The variable part of the peptide chains provides specificity for binding antigen; the constant part is associated with different biologic properties, which vary from one immunoglobulin class to another (Fig. 2–4). In addition, studies of the light chains using the Bence Jones protein (found in a proportion of patients with multiple myeloma) revealed that they could be divided into two groups, called kappa (κ) and lambda (λ). Whereas each immunoglobulin class is associated with a particular type of heavy chain, each myeloma protein studied thus far, whatever its class, has possessed light chains of either kappa or lambda specificity, but never of both together.

These findings provided the following information: (1) The Fc portion of the molecule directs the *biologic activity* of the antibody molecule (*e.g.,* placental transfer of IgG and complement fixing). (2) the Fab portion is involved in antigen binding.

Further studies of the peptide chains have been made by analysis of enzyme digestion products of myeloma proteins. (In the disease known as multiple myeloma, a cell making a particular immunoglobulin repeatedly divides in an uncontrolled way. The patient then possesses enormous numbers of identical cells derived as a clone from the original cell, all synthesizing the same immuno-

General Function of Immunoglobulin

For each molecule of antigen, millions of specific antibody molecules may be produced and secreted into the body fluids. Basically, the function of antibody is to neutralize toxic substances, to facilitate phagocytosis and kill microbes, and to combine with antigens on cellular surfaces and thereby cause the destruction of these cells either extravascularly (outside the blood vessels within the re-

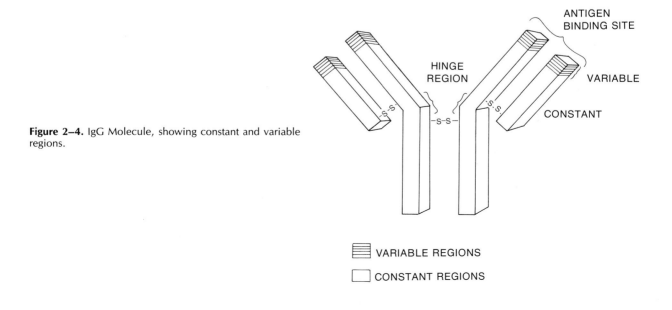

Figure 2–4. IgG Molecule, showing constant and variable regions.

ticuloendothelial system) or intravascularly (within the blood vessels through the action of complement).

Immunoglobulin Domains

The four chains of the immunoglobulin molecule are held together by covalent (disulfide) and noncovalent bonds. The convalent bonds are located mainly in the hinge region (see Fig. 2–4). Additional cystines form interchain disulfide bridges, and their number and position is characteristic for different classes of immunoglobulins. The internal disulfide bridges form loops in the peptide chains that are compactly folded to form globular "domains" (Edelman, 1971; Fig. 2–5) that appear to serve distinct functions, namely, complement activation, antigen binding, adherence to the monocyte surface, and so forth.

The variable region domains (variable light, V_L; and variable heavy, V_H) are responsible for the formation of a specific antigen-binding site. The C_H2 (second heavy chain in the constant region) domain in IgG binds C1q, initiating the classic complement sequence (see Chapter Three). The C_H3 (third heavy chain in the constant region) domain is responsible for adherence to the monocyte surface.

Types of Immunoglobulin (Table 2–1)

IgG (Immunoglobulin G). Of the major classes of immunoglobulins, IgG, which represents about 80 to 85 per cent of the total immunoglobulin, is the best known and the most fully studied. It is also known as γ2-globulin and 7Sγ-globulin, the γ indicating its position in the serum electrophoretic profile, which is actually a rather broad region compared with the albumins. The 7S refers to its $S_{20,w}$ sedimentation coefficient (svedberg coefficient), a number that indicates its sedimentation rate in the analytic ultracentrifuge.

In terms of concentration, IgG occurs in amounts of 1275 ± 500 mg per dl of serum. This high serum level is a reflection of both the rate of synthesis and the rate of elimination of IgG. The immunoglobulin is produced at the rate of about 28 mg per kg of body weight per day and has a half-life of approximately 1 month. IgG has a molecular weight of approximately 150,000, 2.5 per cent of which is in the form of carbohydrate. Most bacterial antibodies, virus-neutralizing antibodies, precipitating antibodies, hemagglutinins, and hemolysins are IgG.

The IgG molecule itself is made up of one basic structural unit known as a monomer (shown in Fig. 2–4), consisting of two heavy chains and two light chains (which may be kappa or lambda, but

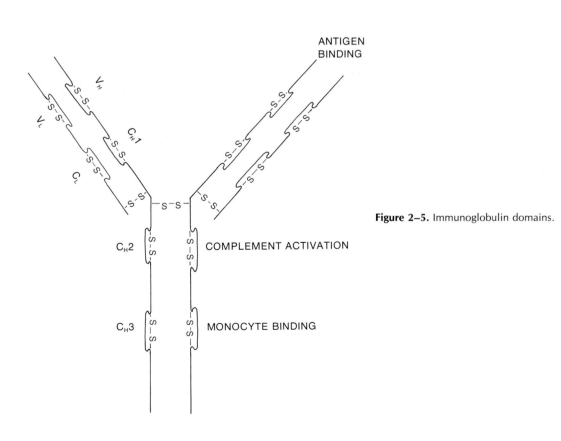

Figure 2–5. Immunoglobulin domains.

Table 2–1. SOME BIOLOGIC PROPERTIES OF THE IMMUNOGLOBULINS

Property	IgG	IgD	IgM	IgE	IgA
Molecular weight	140,000	140,000	900,000	200,000	180,000
Sedimentation coefficient	7S	7S	19S	8S	7S, 9S, 11S
% Carbohydrate	3	13	11.8	10.7	7.5
Normal serum concentration (mg/100 ml)	1275 ± 280	3	125 ± 45	?17–450	225 ± 55
Relative abundance (molecular formula)	$\gamma_2\kappa_2$ or $\gamma_2\lambda_2$	$\delta_2\kappa_2$ or $\delta_2\lambda_2$	$(\mu_2\kappa_2)_5$ or $(\mu_2\lambda_2)_5$	$\epsilon_2\kappa_2$ or $\epsilon_2\lambda_2$	$(\alpha_2\kappa_2)_2$ or $(\alpha_2\lambda_2)_2$
% Intravascular	44	?	70	?	40
Turnover rate (synthesis) mg/kg/day	28	0.4	5–8	?	8–10
Complement fixation	+		+		−
Crosses placenta	+	−	−	−	−
Presence in colostrom	+		−		+
Catabolic rate (%/day)	4–7		14–25		13–34
Half-life (days)	25–35	2–3	9–11	?	6–8

not both). The molecule is capable of changing its shape; free IgG is usually Y-shaped, whereas antigen-bound IgG may adjust its shape to accommodate the antigen. This shape change is facilitated by the so-called hinge region, where the chains are uncoiled, allowing for some considerable flexibility (see Fig. 2–4). The reason for this shape change is not fully understood, although Edelman (1971) suggests that it may serve to expose hidden sites responsible for various functions such as complement fixation.

The latest figures, concluded from x-ray diffraction studies on human IgG molecules, give the breadth as 140Å and the length as 85Å.

So far, four subclasses of IgG have been demonstrated: IgG1, IgG2, IgG3, and IgG4. These subclasses are recognized by antisera produced in animals by injecting purified myeloma proteins and absorbing the resulting antiserum with other myeloma proteins. The average concentrations of these subclasses in normal adult serum (according to Morell *et al.*, 1971) are as follows:

IgG1 = 6.63gm/L
IgG2 = 3.22gm/L
IgG3 = 0.58gm/L
IgG4 = 0.46gm/L

The number and position of the disulfide bonds vary with the IgG subclass. There are two such bonds in IgG1 and IgG4, four in IgG2 (Nisonoff *et al.*, 1975), and 11 in IgG3 (Michaelsen *et al.*, 1977; Fig. 2–6).

Differences within IgG subclasses are recognized by antisera against polymorphic antigenic determinants on gamma chains. These differences constitute the Gm allotypes. There are also differences between the IgG subclasses with respect to the binding of macrophages and to the activation of complement (Table 2–2).

Most of the IgG in the serum of newborn infants is derived from the mother by placental transfer.

A small amount, however, is of fetal origin, as shown by the fact that it may have the father's Gm allotype (Martensson and Fudenberg, 1965). Generally, the amount of IgG starts to increase between 3 and 6 weeks after birth; antibodies are detectable at about 2 months, by which time the immunoglobulin level has reached 2 gm per liter (Zak and Good, 1959).

IgM (Immunoglobulin M). The IgM molecule is made up of five basic structural units in a circular arrangement (Fig. 2–7). It therefore possesses 10 heavy chains and 10 light chains. The heavy and light chains are linked to each other by disulfide (S-S) bonds in the same general manner as IgG, but there are additional disulfide bonds linking the Fc portions of alternate heavy chains so as to produce a molecule with a central circular portion and five radiating arms. The disulfide bonds linking the Fc portions can be broken by reducing agents (*e.g.*, 2-mercaptoethanol, 2-ME; dithiothreitol, DTT).

The heavy chains of the IgM molecule are mu (μ) chains; the light chains, as in the case of IgG, are either kappa or lambda, but not both. A third type of chain, thought to function in the joining or linking together of the molecule's subunits, has been termed the *J* (joining) chain (also found in IgA). This third chain has a molecular weight of about 16,000 and contains about 20 per cent carbohydrate. This J chain is found invariably in association with intact IgM. The structure and function of the J chain in relation to IgM and IgA basic units are not fully elucidated.

Like IgG, the IgM molecule appears to be quite flexible in the region of the "hinge." It is capable of assuming numerous different shapes, from the fully extended form shown in Figure 2–7 to the dumpy, "crablike" form shown in Figure 2–8.

Electron micrographs of IgM molecules show them to be about 300Å in diameter—the arms

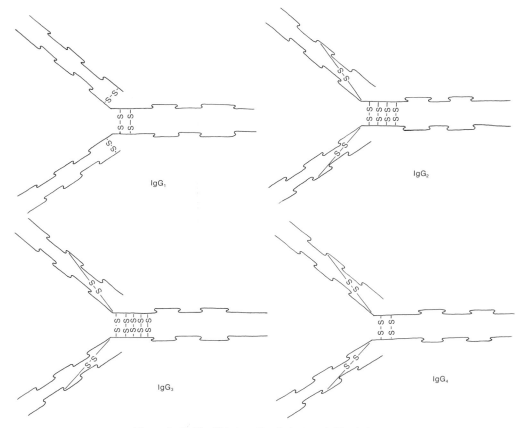

Figure 2–6. Disulfide bonding in human IgG subclasses.

being 25 to 30Å wide and 100Å long, the length of the branched sections being 55 to 70Å. The molecular weight of the molecule is about 900,000.

IgM is the antibody that is often first to appear after a primary antigenic stimulus, the first to appear in phylogeny (*i.e.,* in a given species of animal) and the last to leave in senescence, the condition of growing old, *i.e.,* deterioration). It constitutes 5 to 10 per cent of the total immunoglobulin, with an average concentration of about 1 gm per liter. About 80 per cent of IgM is intravascular; 15 to 18 per cent is catabolized per day (Cohen and Freeman, 1960; Schultze and Heremans, 1966; Brown and Cooper, 1970). During the secondary response (*i.e.,* the response to second or subsequent encounter with the same foreign antigen), synthesis of IgM usually diminishes as the concentration of IgG increases.

Intact IgM is cleaved by trypsin (at 25°C) to give in succession F(ab')$_2$ (molecular weight, MW, 114,000) and Fab (MW 47,000). (See Nisonoff *et al.,* 1975.)

IgM is the antibody most often formed in response to stimulus by gram-negative bacteria. The Wassermann antibodies, heterophil antibodies, rheumatoid factor, cold agglutinins, and allohemagglutinins also characteristically occur as IgM. There is some doubt as to whether all IgM molecules are capable of binding complement. The immunoglobulin is not transported across the human placenta, therefore the concentration in cord serum is fetal in origin and measures between 5 and 10 per cent of that found in adult serum (Franklin and Kunkel, 1958; Polly *et al.,* 1962). Within 2 or 3 days of birth, the concentration of IgM starts to rise and reaches 50 per cent of adult level in 2 to 3 months and 100 per cent at about 9

Table 2–2. SOME CHARACTERISTICS OF IgG SUBCLASSES

	IgG$_1$	IgG$_2$	IgG$_3$	IgG$_4$
Concentration in normal serum (% total IgG)	65	25	6	4
Half-life (days)	22	22	9	22
Complement fixation	yes	yes	yes	no
Cryoprecipitation	yes		yes	
Reactivity with dextrans	yes	yes	yes	no
Staphylococcal antigen	yes	yes	no	yes
DNA	yes	yes	yes	yes

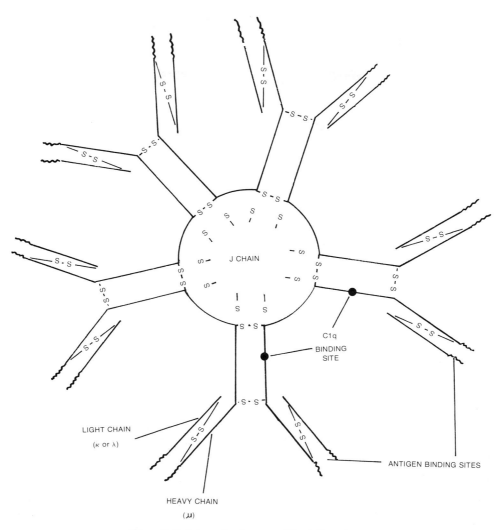

Figure 2–7. Schematic diagram of the IgG pentamer.

months; between the ages of 9 months and 3 years, values remain at the adult level, although between 5 and 9 years, they are at the lower end of the adult range (West *et al.*, 1962).

Two IgM subclasses, IgM1 and IgM2, have been recognized, based on differences in the mu chain. A secretory form of IgM has recently been described. Its distribution in body fluids parallels that of secretory IgA.

IgA (Immunoglobulin A). The main serum component of IgA has been found to have a sedimentation constant of about 7, with minor components at 10, 13, 15, and 17 to 18. This suggests that the molecule can be found in varying degrees of polymerization, ranging from a single structural unit (monomer) to five basic structural units (pentamer). The heavy chains of the molecule are alpha, and the light chains, as in IgG and IgM, may be either kappa or lambda, but not both.

SERUM IgA. The predominant portion of IgA in serum is 7S and represents only 5 to 15 per cent of all serum gamma globulins. This is equivalent to 225 (±55) mg per dl of serum. IgA has a half-life of about 6 days (Tomasi *et al.*, 1965) and is

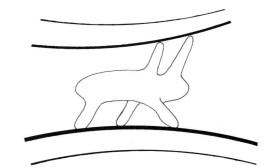

Figure 2–8. Illustration showing one of the possible shape changes of IgM.

synthesized at a rate of about 2 mg per kg of body weight per day.

Two major subclasses of human IgA, IgA1 and IgA2, are known to exist, of which IgA1 accounts for 90 per cent of the total serum IgA. IgA2 is unique in that it is completely devoid of heavy-light interchain disulfide bonding, the two chains being held together strictly by noncovalent linkages of the standard type (Jerry *et al.*, 1970). The two subclasses are therefore distinguished on the basis of antigenic differences (allotypic variation in the alpha chain of IgA2 depends upon the presence of the antigens A2m(1) and A2m(2), whereas the alpha chains of IgA1 do not express allotypic variation) (Kunkel and Prendergast, 1966; Vaerman and Heremans, 1966), as well as striking structural differences (Gray, 1960; see also Barrett, 1983).

Papain and pepsin digestion of serum IgA yields the expected Fab or F(ab')₂ units, but the Fc and Fc' units are difficult to isolate because of their sensitivity to further digestion by papain or pepsin. Certain bacterial proteases cleave only IgA1. Reductive cleavage to release heavy and light chains is also possible.

IgA cannot be detected in cord serum. By the age of 2 months, the amount in serum has reached about 20 per cent of the adult level (West *et al.*, 1962).

SECRETORY IgA. Whereas the ratio of IgG to IgA in serum is 6:1 in the internal secretions (synovial fluid, cerebrospinal fluid, aqueous humor, and so forth) and in the external secretions (*i.e.*, colostrum and early milk, nasal and respiratory mucus, intestinal mucus, saliva, and so forth), IgA is usually present in a much higher concentration than either IgG or IgM. In these external secretions, IgA serves as a first line of defense against microorganism invasion. It is particularly important in preventing gastrointestinal infections of the secreting glands. In contrast to IgG and IgM, the immunoglobulin is synthesized in plasma cells located primarily in the epithelial surfaces of the respiratory tract and intestine and in almost all excretory glands.

Following synthesis, some of the IgA finds its way into the systemic circulation, but most of it passes through or between the epithelial cells to be secreted. This last is known as secretory IgA (SIgA). The SIgA molecule is made up of two basic structural units and a glycoprotein secretory component, which is linked to the respective heavy chains of the molecule by disulfide bonds and may serve to make the molecule more resistant to enzyme attacks. The J chain described in IgM is also found in SIgA and in polymeric forms of serum IgA (Fig. 2–9).

IgA does not fix complement and is not transported across the human placenta.

IgE (Immunoglobulin E). The existence of a heat-labile antibody, originally called *reagin,** in the sera of individuals displaying various allergies was first encountered by Prausnitz and Kustner in 1921. This antibody was noted to have the following characteristics:

1. It was specific for the allergen or antigen that evoked its production.
2. It would not pass the placenta to passively hypersensitize the fetus.
3. It would not give the usual *in vitro* serologic reactions in tests such as precipitation, agglutination, complement fixation, or others associated with the heat-stable immunoglobulins.
4. On passive transfer to a normal individual, it would "fix" in the skin for several days or weeks.

Immunization of rabbits with a reagin-rich fraction prepared by DEAE cellulose ion exchange chromatography and Sephadex gel filtration resulted in an antiserum that would remove the reaginic activity of sera by serologic precipitation. Adsorption of this rabbit antiserum with the four well-known immunoglobulins did not delete the antibody that precipitated reagin. By the extensive use of radioimmunodiffusion experiments, it was shown that reagin was, in fact, a new and distinct immunoglobulin; it was named *IgE*, the E assigned because the reagin most studied was specific for the antigen E of ragweed. IgE now refers to reagin in a general sense, and its specificity for an antigen is designated in the same way as for any other immunoglobulin.

For several years after its discovery, critical biochemical studies of the immunoglobulin were hampered by the fact that it only occurs in minute quantities in normal sera (16–17 μg/ml of serum) and that sera from allergic individuals with elevated IgE levels were not available for testing. This dilemma was resolved by the discovery in

---

*This is separate and different from the reagin of syphilis.

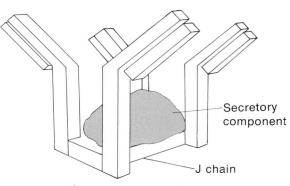

Secretory component

J chain

Figure 2–9. Secretory IgA (sIgA).

Sweden of a patient with a unique myeloma protein, which proved to be identical to IgE. From studies of this protein, the following data have been accumulated. IgE has a molecular weight of 190,000 and is an 8.2S molecule. It has a carbohydrate content of 11.7 per cent, and its concentration in serum is 0.1 to 1.0 mg per dl. It constitutes 1 per cent of the total immunoglobulin and has a half-life of 2.3 days. The rate of synthesis of IgE is 2.3 μg per kg of body weight per day. There are no heavy chain subclasses of IgE, and the heavy chain has four constant domains.

Papain digestion of IgE produces several fragments, including the two Fab units and an Fc unit. In addition, a light chain fragment known as lambda C, an Fc″, and a $7S_{20,w}$ fragment are produced.

The role of IgE in allergic conditions is now clear. Hypersensitivities caused by IgE may assume any of several forms from the life-threatening anaphylactic reactions to the milder discomforts associated with food allergies. Regardless of their severity, these depend upon the presence of an IgE with a serologic specificity for the offending allergen. The combination of the allergen with IgE on the surface of mast cells and basophils releases pharmacologic agents that trigger an immediate physiologic response. (For further discussion, see Barrett, 1983.)

IgD (Immunoglobulin D). IgD was first identified as a unique immunoglobulin in human serum in 1965 as a result of the discovery of a myeloma protein that was found to be antigenically different from other immunoglobulins. Since that time, many other examples of IgD-related myeloma proteins have been reported, although they are now known to occur in only 3 per cent of all myelomas.

IgD occurs in minute quantities in serum (0.03 mg/ml); therefore, the majority of chemical data available with respect to this immunoglobulin have been derived from the gamma D myeloma proteins.

IgD, like all other immunoglobulins, is made up of two heavy chains and two light chains. Both kappa and lambda light chains have been detected, although the lambda-type myelomas predominate (80 per cent, compared with 20 per cent kappatype). The heavy chain of IgD, designated delta (δ), is structurally and antigenically different from the heavy chains of other immunoglobulins, although the kappa and lambda light chains do not differ from their kind in other immunoglobulins. The delta chain (heavy chain) has a molecular weight of 70,000 (approximately 12,000 greater than the gamma chains of IgG). This additional molecular weight has led to the suggestion that the delta chain has a fourth CH unit or that the hinge region may be extended. Because of this high molecular weight of the heavy chain, IgD has an overall molecular weight of 180,000, rather than 160,000. On an average, it occurs as a 6.55S molecule.

Papain digestion results in the expected two Fab and one Fc fragments, but the Fc fragment is rapidly degraded further and, as such, is difficult to isolate intact.

IgD contains about 12 per cent polysaccharide (all of which is attached to the heavy chain), which appears to be divided into three discrete sections, one located at the Fc-Fd interface (hinge region) and the other two in the Fc region.

IgD is synthesized at a rate of 0.4 mg per kg of body weight per day (*i.e.,* about 100 times less than the synthetic rate of IgG) and has a half-life of only 2 to 3 days. The immunoglobulin is heat and acid labile; if stored at 56°C for 1 hour, its amount in serum is reduced by half, and, after 4 hours, only 10 per cent is recoverable. A pH of 3 denatures IgD. IgD aggregates very readily, which can change its biologic activity as well as its structure.

Very little is known about the functional importance of IgD. There is evidence, however, to suggest that IgD may be important as a membrane receptor and is synthesized early in the antigen-independent differentiation of B-cells (discussed later).

CELLS INVOLVED IN SPECIFIC IMMUNITY

It is generally accepted that the "parent" cell of all erythroid, myeloid, and lymphoid cellular elements is the pluripotent hemopoietic stem cell, which migrates from the yolk sac through the fetal liver, spleen, and bone marrow. From these sites, some lymphoid stem cells migrate to the thymus, where further differentiation occurs, resulting in the production of thymus-derived cells (T-cells). Other lymphoid stem cells are independent of the thymus. In birds, they come under the influence of the bursa of Fabricus; in humans and other mammals, a mammalian equivalent such as the fetal liver, bone marrow, or gut-associated lymphoid tissue appears to be involved. These lymphoid stem cells differentiate to become bursa- or bone marrow–derived cells (B-cells).

Both B- and T-lymphocytes, on appropriate stimulation by antigen, proliferate and undergo morphologic changes. The T-lymphocytes become lymphoblasts, which are involved in cell-mediated reactions, and the B-lymphocytes become plasma cells, which are involved in humoral antibody synthesis (Fig. 2–10).

In addition to B- and T-lymphocytes, three other types of immunocompetent cells (null cells, NK cells, and macrophages) are also involved in the immune response. In the discussion that follows,

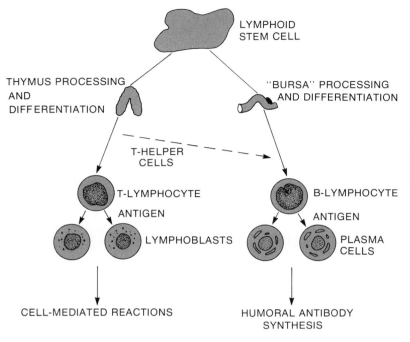

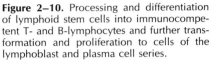

Figure 2–10. Processing and differentiation of lymphoid stem cells into immunocompetent T- and B-lymphocytes and further transformation and proliferation to cells of the lymphoblast and plasma cell series.

their interaction during humoral and cell-mediated immunity is examined.

T-Lymphocytes

As previously mentioned, thymus-derived lymphocytes (T-cells) originate in the bone marrow and mature in the thymus, where they acquire some of their T-cell characteristics. They then move to the lymph node and spleen via the lymphatics and blood stream. Some of these maturation steps are under the influence of thymosin (a thymic hormone), which is produced by the reticuloendothelial cells of the thymus. This hormone has been found to be useful for the treatment of thymic deficiencies (Goldstein, 1975).

About 90 per cent of lymphocytes in the thoracic duct and 70 to 80 per cent in the peripheral blood show T-cell characteristics. The average half-life of most of these circulating T-cells is 2.2 years; they are termed *long-lived* lymphocytes. In fact, some long-lived lymphocytes survive for 20 years or more. In contrast, short-lived lymphocytes, which are mostly B-cells, have a life span of only 3 days.

There are a number of subpopulations of T-cells (Cantor, 1977).

T-"Helper" Cells. T-helper (Th) cells are required to assist B-cells in the production of antibody to most antigens. These cells are believed to concentrate the antigen via specific receptor molecules on the cell surface. These receptors bind the carrier part of the antigen molecule. The

antigen-receptor complex is then picked up by a macrophage and is presented to the potential antibody-forming cells. So-called macrophage independent antigens (discussed later) are thymus independent and do not require the cooperation of Th-cells.

Th-cells also play a role in the cell-mediated immune response. For example, these cells cooperate with the GVH-reactive T-cell in graft versus host reaction (GvHR). Interaction with the Th-cell is required for the proliferation of T-cells or the generation of cytotoxic T-cells in mixed lymphocyte cultures. It is not certain that the Th-cells involved in humoral antibody synthesis are the same cells required for the cell-mediated immune response. Other T-cells may also be required for full expression of helper functions.

The human helper cell represents 40 to 60 per cent of the peripheral blood T-lymphocytes.

T-"Cytotoxic" Cells. The cytoxic T-lymphocytes (Tcx) (also known as T-"effector" cells) are the killer cells in cellular immunity. These cells have highly specific receptors that react with and have the ability to destroy specific antigens or antigen-bearing target cells. Tcx-cells may also render macrophages specifically cytotoxic to tumor target cells. Foreign tissue in the form of transplants, tumor cells, virus-infected host cells, or cells infected by other infectious agents are the best targets. The Tcx-cell contacts the primary antigen and the histocompatibility antigen as the dual recognition signal to initiate cell killing.

T-"Suppressor" Cells. A third subpopulation of

T-cells function as suppressor cells (Ts)(Gershon, 1975). The identification of these cells emerged from several different types of experiments, in which it was found that these Ts-cells can be activated during humoral immunity or in cell-mediated immunity. In one experiment, it was found that thymectomy enhanced the B-cell response to a T-cell–independent antigen, yet, in this instance, the B-cell required no assistance from the Th-cell but was affected by the Ts-cell. In another experiment, it was found that T-cells play a role in tolerance to large doses of antigen.

Although the exact mechanism by which Ts-cells suppress the immune response is not clear, it is possible that it may be via a soluble factor produced by Ts-cells. What is known is that Ts-cells will respond to low doses of antigen, much lower than required to stimulate B-cells. Ts cells exert their action on B-cells, on Th-cells, on Tdh-cells (described below), and on macrophages.

T-"Delayed Hypersensitivity" Cells. The T-delayed hypersensitivity cells (Tdh) have mainly been studied in mice, and little is known about the human Tdh-cell except that its response is antigen specific and that it is the source of several lymphokines, such as migration inhibition factor (MIF) and macrophage chemotaxin, which participate in the hypersensitivity reaction.

T-"Amplifier" Cells. The amplifier T-cell (Ta) has been described only recently. It causes Th-, Ts-, and B-cells to exaggerate their normal activities.

B-Lymphocytes

Bone marrow–derived lymphocytes (B-cells) are the precursor cells in antibody production. B-line stem cells in the bone marrow are the source of the pre–B-cell. This pre–B-cell, even in the animal not yet stimulated by an antigen, synthesizes IgM, the globulin being confined to the cytoplasm of the cell and not secreted (as opposed to the mature B-cell, which does secrete IgM and has it on its surface). From the bone marrow, the pre–B-cell migrates from the bone marrow to the germinal centers of the lymph nodes and spleen. As it does so, it loses some of its cytoplasm and becomes a smaller cell (recognized as an immature B-cell), many of which express surface IgD. At this stage, the B-cell can be identified by surface receptors for complement components, especially C1q, C3b, C3d, and C4b, and receptors for the Fc region of IgG. The I-A and/or I-E proteins are also present in these cells.

This immature B-cell differentiates into a mature B-cell after antigen exposure, after which it secretes a single class of immunoglobulin molecule, which is specific for a single determinant on the antigen. At the same time, there is a morphologic differentiation into a plasma cell, which is the most proficient antibody-forming cell.

In the peripheral blood, approximately 20 to 30 per cent of the circulating lymphocytes are B-cells, identified on the basis of their surface immunoglobulin. Approximately 50 per cent of tonsillar and splenic lymphocytes are B-cells.

Although B-cells have many common features, they can be subdivided into major subsets on the basis of the class of immunoglobulin that they are patterned to synthesize. These are known as Bμ (IgM), Bγ (IgG), Bα (IgA), Bδ (IgD), and Bϵ (IgE). Within each of these subsets, further differentiation is possible, based on the type of light chain involved (kappa or lambda) and on the subclass of the heavy chain.

All B-cells are not necessarily fixed to synthesize just one type of immunoglobulin, because class "switch" from IgM to IgG has been reported. The stimulus for this may be reexposure to antigen and assistance from Th or Ta cells.

The immunoglobulin on the B-cell surface behaves as a specific receptor for antigen. The immunoglobulin has been shown to be randomly distributed over the surface of the B-cell (through histochemical techniques). When antigen is added, the immunoglobulin begins to accumulate in distinct foci that further blend into one agglomerate. This is known as *lymphocyte capping,* after which there is a gradual disappearance of the antigen and the immunoglobulin as the complex moves into the interior of the cell.

Lymphocyte capping is peculiar to B-cells and is not demonstrated by T-cells. It signals a phase of cell differentiation into actively secreting plasma cells and memory cells, the latter of which cannot be described in cytologic terms, but which are responsible for the recognition of antigen on reexposure. Plasma cells, however, are easily recognized both morphologically and functionally.

B-cell transformation into plasma cells is also stimulated by certain so-called *mitogens,* which are polyclonal in their stimulating effect (as opposed to antigen, which is characterized as monoclonal). Polyclonal mitogens stimulate all B-cells regardless of their antigen specificity, which reflects a shared ability of the mitogens to affect the plasticity of the B-cell cytoplasmic membrane in the same manner accomplished by antigen.

The most specific of the commonly used B-cell mitogens is the lipopolysaccharide (LPS) that is extracted from the cell wall of many gram-negative bacteria, where it functions as the somatic or O antigen and is an endotoxin. The lipid portion of LPS is the site of its mitogenic activity. Other mitogens for B-cells include protein A (found on the surface of the bacterium *Staphylococcus au-*

reus), which combines with immunoglobulin on the B-cell by a different mechanism than antigen, but, nevertheless, it stimulates lymphocyte transformation.

The end cell of the B-cell lineage is the plasma cell. This is about the same size as the small lymphocyte (6–10 μm), although not all plasma cells are the same size, and some may approach 20 μm in diameter. The nucleus for the plasma cell is in the center, and the cytoplasm, which is usually sparse in relation to that of other cells, is usually gathered at one side. The nucleus stains darkly, and the lumpy strands of chromatin give it a "cartwheel" appearance. The cytosol of plasma cells is literally filled with rough endoplasmic reticulum. This complex intracellular system consists of two serpentine, parallel membranes, which are laden with ribosomes (see Fig. 2–11). The ribosomes contain considerable RNA and serve as the site of messenger RNA attachment during protein synthesis. It is here that immunoglobulin synthesis occurs.

Null Cells (K Cells)

During certain cell-mediated immune responses, cytoxic cells are found that have been described as "null" cells (*i.e.*, they are neither macrophages nor T- or B-cells), despite their acknowledged role as receptors for immunoglobulin. Currently, it is more common practice to refer to these cells as killer (or K) cells (Perlmann, 1976). They possess Fc receptors for IgG and are capable of killing antibody-coated target cells *in vitro* (antibody-dependent cytotoxic cells, ADCC). K-cells are unable to kill target cells except in the presence of specific antibody and are not major histocompatibility complex (MHC)–restricted (*i.e.*, they are capable of killing cells that do not have the same histocompatibility antigen on their surfaces), as is the case with the cytotoxic T-cell.

The precise role of these K-cells in cell-mediated immunity is not yet clear, but it is understood that they may play a role in autoimmune disorders (Allison, 1976).

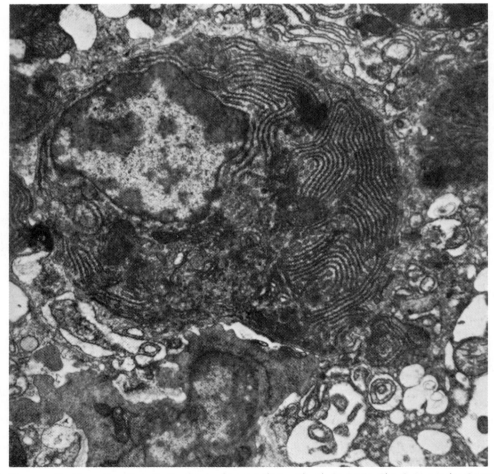

Figure 2–11. Plasma cells. (From Barrett, J. T.: Textbook of Immunology, 4th ed. St. Louis, The C. V. Mosby Company, 1983, p. 95.)

Natural Killer (NK) Cells

The peripheral lymphocytes from nonimmunized individuals or the spleen of nonimmunized mice may also contain a population of cells that are cytotoxic for several targets. These cells do not have markers for B- or T-lymphocytes and are not phagocytic; therefore, they are also "null" cells. Because of their wide-ranging cytotoxic abilities, they are referred to as natural killer (NK) cells.

This natural killer activity may present our first line of defense against neoplastic cells and virally infected cells and may be responsible for immunosurveillance against tumor cells, for which they have a spontaneous cytotoxicity, almost regardless of the target cell source.

The attack of NK cells on their targets is blocked by gangliosides, which may represent their natural receptor.

REVIEW QUESTIONS

MULTIPLE CHOICE

Choose the phrase, sentence, or symbol that completes the statement or answers the question. More than one answer may be correct in each case. Answers are given at the end of this book.

1. The artificial transmission of antibodies, which affords temporary protection against invading antigen, is known as:
   (a) active immunity
   (b) artificial immunity
   (c) host-related immunity
   (d) passive immunity
   (Introduction)

2. The factors that are involved in the *degree* of protection produced as a response to infection or inoculation include:
   (a) the size of the infecting dose
   (b) the route of administration
   (c) the type of infecting agent
   (d) none of the above
   (Introduction)

3. Active immunity follows effective contact with foreign microorganisms or their products. Such contact may be caused by:
   (a) clinical infection
   (b) the injection of live or killed microorganisms or their antigens
   (c) subclinical infection
   (d) the absorption of bacterial products
   (Introduction)

4. The outstanding characteristic of an antibody is its:
   (a) specificity
   (b) nonspecificity
   (c) broad-spectrum of activity
   (d) none of the above
   (Antigens and Antibodies: Introduction)

5. An antigen that is different from that used in the immunization that may or may not react with the antibody formed is referred to as a (an):
   (a) autologous antigen
   (b) heterophile antigen
   (c) heterologous antigen
   (d) isoantigen
   (Antigens)

6. Which of the following is **not** a recognized immunoglobulin?
   (a) IgG
   (b) IgD
   (c) IgF
   (d) IgE
   (Antibodies)

7. The Fab fragment of the IgG molecule, after treatment with the enzyme papain, is composed of:
   (a) one heavy chain and one light chain
   (b) two heavy chains and two light chains
   (c) one light chain and one half of one heavy chain
   (d) two light chains and one half of one heavy chain
   (Structure of Immunoglobulins)

8. Treatment of IgG with the enzyme pepsin results in the following fragments:
   (a) one Fc fragment and one Fab fragment
   (b) two Fc fragments and two Fab fragments
   (c) one $F(ab')_2$ fragment and several smaller fragments
   (d) two $F(ab')_2$ fragments and one Fc fragment
   (Structure of Immunoglobulins)

9. Specificity for binding antigen is the responsibility of:
   (a) the Fab fragment of the immunoglobulin molecule
   (b) the variable region of the immunoglobulin molecule
   (c) the constant region of the immunoglobulin molecule
   (d) the Fc fragment of the immunoglobulin molecule
   (Structure of Immunoglobulins)

10. The basic function of immunoglobulin is:
    (a) to neutralize toxic substances
    (b) to phagocytose antigen
    (c) to facilitate the process of phagocytosis
    (d) to combine with antigens on cellular surfaces and thereby cause the destruction of the cells either extravascularly or intravascularly
    (General Function of Immunoglobulin)

11. The formation of a specific antigen-binding site is the responsibility of:
    (a) the VL and VH domains of the immunoglobulin molecule

(b) the CL and CH domains of the immunoglobulin molecule
(c) the C_H3 domain of the immunoglobulin
(d) the C_H2 domain of the immunoglobulin molecule
(Immunoglobulin Domains)

12. Eighty to 85 per cent of the total immunoglobulin is:
(a) IgG
(b) IgM
(c) IgA
(d) IgD
(Types of Immunoglobulin)

13. IgG has a half-life of approximately:
(a) 24 hours
(b) 1 week
(c) 1 month
(d) 1 year
(Immunoglobulin G (IgG))

14. Which of the following statements, with respect to the concentration of IgG subclass in normal serum, is incorrect:
(a) IgG1—6.63 gm/L
(b) IgG2—9.87gm/L
(c) IgG3—0.58gm/L
(d) IgG4—0.46gm/L
(Immunoglobulin G (IgG))

15. The so-called J chain is found in:
(a) IgG
(b) IgM
(c) IgA
(d) IgG3
(Types of Immunoglobulin)

16. Which of the following immunoglobulins is most often formed in response to gram-negative bacteria?
(a) IgG
(b) IgA
(c) IgM
(d) IgD
(Types of Immunoglobulin)

17. When compared with IgG, IgA has:
(a) a greater carbohydrate content
(b) a lesser carbohydrate content
(c) a different amino acid sequence
(d) the same amino acid sequence in the constant portion of the molecule
(Immunoglobulin A (IgA))

18. IgA1 accounts for:
(a) 20 per cent of the total serum IgA
(b) 50 per cent of the total serum IgA
(c) 90 per cent of the total serum IgA
(d) 1 per cent of the total serum IgA
(Immunoglobulin A (IgA))

19. IgA:
(a) commonly binds complement
(b) does not fix complement
(c) is not transported across the human placenta
(d) is sometimes (though rarely) transported across the human placenta
Immunoglobulin A (IgA))

20. IgE:
(a) was originally known as reagin
(b) will "fix" to the skin for several days or weeks on passive transfer to a normal individual
(c) has a molecular weight of 190,000
(d) has a half-life of 1 month
(Immunoglobulin E (IgE))

21. IgD:
(a) has a higher molecular weight than IgG
(b) is not affected by papain digestion
(c) contains about 12 per cent polysaccharide
(d) is denatured at a pH of 3
(Immunoglobulin D (IgD))

22. About 70 to 80 per cent of lymphocytes in the peripheral blood show:
(a) B-cell characteristics
(b) T-cell characteristics
(c) are "long-lived" lymphocytes, some of which may survive for 20 years or more
(d) have an average half-life of 3 days
(Cells Involved in Specific Immunity)

23. The subpopulations of T-cells include:
(a) T-helper cells
(b) T-cytotoxic cells
(c) T-suppressor cells
(d) all of the above
(T-Lymphocytes)

24. Lymphocyte capping occurs when antigen is added to:
(a) B-cells, but not T-cells
(b) T-cells, but not B-cells
(c) T-helper cells only
(d) T-suppressor cells only
(Cells Involved in Specific Immunity)

25. Null cells (K cells):
(a) are neither macrophages nor B- nor T-cells
(b) possess Fc receptors for IgG
(c) are able to kill target cells in the presence of specific antibody
(d) all of the above
(Null cells [K cells])

ANSWER "TRUE" OR "FALSE"

26. The synthesis and release of free antibody into the blood and other body fluids is referred to as cell-mediated immunity.
(Introduction)

27. Antigens that exit in unrelated plants or animals, but which are either identical or so closely related that antibodies to one will cross-react with antibodies to the other, are known as heterophil antigens.
(Antigens)

28. The Fc portion of the immunoglobulin molecule directs its biologic activity.
(Structure of Immunoglobulins)

29. There are no subclasses of IgM.
(Immunoglobulin M (IgM))

30. T-helper cells are believed to concentrate the anti-

gen via specific receptor molecules on the cell surface.
(T-Lymphocytes)

31. The T-effector cells are the killer cells in cellular immunity.
(T-Lymphocytes)

32. The pre–B-cell synthesizes IgM, even in an animal not yet stimulated by antigen.
(B-Lymphocytes)

33. The pre–B-cell differentiates into an immature B-cell after antigen exposure.
(B-Lymphocytes)

34. All B-cells are fixed to synthesize only one type of immunoglobulin.
(B-Lymphocytes)

35. B-cell transformation into plasma cells is partly stimulated by mitogens.
(B-Lymphocytes)

36. NK cells may represent our first line of defense against neoplastic cells and virally infected cells.
(Natural Killer [NK] Cells)

37. The attack of NK cells on their targets is blocked by gangliosides.
(Natural Killer [NK] Cells)

General References

1. Barrett, J. T.: Textbook of Immunology, 4th ed. St. Louis, The C. V. Mosby Co., 1983.
2. Bellanti, J. A.: Immunology: Basic Processes. Philadelphia, W. B. Saunders Company, 1979.
3. Henry, J. B. (Ed.): Clinical Diagnosis and Management by Laboratory Principles, 17th ed. Philadelphia, W. B. Saunders Company, 1984.
4. Parker, C. W.: Clinical Immunology. Philadelphia, W. B. Saunders Company, 1980.

THREE
COMPLEMENT

Introduction

The term *complement* refers to a complex set of 11 distinct serum proteins (nine components), each of which can be isolated. The general properties of complement, which serve to distinguish it from the immunoglobulins and other serum proteins and their activities, are as follows:

1. Complement plays a role in the cytolytic destruction of cellular antigens by specific antibodies, although not all cellular antigens are susceptible to dissolution by complement and immunoglobulins. In general, those cells that are naturally most fragile (white blood cells, erythrocytes, thrombocytes, and gram-negative bacteria) are the most susceptible to immune cytolysis, whereas yeasts, molds, many gram-positive bacteria, most plant cells, and even most mammalian cells resist complement-mediated cytolysis.
2. Complement activity in antigen-antibody reactions is destroyed by heating sera to 56°C for 30 minutes (see further discussion later in this chapter).
3. IgM and IgG are the only immunoglobulins that react with complement. The subclasses of IgG are not equally potent in this respect. IgG4 fails to operate with the complement system, and IgG3 is the most active in this regard (when compared with the other IgG subclasses). IgA, IgD, and IgE do not function with complement.
4. Provided that the immunoglobulin is of the proper class, complement is bound to all antigen-antibody reactions. This fixation occurs even when complement is not required to display the serologic reaction being studied (*e.g.*, precipitation and agglutination). The classical pathway of complement activation (see later discussion) is initiated by the binding or fixation of complement by complexes of antigen and antibody.
5. Complement is found in all mammalian sera and in the sera of most lower animals, including birds, fish, amphibia, and sharks (elasmobranchs). There is no increase in complement levels (which constitute about 10 per cent of the total globulins) as a result of immunization.
6. Complement from one species will usually react with immunoglobulins of another species from the same taxonomic order and can therefore be considered a nonspecific serologic reagent. Interaction decreases as the taxonomic position of the two species becomes more distant.

7. Portions of the complement system contribute importantly to chemotaxis, opsonization, immune adherence, anaphylatoxin formation, virus neutralization, and other physiologic functions.

8. Complement can be activated by nonserologic reactions (*e.g.,* the properdin activation—see Complement Activation: The Alternative Pathway, page 32). In these alternative pathways, complement activation is initiated by complex polysaccharides or enzymes.

9. Complement is a complex of nine major components that act in consort with one another. All nine of these components are required for "classical" activation, whereas only six (*i.e.,* exclusive of the first three) are required in the properdin activation pathway (see later discussion).

The discovery of complement is credited to Pfeiffer (1894) and resulted from his studies on experimental cholera infections in guinea pigs, although a heat-labile protective activity of blood had been described earlier and named "alexin" by Buchner.

Pfeiffer's experiments were confirmed by Bordet in 1898, who also described immune hemolysis following the mixture of red blood cells with specific antibody and alexin. The term *complement* was proposed by Ehrich at around the same time. The term, which means something that completes or makes perfect was considered more meaningful than the term *alexin,* which means to ward off and has therefore persisted.

Bordet and Gengou (1901) formulated the complement fixation test (described in a later chapter), which, until recently, was the standard serologic test for the diagnosis of syphilis. Because of his many contributions and related studies of immunity and to the understanding of complement, Bordet received the Nobel Prize in 1919.

The Components of Complement (Nomenclature)

As previously mentioned, there are nine basic components in the classical activation sequence of complement; it can be considered that 11 proteins participate in the system. These components are numbered sequentially from C1 to C9. The individual peptide chains of these proteins are designated by greek letters (*e.g.,* C3α, C3β, C4β, and C4γ), in keeping with the biochemical system for identifying the subunit peptides that have a quarternary structure.

When a peptide chain is fragmented by proteolysis, the resulting cleavage peptides are denoted by lower case Arabic letters (*e.g.,* C3a, C3b, C4a and C4b). These difficult lettering systems are

important, because they carry a particular meaning (*e.g.,* C3a and C3b arise from C3α and therefore refer to different things and cannot be used interchangeably. If a fragment loses activity as a result of further proteolysis, the letter "i" is added as a subscript to indicate inactivation (*e.g.,* C3b$_i$).

When a complement component is activated, a horizontal bar over the designation for the protein is usually used, although this practice is gradually losing its popularity. Under this system, C1 becomes $\overline{C1}$ when it acquires esterase activity; when referring to specific fragments, the appropriate letters are used (*e.g.,* $\overline{C4b2a}$).

Recent studies of the alternative (properdin) pathway of complement activation has revealed several additional serum proteins that function with the "later" components of activation (*i.e.,* those that follow C3 in the classical pathway). At least five additional proteins participate in the alternative pathway, and these have recently acquired their own nomenclature. Under this system, there are properdin factor B (formerly known as C3 proactivator), factor D (formerly known as C3 proactivator convertase), C3b,Bb (the C3 activator), cobra venom factor (CVF), and another initiating factor that has not yet been characterized. This raises the number of proteins in the complement system to 14—9 classical pathway molecules plus 5 alternative pathway molecules.

To these 14 molecules, all of which are present in normal serum, must be added those serum proteins that modulate complement-derived activities. At the present time, 5 such proteins are known: C1s inhibitor (C1s INH), C3b,C4b inactivator (C3b,C4b INAC or factor 1), C3a and C5a anaphylatoxin inactivator (Ana ING), C6 inactivator (C6 INAC), and C5b inactivator (C5b INAC). Note: C3b,C4b INAC is identical to conglutinogen-activating factor (KAF, from the German abbreviation).

If plasmin, Hagerman's factor, Hageman's factor fragments, and other molecules are included, the total number of proteins that participate in the complement system can be extended beyond these 19. The complement system, therefore, can be viewed as a highly complex system that may involve as many as 24 molecules whose biologic activities are numerous and closely coordinated.

COMPLEMENT ACTIVATION: THE CLASSICAL PATHWAY

The activation of complement is often referred to as the complement "cascade," which begins when the C1 molecule is activated by certain reactions. From that point, the components C4, C2, and C3 participate (in that order rather than in straight-numerical sequence), followed by the remaining

Table 3–1. CHARACTERISTICS OF THE COMPLEMENT COMPONENTS

Characteristic	C1q	C1r	C1s	C2	C3	C4	C5	C6	C7	C8	C9
Serum concentration (μg/ml)	150	50	50	15	1250	400	80	60	55	55	60
Sedimentation coefficient ($S_{20,w}$)	11.2	7.5	4.5	4.5	9.5	10.0	8.7	5.5	6.0	8.0	4.5
Molecular weight	410,000	83,000	83,000	110,000	180,000	206,000	180,000	130,000	120,000	150,000	79,000
Number of peptide chains	18	2	1		2	3	2	1	1	3	1
Electrophoretic position	γ_2	β	α	β_1	β_2	β_1	β_1	β_2	β_2	γ_1	α

molecules C5 to C9, terminating in cytolysis of certain cellular antigens that initiated the sequence.

C1: The Recognition Unit

C1, the first component of complement, is a macromolecule with a molecular weight of approximately 600,000 and a sedimentation coefficient of 18 (Table 3–1). In its "associated" form, it is a trimolecular complex, held together by calcium ions (Ca^{++}). Removal of calcium (by the use of chelating compounds such as ethylenediaminetetraacetic acid (EDTA) causes C1 to dissociate into three subunits; restoration of calcium causes the reassociation of C1 into trimeric form. The presence of calcium, therefore, can be regarded as essential for the integrity of the complex.

The three subunits of C1 are called C1q, C1r, and C1s, which are different in size and in chemical properties (see Table 3–1). The C1q molecule is by far the largest (molecular weight, MW 410,000) and can be easily viewed under the electron microscope, where it appears as six "globes" held on slender shafts that fuse into a common base (Fig. 3–1). These "globes" are believed to act as the recognition unit that bind to the Fc region of the complement-activating IgM and IgG immunoglobulins. This occurs in the C_H2 domain of IgG and in the C_H4 domain of IgM. For C1q to initiate the cascade, it must attach to *two* Fc fragments. With IgG-coated cells, therefore, two antibody molecules, each of which can contribute only one Fc fragment, must bind to adjacent antigen sites. It appears that if the IgG molecules are attached to nonadjacent sites, the Fc pieces are too far apart to initiate complement activation. IgM, however, has five Fc pieces, and, therefore, one molecule of this immunoglobulin is independently capable of causing complement to be bound. IgA, IgD, and IgE do not bind C1q and therefore cannot initiate the complement cascade.

The other two subunits, C1r and C1s, are similar molecules, each composed of a single peptide chain with a molecular weight approaching 83,000 (see Table 3–1) and containing about 7 to 9 per cent of their protein weight in polysaccharide. C1r is a beta globulin and a proteolytic zymogen (or proenzyme) in its native state. It tends to self-associate to form a dimer (which probably explains why the molecular weight of C1r is frequently given as 180,000). C1s, which is an alpha globulin, is also a proteolytic zymogen (proenzyme) when free. Once bound to C1r, it develops esterase activity.

The exact mechanisms of C1r and C1s activation is uncertain, although it has been suggested that their incorporation into antigen-antibody complexes creates a susceptibility to a naturally existing serum protease such as plasmin or thrombin (Fig. 3–2).

C4: The Activation Unit

Once the C1 complex is attached, the esterolytic site on C1s activates the next complement component, C4 (Fig. 3–3). C4 is a beta globulin with a molecular weight of 206,000, which originates from a pro C4 (MW 210,000), synthesized by macrophages. In human serum, its serum concentration of 400 μg per ml is second only to the serum concentration of C3. The molecule itself consists of three peptide chains, C4α, C4β, and C4γ, which are joined by disulfide bonds. The

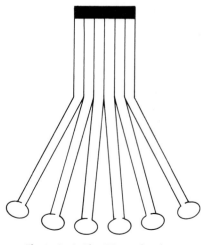

Figure 3–1. The C1q molecule.

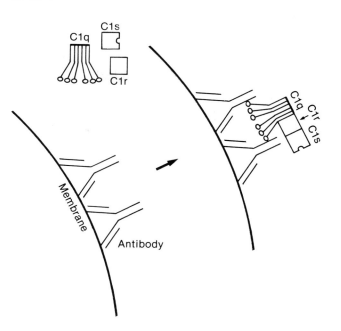

Figure 3–2. Fixation and activation of the first component of complement (C1).

"attack" of C1s on C4 takes place in the alpha chain and releases C4a, a so-called subunit of C4. This C4a subunit, which has a molecular weight of about 9000, is released and appears to play no further part in the complement sequence; however, it has been recognized as an anaphylatoxin, which is able to bind to mast cells and cause them to discharge their cytoplasmic granules. The remainder of the molecule is known as C4b (MW about 198,000). This subunit will attach to erythrocyte surfaces, bacterial cell membranes, and other antigens. It does not attach to C1 on the antigen-antibody complex. C4b can be cleaved by the serum C3b,C4b INAC, which produces C4c (MW 150,000) and C4d (MW 49,000), concomitant with the destruction of C4b activity (shown in Fig. 3–3). The C4c subunit is released into the body fluids, leaving C4d permanently fixed to the cell membrane.

There is evidence that with IgG, only C4 molecules that actually attach to the antibody are able to form C3 convertase (factor D) (Goers and Porter, 1978). On the other hand, C4 molecules do not appear to attach to IgM, in which case it appears that it is the C4 molecules bound to the cell membrane that form C3 convertase (Borsos *et al.*, 1981).

C2: The Second Activation Unit

C2 is also activated by C1s, although probably only after the C1sC4 interaction has taken place. C2 is a beta$_1$ globulin with a molecular weight of 110,000 and occurs in small quantities in serum (15 μg/ml being recorded as the average level). C2 binds with C4b and is cleaved by C1s into C2a and C2b subunits. These subunits have molecular weights of 70,000 and 30,000, respectively. The role of C2b is uncertain at this time, but C2a is known to activate C3 and C5 and may be the critical catalytic portion, C3 convertase (factor D or C4b2a; Fig. 3–4).

C3: The Third Activation Unit

C3 is the complement component that is most abundant in serum (1250 μg/ml; see Table 3–1). It is a beta$_2$ globulin (β$_{1C}$ globulin) with a molecular

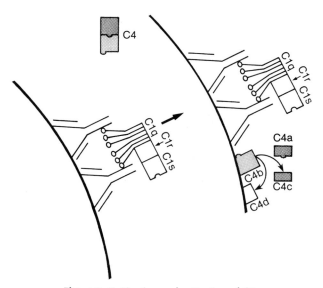

Figure 3–3. Fixation and activation of C4.

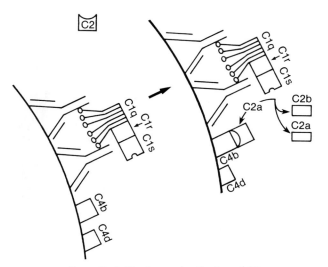

Figure 3–4. Fixation and activation of C4.

Further enzymatic cleavage of C3bi gives rise to the fragments C3c, C3d, and C3e. It is not clear whether the cleavage of C3de to C3d and C3e occurs physiologically in the circulation; in cold agglutinin disease, red cells are coated with C3de and not with C3d alone (Lachmann and Pangburn, 1981).

Similarly, C4b is cleaved in two places by factor I in the presence of C4b-binding protein, first to C4b$_i$ and subsequently to C4c and C4d (Nagasawa *et al.*, 1980).

The new complex $\overline{C4b,2a,3b}$ is known as C5 convertase, which, like C3 convertase, relies on C2a for its enzymatic activity (Fig. 3–6).

C5: The First Membrane Attack Unit

The next component of complement to become involved in the activation cascade is C5, which, in many respects, is like C3 (see Table 3–1). C5 is a beta$_1$ globulin with a molecular weight of 180,000, and, like C3, it is derived from a precursor molecule (in this case pro C5), secreted from macrophages. C5 is also structurally similar to C3, being composed of two peptide chains, alpha and beta, linked by disulfide bonds (Fig. 3–7). C5 convertase ($\overline{C4b,2a,3b}$ complex) cleaves C5 into two subunits, C5a and C5b. C5a is released into the body fluids, where, as anaphylatoxin II, it acts as a mediator of inflammation and as a chemotaxin for granulocytes. C5b, which remained after the removal of C5a, can be further degraded into C5c and C5d, the biologic roles of which are not known. Intact C5b, which attaches to the earlier complement components and to a specific receptor on the cell surface, serves as the activator of C6 and C7 and, therefore, is the first element in the membrane attack complex (Fig. 3–8).

weight of 180,000 and originates from pro C3, secreted by macrophages. C3 consists of two polypeptide chains, alpha and beta, joined by a number of disulfide bonds (Fig. 3–5). C3 convertase hydrolyzes a peptide bond in the alpha chain to produce C3a, a peptide with a molecular weight of 8900, which is an anaphylatoxin. The remainder of the molecule is known as C3b, and it is this subunit that attaches to $\overline{C4b,2a}$.

Factor I (working in collaboration with factor H) produces two splits in the alpha chain of C3b, but the bits of alpha remain covalently bonded to the beta chain (Harrison and Lachman, 1980; Sim *et al.*, 1981). The resulting product is called C3bi (*i.e.*, inactive, indicating the inability to bind to factor B, although one property, the ability to react with conglutinin, is concurrently gained).

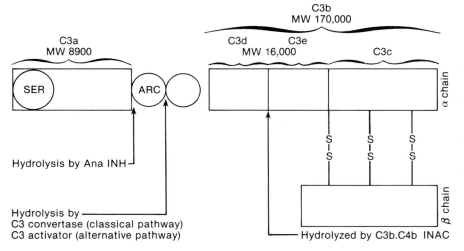

Figure 3–5. The peptide structure of C3. Activation of C3 follows peptide bond cleavage in the alpha-chain by C3 convertase or C3 activator. The anaphylatoxic split product, C3a, is inactivated by removal of its carboxyl terminal arginine by Ana INH. C3b is converted to C3i by C3b.C4b INAC hydrolysis and removal of C3d. (From Barrett, J. T.: Textbook of Immunology, 4th ed. St. Louis, The C. V. Mosby Company, 1983.)

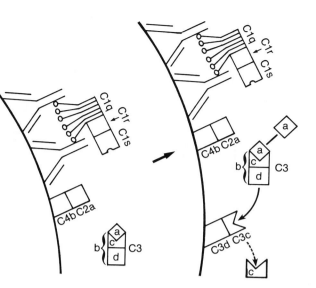

Figure 3–6. Fixation and activation of C3.

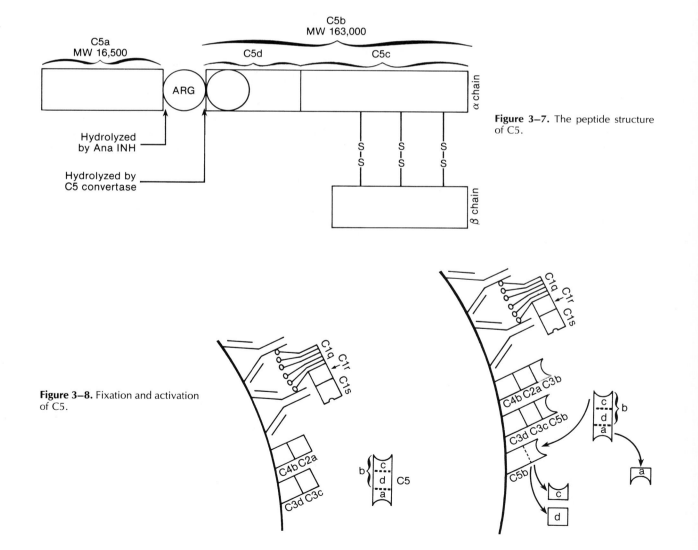

C5a
MW 16,500

C5b
MW 163,000

C5d   C5c

ARG

α chain

Hydrolyzed
by Ana INH

Hydrolyzed by
C5 convertase

S–S   S–S   S–S

β chain

Figure 3–7. The peptide structure of C5.

Figure 3–8. Fixation and activation of C5.

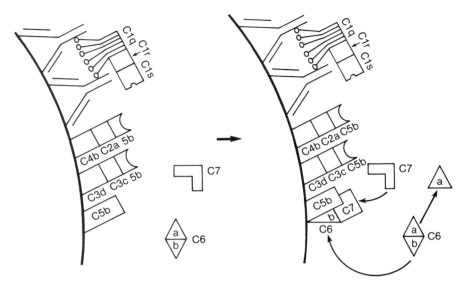

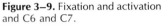

Figure 3–9. Fixation and activation and C6 and C7.

C6 and C7: The Second and Third Membrane Attack Units

Very little is known about C6 and C7 except that both are beta₁C globulins (β_2 globulins) with molecular weights of about 125,000 (see Table 3–1). C6 has a human serum concentration of 60 μg per ml; the level of C7 is 55 μg per ml. C5b cleaves C6 into C6a and C6b. Both C6b and C7 appear to bind to C5b by absorption (Fig. 3–9). The difficulty in obtaining further information about C6 and C7

is probably due to the ease with which they associate with C5 in a trimolecular complex.

C8 and C9: The Final Membrane Attack Units

The next molecule to become involved in the complement cascade is C8, which is composed of three peptide chains, C8α, C8β, and C8γ, two of which are covalently linked to each other (C8γ and

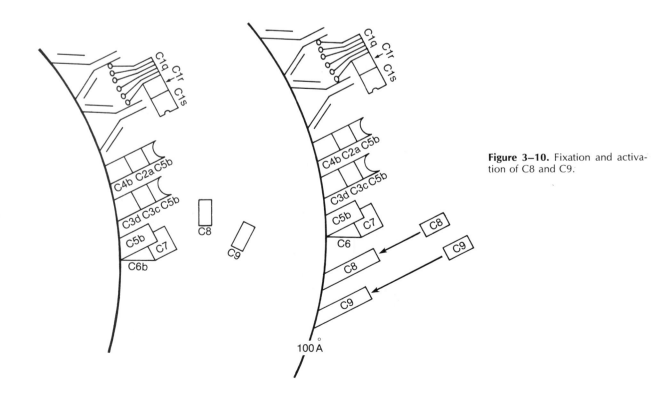

Figure 3–10. Fixation and activation of C8 and C9.

100 Å

C8α) by disulfide bonds, and a third (C8β), which is not covalently joined to the other two. C8 is inserted into the membrane and disrupts it. This disruption of the membrane appears to be irreversible, although the presence of C9 is apparently important in the formation of the membrane defect.

The final complement molecule to interact in the cascade is C9, which is an alpha globulin with a molecular weight of about 79,000. C9 appears to enhance the activity of C8 (Fig. 3–10).

THE EFFECTS OF COMPLEMENT ACTIVATION

The most significant effect of complement activation on sensitized erythrocytes (*i.e.*, those combined with specific antibody) or sensitized gram-negative bacteria is the cytolysis of the antigen. Although it is known that the C5 to C9 complex inserts into the lipid bilayer membrane where it forms a transmembrane protein channel, the exact causative force for the attendant lysis continues to

evade identification. The protein channel is funnel-shaped, being larger in diameter on the exterior surface than on the interior surface. Recent work has revealed that when the C5 to C9 complex is eluted from the lysed cells, an additional molecule (X) of molecular weight 88,000 is also recovered. It is believed that this molecule may be the lytic agent.

In the absence of C9, cells will still undergo lysis, although at a slower rate. When C9 is added, "holes" can be observed on the surface of the cells (Humphrey and Dourmashkin, 1965; Fig. 3–11). These holes have been observed with all cells (*e.g.*, red cells, Krebs ascites tumor cells, bacteria) lysed by the action of complement and have been observed on pseudomembranes formed by the absorption of serum lipids on to a carbon-coated surface; they are also observed when cells are lysed by certain other agents (*e.g.*, saponin; Humphrey and Dourmashkin, 1969). The diameter of these holes is about 80 to 100 μm (8–10nm) and appear to be about the same size (100 Å) regardless of the causative antibody (Rosse *et al.*, 1966).

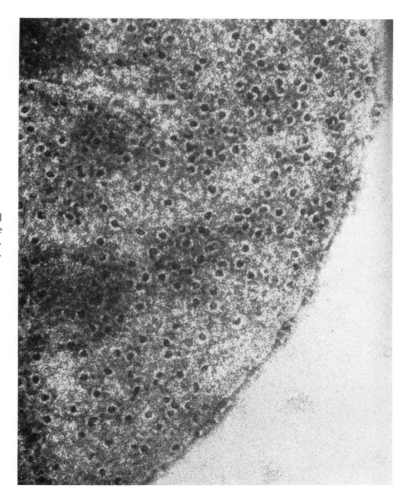

Figure 3–11. Multiple lesions in the cell wall of *Escherichia coli* bacterium caused by the interaction with IgM antibody and complement. Magnification × 400,000. (Courtesy of Drs. R. Dourmashkin and J. H. Humphrey.)

It is interesting to note that the "holes" do not penetrate the membrane and, therefore, should more correctly be described as "erosions" on the membrane. These erosions can be erased with lipid solvents. How they contribute to rapid cell lysis is not known but may be clarified when the role of the molecule X is better understood.

COMPLEMENT ACTIVATION: THE ALTERNATIVE PATHWAY

The alternative complement activation pathway was orginally described by Pillemer *et al.* (1954), who discovered that cell wall preparations from yeast or zymosan would activate complement. This activation was related to the serum globulin, properdin, which was newly discovered, and became known as the "properdin pathway." Since that time, it has been discovered that many complex polysaccharides will activate this alternative pathway (*e.g.,* liposaccharides, bacterial capsules, teichoic acids from bacterial cell walls, inulin, dextran). At least four serum proteins function in the alternative pathway that do not contribute to the classical pathway. These are factor B, factor D, C3b,Bb, and properdin (factor P; Table 3–2).

The initiating factor for the alternative pathway has not yet been clearly identified, but it is *not* properdin, as was earlier believed. The first molecule to be activated is C3, which is acted on by an enzyme complex formed in the alternative pathway (known as C3 activator), which has the same enzymatic activity as C3 convertase of the classical pathway. The formation of the complex in the alternative pathway that generates C3b (and C3a) from C3 is a multistage process that involves several molecules (although exactly how they participate remains uncertain). The alternative pathway, therefore, proceeds to the C3 activator stage without the participation or consumption of C1, C4, or C2 (Bitter-Suermann *et al.*, 1972). Once the C3 activator splits C3a from C3, the activation sequence proceeds to C9 in the same way as in the classical pathway.

BIOLOGIC FUNCTIONS ASSOCIATED WITH COMPLEMENT ACTIVATION

The large number of proteins involved in the complement system and the complexities of their interaction, plus the fact that two separate mechanisms have evolved for the activation of the complement system, suggest that several important biologic activities are associated with this system. Many of these functions (which do not include cell lysis) are now known. Table 3–3 lists the most widely accepted biologic functions of complement components and complement fragments. Although many of these are self-explanatory, it should be mentioned that anaphylatoxic factors cause mast cells to degranulate and release their various mediators in the absence of cytotoxicity. The opsonic properties of the complement proteins appear to depend upon the presence of specific receptors on the surface of phagocytic cells. Foreign materials with opsonically active fragments on their surface interact with these receptors, leading first to membrane adherence and, as a second step, to phagocytosis.

The control of the biologic properties of these complement fragments is the responsibility of specific serum protein inhibitors such as C1 esterase inhibitor (which destroys the enzymatic activity of activated C1); C3b inactivator destroys the integrity of the opsonically active protein C3b. An inactivator of cell-bound C6 is also known to exist, as is an inactivator of the vasoactive material, anaphylatoxin, which destroys the activity of C3a and, to a lesser extent, C5a.

Table 3–2. CHARACTERISTICS OF PROTEINS IN THE ALTERNATIVE COMPLEMENT ACTIVATION PATHWAY

Component	Abbreviation	Serum Concentration (μg/ml)	Sedimentation Coefficient ($s_{20,W}$)	Molecular Weight	Electrophoretic Position	Comment
Properdin	P	25	5.4	184,000	γ_2	Exists as tetramer
C3 (factor A)	C3	1,250	9.5	180,000	β_2	Also intermediate in classic pathway
C3 proactivator convertase (factor D)	C3 PAse	2	3	24,000	α	Trypsin-like enzyme
C3 proactivator (factor B)	C3 PA	200	5–6	93,000	β	Proenzyme
C3 activator	C3 A	Unknown	4	63,000	γ	Cleaves C3 at bond 77–78
Cobra venom factor	CoF, CVF	Not found in serum	6.7	144,000		May be cobra C3b

From Barrett, J. T.: Textbook of Immunology. St. Louis, The C. V. Mosby Co., 1983, p. 182.

Table 3–3. PROPERTIES OF THE COMPLEMENT–DERIVED PEPTIDES

Protein	Source	Molecular Weight	Biologic Activity	Released By
C2b	C2	37,000	Unknown	$C\overline{1}s$
C3a	α chain of C3	8,900	Anaphylatoxic	C3 convertase and C3 activator
C4a	α chain of C4	9,000	Anaphylatoxic	$C\overline{1}s$
C5a	α chain of C5	11,000	Anaphylatoxic and chemotactic	C5 convertase

From Barrett, J. T.: Textbook of Immunology. St. Louis, The C. V. Mosby Co., 1983.

THE DESTRUCTION OF COMPLEMENT *IN VITRO*

Complement components can be destroyed *in vitro* in the following ways:

Anticoagulants. As previously mentioned, ionized calcium (Ca^{++}) is required for the integrity of C1 and is therefore required for the activation of complement via the classical pathway. Similarly, ionized magnesium (Mg^{++}) is required for the formation of the C3 convertases of both the classical and alternative pathways (*i.e.*, C42 and C3b,Bb, respectively). Because of this, all chelators of Ca^{++} and Mg^{++} (also written as Ca^{2+} and Mg^{2+}) will inhibit complement activity. For example, the addition of 2 mg of Na_2H_2EDTA to 1 ml of serum completely blocks the activation of complement.

The anticoagulant heparin is also anticomplementary and, in sufficient quantities, will completely inhibit the cleavage of C4 by $C\overline{1}$.

Heating. The heating of serum to 56°C for 30 minutes completely inactivates C1 and C2. C4 is also damaged (although to a lesser extent) (Bier *et al.*, 1945; Heidelberger and Mayer, 1948). Factor B of the alternative pathway is inactivated by heating to 50°C for 20 minutes.

Normal Serum Inhibitor. Serum normally contains an inhibitor of $C\overline{1}$, which does not interfere with the conversion of C1 to $C\overline{1}$ but directly inhibits the action of $C\overline{1}$ by binding to and removing $C\overline{1}s$ and $C\overline{1}r$ from the $C\overline{1}qrs$ complex.

Storage. On storage, serum regularly becomes anticomplementary—preliminary observations suggest that the alteration may principally affect C4.

COMPLEMENT IN DISEASE STATES

In the majority of disease states, complement functions normally in producing inflammation and tissue damage. In those cases in which complement plays a role in the development of a disease, it is often being activated by an irregular antibody, immune complex for foreign material. The activity of a disease state can often be followed by assessing the level of one or another complement component (see Measurement of Complement Components, Chapter 15).

In addition to the role of complement components in disease states, there is now considerable interest in the detection of decay products in various body fluids. In this respect, C3 decay products have been found in the sera of patients with primary biliary cirrhosis, rheumatoid arthritis, and lupus erythematosus. Because this area is currently under active investigation, it is probable that this list will grow rapidly.

The following is a brief review of the levels of complement in various disease states. The reader interested in more detailed information is referred to the list of general references at the end of this chapter.

Rheumatologic Diseases

Systemic Lupus Erythematosus. In systemic lupus erythematosus (SLE), circulating immune complexes activate complement and are deposited in a variety of tissue sites, leading to tissue damage. It has been suggested that the activity of the disease can be followed by the determination of C3 and C4 levels. As mentioned, C3 decay products have also been found in the sera of patients with this disease.

Rheumatoid Arthritis. Depressed levels of complement have been shown to exist in rheumatoid arthritis as well as a number of other rheumatologic diseases. Normal or elevated serum complement levels are found in juvenile rheumatoid arthritis and in most patients with adult onset rheumatoid arthritis. Depressed CH_{50} and cleavage products of C3 and properdin factor B are thought to represent intra-articular activation in the synovial fluid of almost all patients with seropositive rheumatoid arthritis. This is not true of fluids obtained from patients with degenerative arthritis (Hunder, 1977).

Others. Normal or elevated serum complement levels are also found in patients with paledromic arthritis, pseudogout, gout, Reiter's syndrome, and gonococcal arthritis. Depressed CH_{50} and cleavage products of C3 and properdin factor B

Table 3–4. COMPLEMENT LEVELS IN SELECTED RENAL DISEASES

	C1	C4	C2	C3	P	B
Acute glomerulonephritis	N	D	D	D	D	N or D
Systemic lupus erythematosus	D	D	D	D	N or D	D
Membranoproliferative glomerulonephritis	N	N	N	D	N or D	N or D
Post-streptococcal glomerulonephritis	Normal in initial sera (<10 days) in some studies					
Post-streptococcal glomerulonephritis (later)	D	D slight	D slight	D	D	N or D
Idiopathic nephrotic syndrome	N	N	N	N		D
Anaphylactoid purpura with nephritis	N or D low levels transient	N or D	N	—	N or D	N

Note: The syndrome of partial lipodystrophy may be associated with C3 depression, C3NeF in serum, and membranoproliferative glomerulonephritis.
B = Factor B; D = depressed; N = normal; and P = properdin.
From Henry, J. B. (Ed.): Clinical Diagnosis and Management by Laboratory Methods, 17th ed. Philadelphia, W. B. Saunders Company, 1984, p. 884.

are also thought to represent intra-articular activation in the synovial fluid of many patients with SLE, pseudogout, gout, Reiter's syndrome, and gonococcal arthritis.

Infectious Diseases

Patients with gram-negative septicemia and certain fungal diseases (e.g., cryptococcal septicemia) are often depleted of C3 and components of the alternative pathway of complement activation. It is now known that patients with HB_sAg-positive infectious hepatitis may have an early fall in serum C3, which later returns to normal. This may be associated with signs of immune complex disease (e.g., arthralgia). Complement also appears to play a similar role in a number of parasitic infections, including malaria. In patients with vivax malaria, C1, C4, and C2 may be depressed. C3 may be depressed, in addition to these, in falciparum malaria.

Renal Diseases

Michael (1974) reported that complement is of key importance in glomerular damage in a variety of the glomerulonephritides. This is usually demonstrated through the deposition of C3 and/or other components in the vicinity of the glomerular basement membrane (Table 3–4). Many patients will show activation of the alternative pathway on serum analysis. In interstitial and tubular disease, the role of complement is less clear, although it is believed by some investigators that complement may also have some function in these disorders.

Dermatologic Diseases

Complement is believed to play a role in the ongoing tissue damage in a variety of dermatologic illnesses, including pemphigus vulgaris, bullous pemphigoid, and herpes gestationis. Serum complement levels are usually normal or elevated in these chronic inflammatory states, and the importance of complement is suggested by immunofluorescent analysis of tissue biopsies and by studies of blister fluid.

Hematologic Diseases

Complement plays an important role in opsonization of erythrocytes in many types of autoimmune hemolytic anemia, leading to their clearance by the cells of the reticuloendothelial system. It should be noted, however, that even in those cases in which complement is clearly involved, complement levels are usually normal. Complement is of particular importance in the clearance of cells coated with IgM cold agglutinins of anti-I specificity. In paroxysmal nocturnal hemoglobinuria (PNH), the patient's red cells and other blood cell elements develop a membrane defect that renders them susceptible to complement-mediated lysis. This acquired cellular defect is associated with cytotoxicity and clearance due to activation of the alternative pathway by the cell membrane.

REVIEW QUESTIONS

MULTIPLE CHOICE

Choose the phrase, sentence, or symbol that completes the statement or answers the question. More than one answer may be correct in each case. Answers are given at the end of this book.

1. The term *complement* refers to a complex set of:
   (a) nine distinct components
   (b) eleven distinct components
   (c) eleven distinct serum proteins
   (d) nine distinct serum proteins
   (Introduction)

2. Which of the following cells are most susceptible to immune cytolysis?
   (a) gram-positive bacteria
   (b) gram-negative bacteria
   (c) thrombocytes
   (d) most mammalian cells
   (Introduction)

3. Which of the following immunoglobulins do not function with complement?
   (a) IgA
   (b) IgM
   (c) IgG3
   (d) IgE
   (Introduction)

4. Complement levels are:
   (a) increased as a result of immunization
   (b) decreased as a result of immunization
   (c) not affected by immunization
   (d) depleted as a result of immunization
   (Introduction)

5. A "bar" over the designation for a complement protein (e.g., C$\overline{1}$), indicates:
   (a) that the protein is activated
   (b) that the protein is inactivated
   (c) that the protein participates in the alternative pathway *only*
   (d) that the protein has failed to react in a specific way
   (The Components of Complement)

6. In the alternative pathway of complement activation:
   (a) 9 additional proteins participate
   (b) 5 additional proteins participate
   (c) 12 additional proteins participate
   (d) a total of 14 proteins participate
   (The Components of Complement)

7. The order of activation of the first four components of complement in the classical pathway is:
   (a) C1, C2, C3, C4
   (b) C1, C3, C4, C2
   (c) C1, C4, C2, C3
   (d) C1, C4, C3, C3
   (Complement Activation: The Classical Pathway)

8. The three subunits of C1 are called:
   (a) C1q, C1r, C1s
   (b) C1r, C1s, C1t
   (c) C1a, C1b, C1c
   (d) C1qr, C1rs, C1st
   (C1: The Recognition Unit)

9. Of the three subunits of C1:
   (a) C1q is the largest
   (b) C1q is the smallest
   (c) C1q has the highest molecular weight
   (d) C1q is the least important and does not directly participate in the activation sequence
   (C1: The Recognition Unit)

10. The C4 molecule consists of:
    (a) three peptide chains joined by disulfide bonds
    (b) six peptide chains joined by disulfide bonds
    (c) two peptide chains joined by hydrogen bonds
    (d) a single peptide chain
    (C4: The Activation Unit)

11. The most abundant component of complement in serum is:
    (a) C1
    (b) C3
    (c) C4
    (d) C2
    (Complement Activation: The Classical Pathway)

12. The complement component C5:
    (a) has a molecular weight of 180,000
    (b) is structurally similar to C3
    (c) is a beta$_1$ globulin
    (d) possesses two peptide chains
    (C5: The First Membrane Attack Unit)

13. The diameter of the "holes" observed on all cells subsequent to complement activation is:
    (a) about 80 to 100 μm
    (b) about 100 Å
    (c) about the same size regardless of the causative antibody
    (d) different according to the nature of the causative antibody
    (The Effects of Complement Activation)

14. With respect to the alternative pathway of complement activation:
    (a) the initiating factor is properdin
    (b) the first molecule to be activated is C1
    (c) it does not involve the participation or consumption of C1, C2, or C4
    (d) it is the same as the classical pathway
    (Complement Activation: The Alternative Pathway)

15. Complement components can be destroyed in *in vitro* by:
    (a) anticoagulants
    (b) freezing
    (c) normal serum inhibitor
    (d) storage
    (The Destruction of Complement)

ANSWER "TRUE" OR "FALSE"

(a) IgM and IgG are the only immunoglobulins that react with complement.
(Introduction)

17. Complement is only found in certain mammalian sera and is not found in birds.
(Introduction)

18. Portions of the complement system contribute to chemotaxis.
(Introduction)

19. Only five major components of complement participate in the alternative pathway.
(Introduction)

20. The protein that was originally known as C3 proactivator convertase is now known as factor D.
(The Components of Complement)

21. The C1 complex is held together by calcium ions.
(C1: The Recognition Unit)

22. C1q binds to the Fab region of the complement-activating IgM and IgG immunoglobulins.
(C1: The Recognition Unit)

23. C4a, the subunit of C4, attaches to erythrocyte surfaces.
(C4: The Activation Unit)

24. C3 and C5 are activated by C2a.
(C2: The Second Activation Unit)

25. C6 is cleaved into C6a and C6b by C5b.
(C6 and C7: The Second and Third Membrane Attack Units)

26. The function of C9 appears to be to enhance the activity of C8.
(C8 and C9: The Final Membrane Attack Units)

27. The lytic agent in the effect of complement activation is believed to be a molecule known as X, which has a molecular weight of 88,000.
(The Effects of Complement Activation)

28. The activity of the disease systemic lupus erythematosus can be followed by the determination of C8 and C9 levels.
(Complement in Disease States)

29. Patients with gram-negative septicemia are often depleted of components of the alternative pathway of complement activation.
(Complement in Disease States)

30. In cases of autoimmune hemolytic anemia, complement levels are usually well below normal.
(Complement in Disease States)

General References

Barrett, J. T.: Textbook of Immunology, 4th ed. St. Louis, The C.V. Mosby Co., 1983.

Bellanti, J. A.: Immunology: Basic Processes. Philadelphia, W. B. Saunders Company, 1979.

Henry, J. B. (Ed.): Clinical Diagnosis and Management by Laboratory Principles, 17th ed. Philadelphia, W. B. Saunders Company, 1984.

Parker, C. W.: Clinical Immunology, Philadelphia, W. B. Saunders Company, 1980.

FOUR

THE IMMUNE RESPONSE

Introduction

When foreign antigen gains entry into the body, several important changes may be initiated, collectively known as the *immune response,* which result in the elimination of the alien antigen. A remarkable feature of this phenomenon is the ability of the adult mammal to distinguish between its own antigens (known as "self" antigens) and those of external or foreign origin (known as "nonself" antigens). This means that, as a general rule, antibody is *selectively* produced in response to foreign substances, yet it is not produced to antigens that are recognized as "self."

The immune response is presumed to have been evolved by animals as a means of self-protection in a world teeming with microorganisms; yet, whereas the self-nonself response is selective, the reaction to foreign substances is not, and antibodies are formed regardless of whether or not these substances are bacterial products.

Under certain circumstances, these antibodies can react with foreign material if it is reintroduced and can produce severe damage to tissue compo-

nents (the phenomenon known as *hypersensitivity*). It is evident that the immune response is not only concerned with immunity to infection but that it is also involved in many disease processes, and, under certain circumstances, it *causes* hypersensitivity (see further discussion later in this chapter).

As previously mentioned, the immune response results in the formation of antibodies, these being either immunoglobulins or cell-bound.

THE FORMATION OF IMMUNOGLOBULIN

The immune response, following the entry of foreign antigen into the body, is preceded by a period of antigen elimination, after which a primary response occurs—or a secondary response if the antigen has previously been encountered.

Antigen Elimination

If foreign antigen is injected intravenously, three phases of antigen removal are easily detected:

The First Phase. This takes about 10 to 20 minutes if particulate antigens are used and represents the time required for equilibrium of the antigen with tissues and fluids. Almost 90 per cent of the antigen is removed from the circulation in the first passage through the liver, lung, and spleen through extensive phagocytosis. Soluble antigens are not removed from the blood quite so quickly because of their slower pinocytic uptake by cells. If the antigen is aggregated, it is removed faster, indicating that size is important in phagocytosis and pinocytosis.

The Second Phase. This is a gradual catabolic degradation and removal process, which continues over a period of 4 to 7 days and represents the gradual enzymatic hydrolysis and digestion of the antigen. The limits of this period are regulated by the enzymatic capability of the host for the particular type of substrate that the antigen represents. In hosts that fail to produce antibody (*i.e.*, become tolerant to the antigen), this phase is extended for several weeks and represents the last phase of antigen elimination.

The Third Phase. In this final phase of antigen elimination, there is, once again, accelerated removal of antigen. The phase is sometimes known as the immune elimination segment and is the result of the newly formed antibody molecules combining with the antigen, enhancing phagocytosis, digestion, and removal. The absolute removal of all antigen, however, may take many months or even years (Fig. 4–1).

The Primary Response

Following the first injection of antigen, there is a lag of several days before antibody is detected in the serum. This latent period (also known as the "induction" period) varies from several hours to several days, depending upon the kind of antigen involved, the amount of antigen given, the route of administration, the species of animal and its health, and the sensitivity of the test used to detect the antibody. On the average, antibody usually appears from the fifth to the tenth day after injection of antigen.

It should be noted that the latent period is *not* a reflection of the amount of time it takes for antibody production to begin at a cellular level. In fact, when antibody-forming cells are removed from an immunized animal, antibody synthesis can be detected within 20 minutes after exposure to the antigen. Because only a few cells are involved in antibody production at this time, it may take several days before the antibody is detectable in the serum. Another consideration is that the first antibody molecules to appear in the serum may find residual antigen still in the circulation and

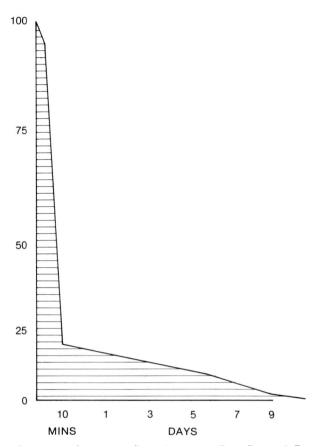

Figure 4–1. The antigen elimination curve. (From Barrett, J. T.: Textbook of Immunology, 4th ed. St. Louis, The C. V. Mosby Company, 1983, p. 142.)

may combine with it, making the detection of the antibody difficult by usual serologic tests. These antigen-antibody complexes are secreted rapidly, so that the first evidence of *free* antibody is not until a few days after the first antibody molecules are liberated into the serum. In this way, very large injections of antigens may tend to extend the latent period.

At the end of the latent period, the primary antibody response becomes visible. The titer of the antibody gradually increases over a period of a few days to a few weeks, reaches a plateau, then begins to drop. The general shape of the primary response curve is that of the typical signoid curve, with an extended decay phase. A typical primary response curve is given in Figure 4–2, although it should be noted that the exact shape of the curve will be dictated by the variables already stated.

The Secondary Response

After second (or subsequent) exposure to a foreign antigen, the response of the host differs dramati-

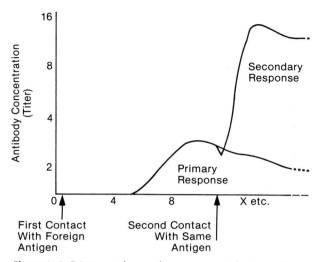

Figure 4–2. Primary and secondary response to foreign antigen.

to the involved foreign antigen is reached. This may not occur until three to five booster injections of the antigen have been given.

The secondary response may be induced by cross-reactive antigens. The degree of response in these cases can be correlated with the similarity of the two antigens—the more alike they are, the better the response is likely to be.

In some cases, so-called negative anamnesis may occur. This can result from the treatment of the immunized host, which may cause lysis or hyperplasia of the antibody-forming cells. It should be noted, however, that the response in these cases is usually minimal.

After the secondary response, the decrease in antibody titer seems to be more gradual than it is after the primary response. This is probably the result of two factors:

1. More cells are involved in antibody production in the secondary response. If some of these cells are long-lived and continue to function, antibody will be formed over a longer period of time after the secondary response than after the primary response.
2. The antiserum in the secondary response is qualitatively different from that of the primary response, containing more IgG, which has a half-life of 25 to 35 days. The primary antiserum is relatively rich in IgM (which has a half-life of only 8 to 10 days). IgG has been referred to as the "memory component," implying that IgM anamnesis does not occur. This is true in a relative sense only, because secondary IgM levels are in fact somewhat greater than primary levels.

When soluble antigens or autocoupling haptens are used for reactivation of the immunoglobulin, a certain danger exists in that a proportion of the antibody produced after the primary antigenic exposure has the capacity to fix to tissue cells, and these cell-bound antibodies can attach to the injected antigen while still attached to the tissue cells. In some cases, this *in vivo* cell-bound antigen-antibody reaction can trigger a set of reactions that may be lethal to the host. This syndrome is known as anaphylactic shock and, under certain conditions, must be considered as a hazard to reimmunization. (See further discussion under *Hypersensitivity*.)

The secondary response, as previously mentioned, occurs as a result of "immunologic memory," carried by the small lymphocytes. This means that the small lymphocytes retain information regarding the challenging antigen. Immunologic memory can be transferred from one animal to another. Small lymphocytes from a rat that has already given a primary response to an antigen

cally from that of the primary response. At first, there is a sharp drop in the amount of circulating antibody, because it is complexing with the newly injected antigen. Immediately thereafter (usually within 2 or 3 days under normal conditions and circumstances), the level of antibody in the blood increases markedly. This increase continues for several days, and, ultimately, the titer of the antibody far surpasses that attained in the primary response. The secondary response is also known as the memory, anamnestic, or booster response. It is as though the host is now primed for that particular antigen and is able to respond to it in an accelerated way (see further discussion that follows).

All the variables that affect the primary response also, to some extent, affect the secondary response, although the latent period is briefer, there is a heightened titer, and the duration of detectable antibody in the blood is extended.

It should be noted that the rapid response seen is not the result of the release of *stored* antibody, but rather the result of bulk synthesis of the new antibody. This has been proved through experiments with radio-labeled amino acids that were injected at the same time as the antigen. When the antibody was studied after a few days, it was found to be heavily labeled with isotope, indicating recent production.

There is no time limit for the secondary response—it may be induced at any time after the primary response, even many years later when the primary titer has dropped to zero. If the secondary response is nearer to the time of the primary response, however, it is usually more striking than it would be after several years.

The secondary response may be repeated many times until the physiologic limit of the host reaction challenge can be injected into another rat with no previous contact with that antigen. Subsequent challenge to the recipient rat with the antigen results in a secondary-type response, with rapid production of high-strength antibodies.

THE EFFECTS OF IMMUNOGLOBULIN *IN VIVO*

Immunity

The primary effect of immunoglobulin *in vivo* is to provide immunity for the host against reinfection. In the case of most infective agents, antibodies that are produced in response to infection are directed against the antigenic components of the organism itself and are called *antibacterial, antiviral,* or *antifungal* antibodies. In general, since the organisms have many antigenic determinants, antibodies are produced that have different specificities.

Some of these antibodies play a protective role against reinfection (*i.e.,* provide immunity), whereas others appear to have no protective activity. These nonprotective antibodies, through their detection in the blood are, however, useful in diagnosis (*e.g.,* in cases of typhoid fever or secondary syphilis; see Chapter six).

Active immunization is carried out through the injection of a suspension of the invasive organism (either living or dead) or through the injection of a *toxoid* (*i.e.,* a chemically altered preparation of bacterial toxin). In addition, passive antibacterial immunity can be achieved by injecting human or animal sera containing specific antibodies, although the discovery of potent antibiotics has made their use unnecessary. Passive immunization against *viral* infections, however, still has a useful role (*e.g.,* anti-measles serum is used to prevent very young children from contracting this infection).

Antibacterial antibodies provide immunity to infection in a variety of ways—some may act as opsonins and aid phagocytosis, others activate complement and lead to lysis of the organism. The activation of complement also releases factors such as C3b, for example, which acts as an opsonin. The spread of infection is limited by anaphylatoxins and chemotactic factors (which augment the inflammatory response) or by agglutinins, although the role of the latter in this is probably minor.

Globulin antibodies are generally named according to the nature of the test used to detect them (*e.g.,* antitoxin, precipitin), although some antibodies are capable of performing several functions, depending upon the conditions under which it is examined. For example, diphtheria toxin, which is capable of neutralizing toxin in an *in vivo* experiment is rightly known as an "antitoxin"; however, *in vitro,* it can produce a precipitin with its corresponding antigen and can, in this instance, be called a "precipitin." Some antibodies (*e.g.,* those directed against certain red cell antigens) produce agglutination in the absence of complement (agglutinins) and lysis when complement is fixed (lysin).

Hypersensitivity (Table 4–1)

There are three distinct ways in which immunoglobulins can produce hypersensitivity: anaphylaxis, cytotoxic, and immune-complex reactions.

Anaphylaxis (Type I hypersensitivity). This type of reaction, also known as *generalized anaphylactic shock,* is rare in humans yet is encountered in three circumstances:

a. When horse gamma globulin is given to patients who are sensitized to horse protein (*e.g.,* in passive immunization against diphtheria and tetanus, whether prophylactic or therapeutic).

b. Through the injection of a drug that is capable of acting as a hapten into a patient who is sensitive to it (*e.g.,* penicillin).

c. Following a wasp or bee sting in highly sensitive individuals.

The manifestations of anaphylaxis include bron-

Table 4–1. TYPES OF CLINICAL HYPERSENSITIVITY

Type	Reaction	Antibody	Clinical Examples
I	Anaphylactic	IgE	Asthma, hay fever, helminth infestation
II	Cytotoxic	IgG, IgM	Antibacterial antibodies, autoimmune disease (Hashimoto's thyroiditis, antigastric antibodies in pernicious anemia, hemolytic anemia, etc.), viral disease prevention
III	Immune complex	IgG, IgM	Serum sickness, glomerulonephritis, and immune complex disease
IV	Delayed hypersensitivity	Sensitized lymphocytes	Tuberculin skin test (also fungal skin tests, Frei antigen, etc.), rejection of allografts or xenografts, "resistance" to viral disease

Modified from Raphael, S. S.: Lynch's Medical Laboratory Technology, 4th ed. Philadelphia, W. B. Saunders Co., 1983.

chospasm, edema (due to generalized increase in vascular permeability), pallor, and low blood pressure. The reaction in humans is due to the formation of sensitized IgE, which has a great affinity for certain cells (particularly mast cells) to which it becomes firmly attached, causing *hystamine* to be liberated, which causes the manifestations described.

Dust and Food Hypersensitivity. This type of reaction occurs after the ingestion of certain foods and the inhalation of pollen or dust. The offending agent may be an antigen or a hapten, and the symptoms appear to be related to the route of absorption.

The inhalation of antigens such as dust or pollen usually produces watering of the eyes or symptoms involving the respiratory tract (congestion of the nasal mucosa, *e.g.*, allergic rhinitis or hay fever, and bronchial asthma), whereas ingestion of certain foods produces either gastrointestinal symptoms or urticarial skin rashes. This type of hypersensitivity appears to be genetically determined in some families (such individuals are termed *atopic*). Attempts to desensitize these atopic individuals are sometimes made using small doses of the offending antigen at weekly intervals, with gradual increases of the dose in an attempt to produce an excess of IgG antibody in the blood, which will intercept the antigens before they reach the cells sensitized by IgE. This procedure, unfortunately, is not uniformly successful.

Cytotoxic (Type II hypersensitivity). This type of reaction is manifested by the production of antibodies that are capable of destroying cells. Although this is an uncommon type of hypersensitivity, it is occasionally seen with penicillin therapy when the drug, acting as a hapten, attaches to the red cell membrane causing antibodies to be formed that react with the penicillin and lead to red cell damage through the activation of complement on the red cell surface. This type of reaction then leads to a hemolytic anemia.

Immune–Complex Reactions (Type III hypersensitivity). Certain types of antibodies have the ability to combine with their corresponding antigens to form complexes that can activate complement. This results in the liberation of chemotactic factors and polymorphs, which are attracted to the complexes and release damaging lysosomal enzymes. Examples in which these immune complexes produce disease include the Arthus reaction, serum sickness, and chronic immune complex disease.

The Arthus Reaction. If subcutaneous injections of an antigen are given to an animal on a weekly basis, progressively more severe local reactions are observed. Swelling and redness appear within 1 hour, and over the next few hours, hemorrhage

and necrosis develop. The pathogenesis is as follows:

1. The injected antigen diffuses into the vessel walls and encounters the specific IgG that is present in the blood.
2. The antigen-antibody complexes activate complement in the vessel wall.
3. Polymorphs accumulate and release their lysosomal enzymes.
4. The cell wall is damaged, and thrombosis follows (Fig. 4–3).

The Arthus reaction is believed to be the explanation for some types of vasculitis in man, such as that seen in gonococcal septicemia.

Serum Sickness. Serum sickness can occur in individuals who have had no previous contact with the offending antigen (primary serum sickness) or in those who have been previously sensitized with the offending antigen (accelerated serum sickness). In both cases, the pathogenesis is the same, although in accelerated serum sickness, the onset of symptoms is more immediate.

Pathogenesis. Following the injection of a large dose of antigen, antibody is produced, which enters the blood stream in increasing amounts over a period of days (in the primary syndrome) or as soon as a few hours (in the accelerated syndrome). If the antigen is still circulating by the time that there is a sizable amount of circulating antibody, antigen-antibody complexes are formed and are rapidly eliminated by the activity of the reticuloendothelial system. The complexes are deposited on a sensitive membrane such as beneath the glomerular endothelium, skin, and joints. Complement is then activated, polymorphs accumulate, and inflammatory products that cause tissue damage are released.

In both the primary and accelerated syndromes, there may be production of IgE as well as IgM and IgG, and, in these instances, anaphylactic symptoms may occur. The syndrome is characterized by fever, joint pains, and urticarial eruptions, which occur within the time limits given.

The course of the illness is variable, depending upon the type, extent, and severity of the lesions, which may involve the joints (arthritis), kidney (glomerulonephritis), heart (myocarditis), and skin (vasculitis). In general, as immune complexes are catabolized, the symptoms of the illness subside and free antibody appears in the blood (Fig. 4–4).

Serum sickness provoked by drugs forming haptens with body protein antigens (*e.g.*, penicillin, streptomycin) is well known.

Chronic Immune–Complex Disease. A number of naturally occurring diseases are believed to be caused by deposits of immune complex and complement in the tissues (*e.g.*, systemic lupus erythe-

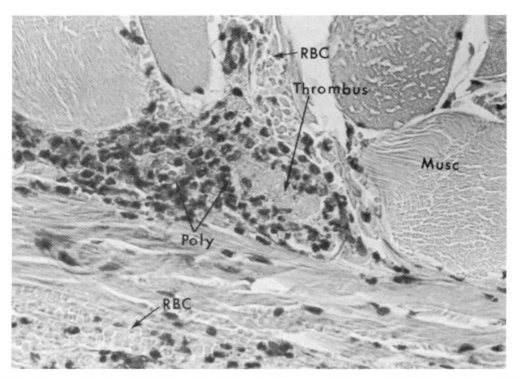

Figure 4–3. The Arthus reaction in a rabbit. This section is from the subcutaneous tissues and includes striated muscle (Musc). The blood vessel in the center is sectioned obliquely and shows occlusion of its lumen by thrombus. Its walls are heavily infiltrated by polymorphs (Poly), many of which are degenerating. Free red cells (RBC) in the tissues bear witness to the severity of vascular damage (× 550). (From Walter, J. B.: An Introduction to the Principles of Disease, 2nd ed. Philadelphia, W. B. Saunders Company, 1982, p. 127.)

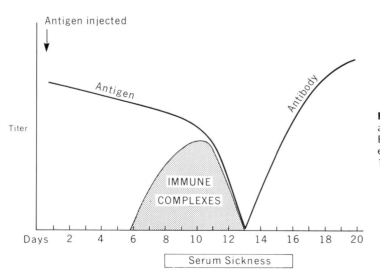

Figure 4–4. A graph showing changes in antigen and antibody titer during serum sickness. (From Walter, J. B.: An Introduction to the Principles of Disease, 2nd ed. Philadelphia, W. B. Saunders Company, 1982, p. 147.)

matosus (SLE), acute diffuse glomerulonephritis, rheumatic fever, rheumatoid arthritis, and periarteritis nodosa). As in serum sickness, these diseases show some or all of the features of arthritis, carditis, glomerulonephritis, and vasculitis.

CELL–MEDIATED IMMUNITY

Cell-mediated immunity is probably a factor in immunity to all infections, but it is of particular importance with respect to infections with viruses, fungi, and acid-fast bacillary infections such as tuberculosis and leprosy.

The manifestations of cell-mediated immunity are as follows:

Following the injection of antigen (particularly if combined with Freud's adjuvant or in the form of a living organism), specifically sensitized T-lymphocytes or specific cell products are formed, which react specifically with antigen and release a number of agents known as *lymphokines*, which have been named according to their specific demonstrable activity. These include *migration-inhibition factor (MIF)*, which makes cells more phagocytic and better able to kill organisms; *transfer factor,* which transfers sensitization to previously uncommitted lymphocytes and therefore recruits new cells to the site of infection; *lymphotoxin,* which has the ability to destroy cells; *skin reactive factor*, which is believed to be responsible for some of the phenomena of the Mantoux test (see later in this chapter); *chemotactic factor,* which can attract neutrophils, monocytes, or eosinophils; *mitogenic factor, which causes blast transformation of lymphocytes and stimulates mitosis; and interferon,* which prevents intracellular viral replication and *immunoglobulin.*

The presence of cell bound antibody is, like the humoral immune response, associated with either immunity to infection or hypersensitivity. Neither cellular immunity nor hypersensitivity, however, can be transferred to another animal by transferring serum; it can only be affected by the transfer of lymphocytes.

There is no simple way of measuring or assessing cell-mediated immunity; only the response to challenging infection can reveal its presence.

Hypersensitivity in Cell–Mediated Immunity (see Table 4–1)

Cell-mediated hypersensitivity is also known as Type VI, or *delayed hypersensitivity*. It is mediated by cells; circulating antibody and complement are not involved. Many reactions to immunologic insult involve both cellular and humoral components; those that may be used as examples of this type of response include The Tuberculin Skin Reaction and autoimmune disease.

The Tuberculin Skin Reaction (The Koch Phenomenon). If tubercle bacilli are injected into a normal guinea pig, a nodule appears at the site of injection after an incubation period of 10 to 14 days, followed by ulceration. The bacilli spread to local lymph nodes, and finally they reach the blood stream, resulting in the death of the animal within 6 to 12 weeks. The injection of more tubercle bacilli into a different site in the same animal infected 4 to 6 weeks previously elicits a completely different response: the nodule appears within 1 or 2 days, ulcerates, and then heals, and the bacilli tend not to spread to local lymph nodes. The details of this second type of response were introduced at the end of the nineteenth century by Robert Koch, who produced a crude filtrate of a broth culture of *Mycobacterium tuberculosis* called *old tuberculin*, which, although valueless as a therapeutic agent (the purpose for which it was originally introduced), it was nevertheless found to be of value as a diagnostic tool. Koch's old tuberculin has now been replaced by the purified protein derivative of tuberculin (PPD). When given intradermally in considerable dilution (1:1000 to 1:10,000) in 0.1-ml amounts, an area of induration of 5 mm or more in diameter at the site of injection surrounded by erythema observed after 48 hours is considered a positive response in individuals who have a hypersensitivity to tuberculoprotein (*i.e.,* those who have been sensitized by previous or present tuberculosis). The test is known as the *tuberculin* or *Mantoux test*. It should be noted that this test, although indicative of sensitization, does not indicate the clinical activity of the disease. The exact relationship between skin sensitivity and the level of cellular immunity is not clear, but it is likely that such a relationship exists.

Other skin tests used similarly include histoplasmin, coccidioidin, blastomycin, and the Frei test.

The characteristics of the Koch phenomenon are:

1. The reaction is delayed, taking at least 12 hours to develop. This is unlike other types of hypersensitivity reactions, which generally take only a few minutes.
2. There is an accumulation of lymphocytes and macrophages (giving a *mild* inflammatory reaction) rather than polymorphs at the site of insult.
3. The reaction is not mediated by histamine (or by any other mediators of acute inflammation) and is not blocked by antihistaminic drugs.
4. Immunoglobulins are not involved in the reaction.
5. The sensitivity to a particular antigen may be

transferred from a sensitive to an insensitive individual by the transfer of T-lymphocytes but not by the transfer of serum. If T-lymphocytes are transferred, passive hypersensitivity persists for as long as the injected cells live in the new host, and, in some way, the transplanted cells alter the new host's own lymphocytes, so that these also take part in the delayed type of skin reaction that is subsequently elicited. Not only living cells but also *extracts* of lymphocytes from responsive individuals can be used to transfer delayed hypersensitivity through the action of a substance known as *transfer factor*, which is one of the lymphokines. The action of this substance is not fully understood; it is evidently very potent, however, because a single injection can bestow hypersensitivity on a recipient for many months.

Cell-mediated immune reactions are of great importance in the transplantation of tissues, in immunity to viral diseases, in forms of contact sensitivity, and in autoimmune disease (see Chapter 12).

IMMUNOGLOBULIN DEFICIENCY DISEASES

The immunoglobulin deficiency diseases can be considered under three headings: (1) the primary immunodeficiency syndromes, (2) the secondary immunodeficiency syndromes, and (3) the acquired immunodeficiency syndrome.

1. Primary Immunodeficiency Syndromes. The primary immunodeficiencies are those conditions in which, as a primary hereditary condition, the cellular, humoral, or both immune mechanisms are deficient. At one extreme, therefore, there may be agammaglobulinemia or dysgammaglobulinemia in which one or several immunoglobulins are absent because of B-cell deficiency—or, at the other extreme, thymic dysplasia will produce T-cell deficiency with lack of cell-mediated immune mechanisms. In the Wiskott-Aldrich syndrome, combined deficiencies occur in which deficiency of immunoglobulin(s) is combined with loss of cell-mediated responses.

Primary immunodeficiencies should also, for the sake of completeness, include disorders of phagocyte functions, such as Chédiak-Higashi syndrome, and a group of derangements of the complement system, discussed in Chapter 15.

2. Secondary Immunodeficiency Syndromes. The secondary immunodeficiencies result from involvement of the immunogenetic system in the course of another disease. Such diseases include tumors of the lymphoid system involving B- or T-cells (causing inadequate function) as well as hematologic disorders in which phagocytes are quan-

titatively or qualitatively deficient (*e.g.,* leukemia). Protein-losing conditions (*e.g.,* nephrotic syndrome) deplete the body of immunoglobulins, and there are mechanisms that are not as well understood that affect patients with diabetes mellitus and renal failure who exhibit diminished resistance to infection.

Immunologic function is also affected by drugs (*e.g.,* cortisone and cytotoxic agents) as well as by x-irradiation used in cancer therapy. In contrast, many drugs are used therapeutically as immunosuppressives, particularly in transplant surgery, glomerulonephritis, and so forth.

3. Acquired Immunodeficiency Syndrome. Acquired immunodeficiency syndrome (AIDS) is a condition in which T-cell dysfunction results from a viral agent transmitted sexually or through exposure to blood or blood products. This loss of T-cell activity renders the patient susceptible to such diseases as *Pneumocystis carinii* pneumonia and Kaposi's sarcoma and to other conditions such as cryptococcosis, strongyloidosis, candidiasis, and cryptosporidiosis. In 1984, 3,452 cases of AIDS occurring in the United States were reported to the Centers for Disease Control as opposed to 1642 cases in 1983. About 75 per cent of the cases occurred in homosexual or bisexual individuals (mostly male). Among the 25 per cent of heterosexual males or females who contracted the condition, 60 per cent used intravenous drugs. Cases have occurred in individuals with hemophilia A (due to cryoprecipitate, Factor VIII, therapy) and in a relatively large proportion of Haitians (which is probably connected with religious rituals related to blood).

Considerable research has been conducted regarding the cause of the disease, and, on April 23, 1984, it was announced that the probable cause had been found—a variant of a known human cancer virus called *HTLV-III.* A spokesperson for the Health and Human Services reported that a blood test, which should be widely available for use within 6 months, had been developed for AIDS. The development of a vaccine for AIDS has been predicted to be available within 2 to 3 years.

THE IMMUNE RESPONSE: FUNCTIONAL ASPECTS

The functions of the immune response are as follows:

1. Recognition. Since, as previously mentioned, an individual does not generally produce antibodies to antigens regarded as "self," it follows that a mechanism must exist for recognizing an antigen as foreign. Moreover, the system must have a memory so that the same antigen can be recognized after reexposure. Morphologically, the small lymphocytes are the "recognition" cells, which *initiate* the immune response, and, as such, are termed *immunologically competent cells.*

2. Processing. Subsequent to recognition as foreign, an antigen's determinants must be processed in such a way that a *specific* antibody can be produced. The macrophages are believed to perform this function, because they ingest antigen and appear to release factors that act on the antibody-producing cells.

3. Production. The final phase of the immune response is the production of antibody, which involves the synthesis of a range of specific proteins as well as the formation of immune lymphocytes. This manufacturing system must be regulated in some way so that the immune response can be discontinued when the antigen stimulation is withdrawn.

Two distinct theories have been postulated to explain the production of antibody, both in terms of the role played by antigen and the extraordinary specificity of the antibodies.

The *Instructive Theory* postulates that antigens play an instructive role, acting as moulds or templates during antibody synthesis. The primary drawback of this theory is that it assumes that antigen remains in the body throughout the period of antibody production (an assumption for which there is little direct evidence, because the immune response is responsible for their rapid elimination). In addition, it is difficult to envisage how a protein molecule (or its determinants) could modify the synthesis of a specific globulin in a cell, although this has been explained through the theory that contact with antigen produces a *permanent* modification of the antibody-producing cell. The explanation is still unsatisfactory, however, because it suggests a change of a self-replicating nature, being handed down to the progeny of the cells for many generations.

The *Selective Theory (Germ Line Theory)* postulates that cells exist in the adult that are capable of mounting an immune response against *any* "nonself" antigen that the host is likely to encounter. The antigen *selects* these cells and stimulates them to grow and produce antibody, thereby determining the quantity of antibody produced, but not its specificity.

The *Somatic Mutation Theory* postulates that during embryonic development, many somatic mutations in the immunologically competent cells result in the formation of a *range* of cells that are capable of mounting an immune response for any encountered foreign antigen. In adults, such contact stimulates growth of these cells, thus producing bodies of cells or "clones" (the name given to a group of cells of like hereditary constitution that

has been produced asexually from a single cell. Gr. *Klon* = a cutting used for propagation). As the size of the clone increases, so does the intensity of antibody production.

If somatic mutation occurs so frequently, obviously cells are produced that can manufacture antibody against all possible antigens, and, inevitably, some mutations will result in cells capable of forming antibodies against the embryo's own developing tissues. The fact that this does not occur lends support to the theory that some mechanisms must exist, activated during embryonic development, for the destruction of these so-called *forbidden clones*, so that any antigen present in the embryo is recognized as "self" and that at birth no cells are present that are capable of producing antibody to it.

(Note: Current thought is that both germ line and somatic mutation are responsible for the observed diversity of immunoglobulin specificity.)

IMMUNOLOGIC TOLERANCE

Immunologic tolerance refers to the situation in which, under certain conditions or circumstances, a foreign antigen fails to elicit the formation of antibody in the recipient. Studies of immune tolerance stem from the work of Owen (1945), who made the observation that dizygotic twin cattle (*i.e.,* nonidentical), which shared the same placental circulation and whose circulations were thereby linked, progressed through life with appreciable numbers of each other's red cells in their blood. Conversely, if they had not shared the same circulation, red cells from one twin injected into the other rapidly provoked an immune response. On the basis of this information, Burnet and Fenner (1941) postulated that an animal would be tolerant toward antigens encountered during embryonic life. This was considered the basis whereby the antigens indigenous to the body (*i.e.,* "self" antigens) were recognized and therefore did not provoke immune responses, whereas foreign antigens (*i.e.,* "nonself" antigens) did. This hypothesis was put to the test by Billingham *et al.* (1953) by injecting embryonic mice with adult cells and showing that after birth, the infant mice were tolerant toward skin from the same adult donors.

Tolerance can also be induced using soluble antigens. For example, rabbits injected at birth with bovine serum albumin fail to make antibodies on later challenge with this protein.

It is now realized that tolerance can be induced in the adult as well as in the neonate. T-cells are involved in tolerance at low antigen levels, whereas both B- and T-cells are made unresponsive at high antigen dose.

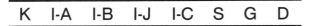

| K | I-A | I-B | I-J | I-C | S | G | D |

Figure 4–5. Schematic diagram of the mouse MHC region.

GENETIC CONTROL OF THE IMMUNE RESPONSE

The immune response is controlled by a small region on chromosome number 6 in man and chromosome number 17 in mice. The major histocompatibility complex (MHC) in the mouse (also known as the H-2 complex) is subdivided into 5 regions: K, I, S, G, and D (Fig. 4–5). The regulation of the production of serologically defined (SD) antigens is the responsibility of the K and D regions, which are located at each side of the MHC. The lymphocyte-activating antigens (LaD, or LD), which control the proliferation of lymphocytes, are regulated by genes located in the I region, which is just to the right of the K region. The strength of the immune response is also controlled by the I region. The S locus, which is situated to the right of the I region, controls the concentration of some serum proteins, including complement. To the right of this and bordering the D region on the far right is the G region, which determines some of the antigens expressed on red cells.

In humans, the MHC (known as HLA), was redefined by a committee organized by the World Health Organization in 1975. It consists of loci A, B, C (the alleles of which control the production of SD antigens) and D (the alleles of which control the production of LaD antigens; Bach, 1976).

There is evidence to suggest that the susceptibility to some diseases is under the control of the MHC. In mice, for instance, the genes that influence the development of virally induced leukemia map at the K end of the H-2 complex. In humans, an association has been reported between HLA-SD antigens and some lymphomas or leukemias

and some types of autoimmune and infectious diseases (Albert, 1977).

AUTOIMMUNITY

As previously stated, under normal conditions and circumstances, an individual does not produce antibodies to antigens regarded as "self." In certain cases, however, the mechanisms that prevent their formation may break down, giving rise to the production of "self-antibodies," or *autoantibodies*, which are directed against the individual's own tissues.

There are, theoretically, three circumstances under which autoantibodies are produced:

1. If the antigenicity of tissue proteins is altered due to *degenerative lesions* (*i.e.*, following necrosis of tissue, such as in skin burns) or the attachment of a hapten (in which case the antibodies are directed against the hapten rather than against the normal tissue proteins).
2. If a tissue antigen is anatomically isolated from the immunologically competent cells (and therefore not recognized as "self"), the release of this antigen into the tissues following injury or disease results in the formation of autoantibodies.
3. If a "self" protein is no longer recognized due to altered reactivity of the immune mechanism. This last condition is known to occur in cases of lymphocytic leukemia. In cases such as this, autohemolysins are sometimes produced, giving rise to a hemolytic anemia.

Autoantibodies may be immunoglobulin or cellular. The immunoglobulin might be of any class and may be *organ specific* (*i.e.*, directed against a determinant present in one organ) or *nonorgan specific* (*i.e.*, directed against DNA, mitochondria, and immunoglobulin determinants).

Further discussion of autoantibodies and autoimmune diseases can be found in Chapter 12.

REVIEW QUESTIONS

MULTIPLE CHOICE

Choose the phrase, sentence, or symbol that completes the statement or answers the question. More than one answer may be correct in each case. Answers are given at the end of this book.

1. The immune response:
   (a) is concerned with immunity to infection
   (b) is involved in many disease processes
   (c) is not involved in disease processes

   (d) under certain circumstances, causes hypersensitivity
   (*Introduction*)

2. The first phase of antigen elimination:
   (a) occupies about 1 hour if particulate antigens are used
   (b) results in 20 per cent of the antigen being removed from the circulation
   (c) occupies about 10 to 20 minutes if particulate antigens are used
   (d) results in almost 90 per cent of the antigen being

removed from the circulation in the first passage through the liver, lung, and spleen through extensive phagocytosis
(Antigen Elimination)

3. The latent period of the primary response varies from several hours to several days. This variation in time is dependent upon:
   (a) the kind of antigen involved
   (b) the amount of antigen given
   (c) the route of administration of the antigen
   (d) the species of animal and its health
   (The Primary Response)

4. In the primary response, antibody production begins:
   (a) within 20 minutes after exposure to the antigen
   (b) within 24 hours after exposure to the antigen
   (c) within 5 to 120 days after exposure to the antigen
   (d) at the end of the latent period
   (The Primary Response)

5. The secondary response to foreign antigen:
   (a) is rapid as a result of the release of stored antibody
   (b) must occur within 1 year after the primary response
   (c) may be induced by cross-reactive antigens
   (d) will occur only once and cannot be repeated
   (The Secondary Response)

6. The antibodies formed in response to infection:
   (a) may play a protective role against reinfection
   (b) may have no protective activity against reinfection
   (c) are directed against the antigenic components of the organism itself
   (d) may have different specificities
   (Immunity)

7. Generalized anaphylactic shock can occur in humans:
   (a) in passive immunization against diphtheria and tetanus
   (b) through the injection of penicillin
   (c) following a wasp or bee sting in highly sensitive individuals
   (d) all of the above
   (Hypersensitivity)

8. The type of hypersensitivity manifested by the production of antibodies that are capable of destroying cells is known as:
   (a) type I hypersensitivity
   (b) type II hypersensitivity
   (c) cytotoxic hypersensitivity
   (d) the Arthus reaction
   (Hypersensitivity)

9. The condition known as serum sickness:
   (a) can occur in individuals who have had no previous contact with the offending antigen
   (b) only occurs in individuals who have been previously sensitized with the offending antigen
   (c) has antigen-antibody complexes formed that are deposited on a sensitive membrane and can lead to tissue damage

(d) involves IgE as well as IgM and IgG production
(Hypersensitivity)

10. The effector cells in cell-mediated immunity:
    (a) react specifically with the offending antigen
    (b) release a number of agents known as lymphokines
    (c) morphologically resemble the large lymphocytes of the blood
    (d) all of the above
    (Cell-Mediated Immunity)

11. Type VI hypersensitivity
    (a) is mediated by immunoglobulin
    (b) does not involve circulating immunoglobulin
    (c) usually involves complement
    (d) is also known as *delayed hypersensitivity*
    (Hypersensitivity in Cell-Mediated Immunity)

12. The tuberculin skin reaction:
    (a) indicates the clinical activity of tuberculosis
    (b) involves "old tuberculin," which has value as a therapeutic agent
    (c) is of value as a diagnostic tool
    (d) is also known as the Koch phenomenon
    (Hypersensitivity in Cell-Mediated Immunity)

13. Cell-mediated immune reactions are of great importance in:
    (a) the transplantation of tissues
    (b) the immunity to bacterial diseases
    (c) forms of contact sensitivity
    (d) autoimmune disease
    (Hypersensitivity in Cell-Mediated Immunity)

14. Secondary immunodeficiency syndromes:
    (a) result from involvement of the immunogenetic system in the course of another disease
    (b) include tumors of the lymphoid system involving B- or T-cells
    (c) occur in diseases such as leukemia
    (d) all of the above
    (Immunoglobulin Deficiency Diseases)

15. Acquired immunodeficiency syndrome (AIDS):
    (a) is a condition that is caused by bacterial contamination
    (b) occurs only in homosexual or bisexual males
    (c) results from a viral agent known as HTLV-III
    (d) can be treated with large doses of penicillin
    (Immunoglobulin Deficiency Diseases)

16. The so-called recognition cells, which initiate the immune response:
    (a) are the small lymphocytes
    (b) are phagocytes
    (c) are termed *immunologically competent cells*
    (d) are unable to differentiate between "self" and "nonself" antigens
    (The Immune Response: Functional Aspects)

17. The "selective" theory of antibody production:
    (a) postulates that antigens act as moulds or templates during antibody synthesis
    (b) postulates that cells exist in the adult that are capable of mounting an immune response against any "nonself" antigen that the host is likely to encounter

(c) assumes that antigen must remain in the body throughout the period of antibody production

(d) postulates that some mechanism must exist for the destruction of forbidden clones

(The Immune Response: Functional Aspects)

18. Immunologic tolerance:
    (a) refers to the situation in which a foreign antigen elicits the formation of antibody in the recipient
    (b) can be induced using soluble antigens
    (c) can be induced in adults as well as in neonates
    (d) involves both B- and T-cells at low antigen levels
    (Immunologic Tolerance)

19. The immune response:
    (a) is controlled by a small region on chromosome number 17 in humans
    (b) is controlled by a small region of chromosome number 6 in humans
    (c) is controlled by a small region on chromosome number 17 in mice (known as the H-2 complex)
    (d) is controlled by a small region of chromosome number 1 in mice and in humans
    (Genetic Control of the Immune Response)

20. Autoantibodies:
    (a) are directed against an individual's own tissues
    (b) may be produced if a "self" protein is no longer recognized due to altered reactivity of the immune mechanism
    (c) may be immunoglobulin or cellular
    (d) may be of any class of immunoglobulin
    (Autoantibodies)

ANSWER "TRUE" OR "FALSE"

21. The immune response is not only concerned with immunity to infection, but is also involved in many disease processes.
    (Introduction)

22. Following the entry of foreign antigen into the body, the immune response is preceded by a period of antigen elimination.
    (The Formation of Immunoglobulin)

23. In the primary response, antibody usually appears in the serum (*i.e.,* free antibody) within 1 day after injection of antigen.
    (The Primary Response)

24. The antiserum in the secondary response contains IgG and no IgM.
    (The Secondary Response)

25. The anaphylactic reaction in humans is due to the formation of sensitized IgE, which becomes firmly attached to certain cells causing hystamine to be liberated.
    (Hypersensitivity)

26. Type II hypersensitivity is occasionally seen with penicillin therapy.
    (Hypersensitivity)

27. Serum sickness can be provoked by drugs forming haptens with body protein antigens.
    (Hypersensitivity)

28. The "effector" cells in cell-mediated immunity are known as lymphokines.
    (Cell-Mediated Immunity)

29. The Koch phenomenon is mediated by histamine and is blocked by antihistaminic drugs.
    (Hypersensitivity in Cell-Mediated Immunity)

30. In humans, the MHC is known as HLA.
    (Genetic Control of the Immune Response)

General References

Barrett, J. T.: Textbook of Immunology, 4th ed. St. Louis, The C. V. Mosby Co., 1983.

Bryant, N. J.: An Introduction to Immunohematology, 2nd ed. Philadelphia, W. B. Saunders Company, 1982.

Henry, J. B. (Ed.): Clinical Diagnosis and Management by Laboratory Methods, 17th ed. Philadelphia, W. B. Saunders Company, 1984.

Walter, J. B.: An Introduction to the Principles of Disease. Philadelphia, W. B. Saunders Company, 1977.

FIVE

THE ANTIGEN-ANTIBODY REACTION *IN VITRO*

Introduction

The fundamental reaction between antigen and corresponding antibody is simply one of *combination,* followed by secondary or tertiary reactions.

There are several types of reaction of antigen-antibody complexes *in vitro*. Each will be considered here in turn, but first, it is necessary to study the basic reaction, the simple combination of antigen and antibody both *in vivo* and *vitro*, known as *sensitization*.

Sensitization. An antigen and its specific antibody possess complementary corresponding structures that enable the antigenic determinants to come into very close apposition with the binding site on the antibody molecule where the two are held together by weak intermolecular bonds, believed to include opposing charges on ionic groups, hydrogen bonds, hydrophobic (nonpolar) bonds, and Van der Waals forces. This is not a covalent bond and, in fact, is about one tenth as powerful as that of a covalent bond.

The antigen-antibody reaction, which is reversible in accordance with the law of mass action, may be written thus:

$$Ab + Ag \underset{k_2}{\overset{k_1}{\rightleftharpoons}} AbAg$$

where k_1 is the rate constant for the forward reaction and k_2 is the rate constant for the reverse action.

According to the law of mass action (see Hughes Jones, 1963):

$$\frac{(AbAg)}{(Ab) \times (Ag)} = \frac{k_1}{k_2} = K$$

where (Ab), (Ag), and (AbAg), respectively, are the concentrations of antibody, antigen, and antigen-antibody (the combined product), and K is the equilibrium or association constant, which can be looked upon as a measure of the "goodness of fit"

49

of the antibody to the corresponding antigen. The value of K is ultimately dependent upon the strength of the antigen-antibody bonds, and, because all antisera contain populations of antibody molecules with a variety of binding strengths, the K value of the serum for any specific reaction is a measure of the *average* binding strength of all antibody populations present.

At equilibrium

$$\frac{(AgAb)}{(Ab)} = K(Ag)$$

That is to say, the higher the equilibrium constant, the more will be the amount of antibody combining with antigen at equilibrium. Assuming that a certain minimum number of antibody molecules must be bound to each red cell (for example) for agglutination to occur, the ratio of (AgAb) to (Ag) at equilibrium should be as high as possible. In practical terms, this means that a high ratio of serum to cells increases test sensitivity.

TYPES OF IMMUNOLOGIC REACTIONS

Antigen-antibody tests can be classified as *primary, secondary,* or *tertiary*, according to whether the test is dependent merely upon the interaction between the antigen and its corresponding antibody or whether it is based on a secondary manifestation such as precipitation, flocculation, agglutination, complement fixation, and so on, following the primary interaction. Tertiary manifestations occur as *biologic* reactions (*e.g.,* the biologic effects of complement activation such as opsonization, phagocytosis, chemotaxis).

Primary Reactions. The primary reaction can simply be viewed as the specific recognition and combination of the antigenic determinant with the binding site of its corresponding antibody. In general, primary tests are more sensitive than secondary or tertiary tests and are not dependent upon the variables that control the latter (discussion follows). The quantitative tests that involve the primary reaction include immunofluorescence, radioimmunoassay, and immunoenzymatic assays. In general, these tests require either a purified antigen or an antibody preparation, a technique to quantitate the antigen or antibody with the use of a radioisotope, enzyme or fluorescent label, or a method to separate the antigen-antibody complex from free antibody or antigen in solution.

Secondary Reactions. These include precipitation in solution or in gel, direct agglutination or hemagglutination (*i.e.,* involving erythrocytes or other particles coated with antigen or antibody), and complement fixation.

Tertiary Reactions. These include phagocytosis, opsonization, chemotaxis, immune adherence, and cellular degranulation.

At a basic level, antibody molecules are considered to be capable of recognition, binding, and complexing with specific antigen, yet many variables exist within the confines of this basic concept, because not all antigens or antibodies are subject to the same type of behavior. The reaction of specific IgG with a hapten antigen, for example, usually produces the complexes (hapten)$_2$ = (antibody)$_1$. Further, in the case of multivalent protein antigens, complexes of varying size may be formed in proportion to the antigen and antibody concentrations. Immune complexes of varying sizes have varying degrees of solubility; their ability to localize along vascular basement membrane and fix complement *in vivo* is responsible for a wide range of immune complex–mediated hypersensitivity diseases. As will be clear from this, the application and understanding of immunologic tests involve a knowledge of this variability, in terms of type, specificity, affinity, antibody and antigen concentration, and, finally, of biologic activity.

The Specificity and Sensitivity of Immunologic Tests

As knowledge has accumulated with respect to the variation of behavior of different antibodies, a broad spectrum of different immunologic methods has been developed, some of which are considerably more sensitive than others. Antigen-antibody binding assays, for example, are sensitive in the nanogram to picogram per milliliter range, whereas the agar gel test for alpha-1 fetoprotein is in the range of 3000 ng per ml. These varying levels of sensitivity are well illustrated by the different tests for hepatitis B–associated surface antigen (HbsAg; Chapter Seven). The agar gel diffusion test, for example, is 10 times *less* sensitive than the cross electrophoretic or electroimmunodiffusion methods and 10,000 times less sensitive than the radioimmunoassay procedure. The relative sensitivity of immunologic tests involving secondary manifestations of antigen-antibody reactions with respect to the minimum amount of antibody detectable or needed for reaction is given in Table 5–1.

The variation in standardization and specificity of immunologic methods is a common problem. This is because certain antibodies that have a high affinity and are potent may give unwanted cross-reactions, whereas weak antisera may be specific but not sensitive. False reactions (*i.e.,* caused by

Table 5–1. RELATIVE SENSITIVITY OF IMMUNOLOGIC
TESTS INVOLVING SECONDARY MANIFESTATIONS
OF ANTIGEN-ANTIBODY REACTIONS

Immunologic Test	Minimum of Antibody N (μg) Detectable or Needed for Reaction
Precipitation	
Tube precipitation	0.1
Immunodiffusion	0.1–0.3
Agglutination	
Qualitative	0.5
Quantitative	0.2–0.1
Hemagglutination, passive	0.001
Hemagglutination-inhibition	0.001
Coombs' reaction	0.01
Complement fixation	0.05

From Henry, J. B. (Ed.): Clinical Diagnosis and Management by
Laboratory Methods, 17th ed. Philadelphia, W. B. Saunders
Company, 1984, p. 895.

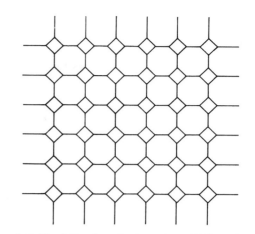

Figure 5–1. The lattice hypothesis: antigen (◇) bound to antibody (—) to form a lattice.

factors other than those expected or desired) are
also a problem in this respect.

Precipitation

Precipitation involves the interaction of antigen
with antibody in "correct" proportions, resulting
in a visible precipitate. The soluble antigens used
in the precipitin reaction are solutions of molecules, which are usually protein or carbohydrate
in nature. The simplest form of the precipitin
reaction would be the layering of antigen in solution over a small volume of antiserum. Precipitation occurs at the interface of the two reagents,
forming a ring.

A concept of the reaction between antigen and
antibody resulting in precipitation was described
by Marrack (1938). This concept, sometimes

known as the *lattice hypothesis*, is based on the
fact that antibody has more than one valence and
therefore may be found with antigen to form a
coarse "lattice" (Fig. 5–1).

This reaction is influenced by the quantities of
antigen and antibody present. To understand the
events that occur, one must assume that an antibody molecule has only two reactive sites, whereas
antigens have multiple sites that can react with
antibody. When a relatively small amount of antigen is added to an excess of antibody, all the
valences of the antigen are satisfied, and complexes
are formed that are composed of much antibody
and little antigen (Fig. 5–2, *1*). As increasing
amounts of antigen are added to the same amount
of antibody, the proportions change (Fig. 5–2, *2*)
until a point of optimal proportion is reached (Fig.
5–2, *3*). This point is known as the *equivalence*

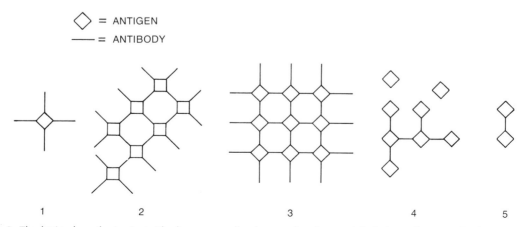

◇ = ANTIGEN

—— = ANTIBODY

1　　　　　2　　　　　3　　　　　4　　　　　5

Figure 5–2. The lattice hypothesis. *1*, Antibody excess—all valences of antigen satisfied; *2*, moderate antibody excess; *3*, optimal
proportions; *4*, antigen excess; *5*, extreme antigen excess—both valences of antibody satisfied. (Modified from Pauling, L. : The
theory of the structure and process of formation of antibodies. J. Am. Chem. Soc. *62*:2643, 1940.)

zone. Further addition of antigen would shift the reaction into the area of antigen excess (Fig. 5–2, *4* and *5*). The largest amount of precipitate is found at the equivalence zone, and excess of either reactant may produce false-negative results (Fig. 5–3). The reaction is rarely used now, but it can provide a fairly good quantitative estimate of the amount of antigen or antibody in an unknown; the equivalence zone of the unknown is determined and compared with that of a standard.

It should be noted that a so-called prozone phenomenon is sometimes observed, in which an antibody apparently reacts more strongly when it is diluted than when it is undiluted. The phenomenon has often been attributed to lack of optimal proportions between antigen and antibody, although according to Wiener (1970), it may actually occur in one of two ways:

1. It may be due to the use of fresh serum containing complement. This can be proved by inactivating the serum and re-titrating, whereupon the prozone disappears.
2. It may be due to the presence of both IgM (agglutinating) and IgG (blocking) antibodies in the same serum. This prozone will disappear if the tests are carried out in a high-viscosity medium (*e.g.,* human AB serum, bovine albumin) in place of saline.

The precipitin reaction is of practical use in the laboratory when it takes place in agar gel or other semisolid media through which soluble molecules can diffuse. The location and density of the precipitin bands in the reaction are determined by differences in the concentration and rates of diffusion of the different molecules. This allows for easier identification of multiple components in mixtures

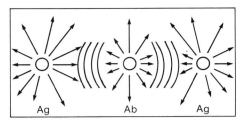

Figure 5–4. A test sample containing several antigens, giving rise to several precipitation lines.

of antigens and antibodies. Thus, a preparation containing several antigens will give rise to multiple precipitation lines (Fig. 5–4), whereas a preparation containing only one antigen will give rise to one precipitation line with its corresponding antibody (Fig. 5–5). Note that when reagents are present in optimal proportions, the precipitation line formed will generally be concave to the well containing the reactant of higher molecular weight, whether it be antigen or antibody. This is caused by the slower diffusion rate of larger-sized molecules.

Immunoelectrophoresis. This is a useful procedure for the differentiation of antigens within a mixture, although so-called double-diffusion tests can also be used. Immunoelectrophoresis combines the principles of gel diffusion and electrophoresis and is especially useful for the study of proteins. The principle of the method is as follows: Under an electrical current, antigen migrates through a gel medium (*e.g.,* agar; Fig. 5–6). The current is then stopped. A trough is cut in the agar and filled with antibody. A precipitin arc is then formed. Because antigen (theoretically at a point source) diffuses radially and antibody from a trough diffuses with the plane front, the reactants meet in optimal proportions for precipitation along an arc. The arc is closest to the trough at a point where antigen is in highest concentration. This technique may be used in two-dimensional or multi-dimensional forms; antigens are then separated on the basis of their electrophoretic mobility. The precipitin reaction is relatively insensitive when used for

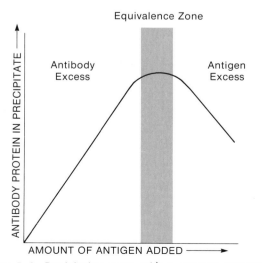

Figure 5–3. Precipitation curve with a constant amount of antibody.

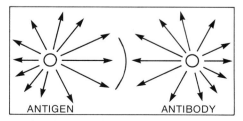

Figure 5–5. A precipitation test showing a single antigen and its corresponding antibody, resulting in a single line of precipitation.

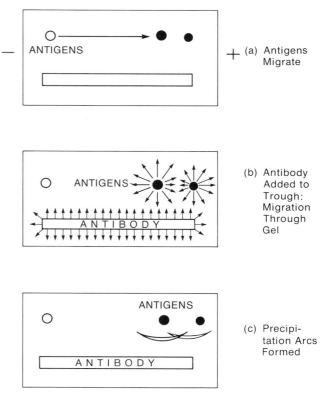

Figure 5–6. The principle of immunoelectrophoresis.

detecting antibody when less than 10 ng per ml of serum is present.

Agglutination

Agglutination reactions are similar to precipitin reactions except that the union of antibody occurs with suspended particulate antigens rather than with soluble antigens. The particles involved are cells (bacteria, yeast, erythrocytes) or latex particles, which, in general, are large enough for direct observations. When these antigens combine with their specific antibodies, aggregation (or clumping) of the particles is seen. If one of these reactants is of known specificity, the clumping may be used for the identification of the corresponding reactant. Several factors influence the reaction, including elevation or decrease of temperature, motion (shaking, stirring, centrifugation), and pH. Agglutination is also used as a semiquantitative test with doubling dilutions of antisera. The strength of the antibody (*i.e.,* the "titer") is then used as the reciprocal of the highest dilution that gives a distinctly positive reaction (see Titration later in this chapter).

Agglutination results from the cross-linking of the cells or particles by antibody molecules, although antibody-induced changes in the electrical charge may also be important.

The range of usefulness of the agglutination reaction has been considerably extended in recent years. This was made possible by the observation that erythrocytes can absorb various polysaccharides and that after treatment with tannic acid (acting as a mordant), they can also absorb many protein antigens (*i.e.,* in passive hemagglutination).

In addition, polystyrene latex suspensions have become available, and the latex particle agglutination test has become a useful tool for the detection of rheumatoid factor and is helpful in the diagnosis of rheumatoid arthritis (see Chapter 12). Passive agglutination tests can also be used for the detection of soluble antigen. In the agglutination inhibition test, antiserum is first combined with antigen, and then the indicator red cells or latex particles coated with the same antigen are added. Inhibition indicates the presence of both antigen and specific antibody.

Reactions Involving Complement

The Complement Fixation Test. The complement fixation test is based on the fact that when an antigen combines with an antibody in the presence of complement, the complement is "fixed" by the antigen-antibody complex and is unable to react with cells sensitized with other antigen-antibody complexes. As an indicator of the presence of "unfixed" complement, erythrocytes sensitized with specific antibodies are used. Lysis of these erythrocytes indicates the presence of unfixed complement; alternatively, the lack of hemolysis indicates that the complement has reacted with the test antigen-antibody complex (Fig. 5–7).

The test is of limited usefulness, because it is applicable to IgM antibodies only. In addition, the antigen must be free of "anticomplementary" activity. It is useful, however, in the diagnosis of syphilis and some parasitic diseases.

Immune Adherence Reaction. Another reaction involving complement is the immune adherence reaction, although this, too, is of limited usefulness. This reaction is based on the fact that, following the primary specific antigen–antibody reaction, the antigen-antibody complex develops an ability to adhere to particles such as erythrocytes, silica, starch granules, and bacteria. Early *in vitro* tests of this phenomenon revealed that complement was an essential part of the reaction. Practically speaking, the test has little application in the clinical laboratory, although it has been successfully used for the antigenic differentiation of species of trypanosomes and leptospires, and for the diagnosis of human trypanosomiasis and of syphilitic infection.

Neutralization of Toxins and Viruses

Neutralization tests are often useful when neither precipitation nor agglutination succeeds in demonstrating an antigen-antibody reaction. Moreover, in work with viral agents, neutralization is a useful technique. One should note that the neutralization of toxins or viruses is the essence of a major protective mechanism in several disease states (*e.g.*, diphtheria, tetanus).

The principle of the test is simple. In the case of viruses, a dose of virus known to be lethal to a test animal is mixed with the serum to be tested for antibody against the virus. The mixture is injected into the test animal, which is observed for reaction. If the lethal dose fails to kill the test animal, neutralizing antibody is known to be present in the test serum. In the case of toxins, an individual who has been exposed to toxin-producing bacteria is injected with antitoxin. The toxin-antitoxin reaction *in vivo* then protects the recipient by neutralization of the toxin. This toxin-inactivating ability of antiserum can be assayed by observing the *in vivo* neutralization of the toxin in laboratory animals. Failure to protect the animal means that the test serum has no protective antibodies against that particular toxin. Antitoxin potency can also be measured by precipitation and by flocculation techniques *in vitro*.

Fluorescent Antibody Reactions (Immunofluorescence)

Immunofluorescence was first developed almost 30 years ago by Coons (1956, 1958, 1961), yet its true value and potential have only recently been exploited. The technique involves the study of antigens in tissue sections by the use of specific antibody that has been labeled with color and is applied over a section of tissue so that a microprecipitate is formed at the site of the antigen. The fluorescent dye usually used, fluorescein isocyanate or isothiocyanate, is linked with serum antibody and yields a blue-green fluorescent substance, which is detected in a fluorescent microscope when illuminated with ultraviolet light.

The simplest application of the technique, using a single treatment with labeled antibody and a subsequent wash in physiologic buffer saline to

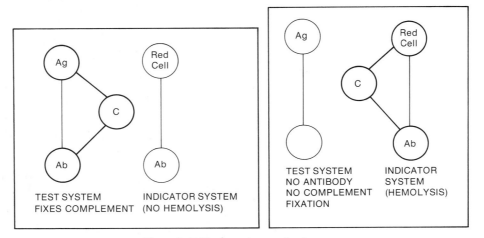

Figure 5–7. The complement fixation test.

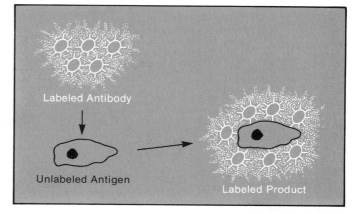

Figure 5–8. Single-layer (or "direct") fluorescent antibody procedure.

remove the excess of uncombined labeled antibody, is known as the single-layer or direct technique. The purpose of the technique is to identify unknown antigen by using known fluorescein-labeled antibody. It consists of exposing the unknown antigen to the known labeled antibody and washing and examining the mixture with the fluorescent microscope (Fig. 5–8).

The method has been used for the identification of foreign antibodies in tissues (*e.g.,* particulate viruses and their soluble antigens and bacteria, protozoa, and fungal antigens).

Several modifications of this technique exist, including the following:

1. *Indirect or double-layer technique:* This procedure is used for the detection of antibody in unknown sera. Unlabeled antibody is exposed to antigen, and this is followed by the addition of labeled antiglobulin sera, directed against the globulin of the species used in the initial exposure. Fluorescence in this case indicates that reaction between the antigen, the unknown antibody, and the labeled antiglobulin has taken place (Fig. 5–9).
2. *Complement staining technique:* This procedure is similar to the indirect procedure except that the antiglobulin conjugate is direct against the species supplying the complement. The main

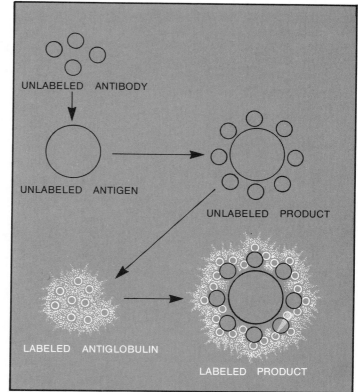

Figure 5–9. Indirect (or double-layer) fluorescent antibody procedure.

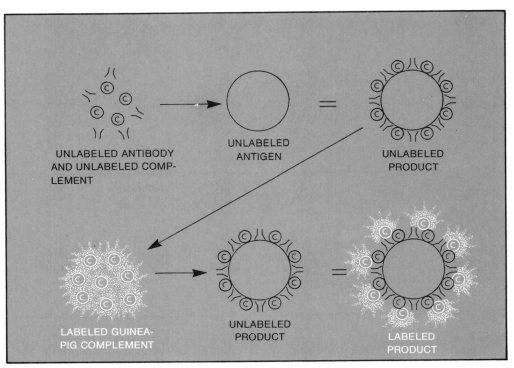

Figure 5—10. Complement staining technique.

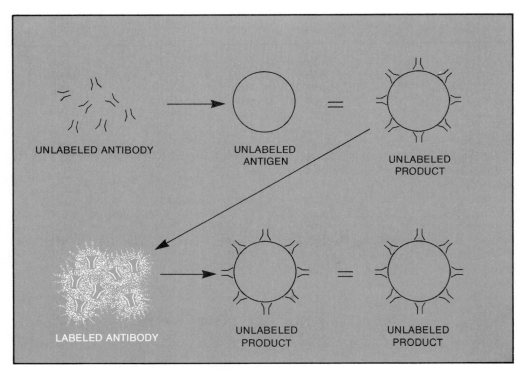

Figure 5—11. Inhibition techinque.

advantage of this technique over the indirect method is that a single conjugate (*e.g.,* anti–guinea-pig complement) may be used to test serum from any species. The test procedure is as follows:

    a. Heat-inactivated unknown antibody and a fixed amount of guinea-pig complement are added simultaneously to known antigen.

    b. After incubation and washing, labeled antibody (anti–guinea-pig complement) is added, and the mixture is incubated again.

Fluorescence indicates that a reaction has occurred between the unknown antibody and the antigen, resulting in the fixation of complement to the complex, and that a subsequent reaction has occurred between the guinea-pig complement and the anti–guinea-pig complement (Fig. 5–10).

3. *Inhibition technique:* The inhibition technique is based on the procedure of blocking specific antigen-antibody reactions by initial exposure to a different aliquot of homologous antibody. In this way, unlabeled antibody is added to antigen, saturating the antigen. Subsequently, labeled antibody is added. No fluorescence is seen, and the test remains nonreactive, because no antigen sites remain to react with the labeled antibody (Fig. 5–11).

Enzyme–Linked Immunoassays

Enzyme-linked immunoassays (ELISA) are rapidly supplementing and, at times, replacing radioimmunoassays and immunofluorescence for the identification of specific antibody. In fact, the principle of ELISA is similar to that of immunofluorescence in that a purified enzyme is linked in a stable manner to a specific antibody.

Horseradish peroxidase and alkaline phosphatase are two commonly used enzymes in the ELISA technique, although other enzymes can be used. The requirements of the utilized enzyme with respect to the technique are as follows:

1. The enzyme activity should be easily detectable either by a cytochemical method or by a change in absorbance at a specific wavelength.

2. For cytochemical uses, the enzyme substrate should not be readily diffusible; in fact, it is preferable if a precipitate results from the reaction.

3. In tissue work, it is useful if the optimum pH of the enzyme is at, or close to, neutral.

4. The enzyme should not affect tissue structure.

5. The active enzyme should be available in pure form, because, if it is not, immunoglobulins could be labeled with "inactive" materials and could decrease the sensitivity and specificity of the reaction.

6. Enzyme activity is often decreased when bound to antibodies, but this activity should not be abolished.

7. The enzyme must be stable for storage purposes.

8. A small enzyme is less likely to interfere with antigen-antibody reactions by steric hindrance and is more likely to penetrate tissue.

In performing ELISA techniques, there should be no natural substrates in tissue or in the clinical specimen.

Two main ELISA methods have been used for toxicology, viral antibody studies, electron microscopy, and light microscopy for the identification of antigens and antibodies: namely, the enzyme-conjugate method and the so-called unlabeled–antibody-enzyme method. The enzyme-conjugate method is considered to be less sensitive than radioimmunoassay or immunofluorescence, sensitivity being lost by the preparation of the conjugate and competition from unlabeled immunoglobulins. The unlabeled–antibody-enzyme method, which usually utilizes soluble enzyme–anti-enzyme complexes is considered to be more specific and is more sensitive, the sensitivity being gained by saturation of all the tissue antigen sites with specific antibody and allowing little excess enzyme or anti-enzyme in the mixture (Sternberger, 1974).

ELISA methods can be automated, are stable, and do not carry the potential hazards of radioisotopes. Tissue preparations do not fade as they do with fluorescent work, and light microscopy may be used.

Titration

In clinical serology, the titer of a substance refers to the number of antibody molecules per unit volume of the original serum. This gives an indication of the antibody concentration in a patient's serum. The titer is read at the highest dilution of serum that gives a reaction with antigen. For example, if the last tube showing a reaction contains a volume of 1 ml and the serum in this tube is 1 part in 1000 parts, the titer is given as 1000 units per milliliter.

REVIEW QUESTIONS

MULTIPLE CHOICE

Choose the phrase, sentence, or symbol that completes the statement or answers the question. More than one answer may be correct in each case. Answers are given at the end of this book.

1. An antigen and its specific antibody possess complementary corresponding structures that enable the antigenic determinants to come into very close apposition with the binding site on the antibody molecule where the two are held together by:
   (a) powerful intermolecular bonds
   (b) hydrogen bonds
   (c) Van der Waals forces
   (d) hydrophilic bonds
   (Introduction)

2. The precipitation test can be classified as:
   (a) a primary test
   (b) a secondary test
   (c) a tertiary test
   (d) all of the above
   (Types of Immunologic Reactions)

3. The agar gel diffusion test, when used for the detection of hepatitis B–associated surface antigen:
   (a) is more sensitive than cross electrophoresis
   (b) is less sensitive than cross electrophoresis
   (c) is more sensitive than radioimmunoassay
   (d) is more sensitive than electroimmunodiffusion
   (The Specificity and Sensitivity of Immunologic Tests)

4. In the precipitation test, the largest amount of precipitate is found:
   (a) at the equivalence zone
   (b) in the area of antigen excess
   (c) in the area of antibody excess
   (d) none of the above
   (Precipitation)

5. Agglutination reactions may involve:
   (a) erythrocytes
   (b) latex particles
   (c) bacteria
   (d) yeast
   (Agglutination)

6. The immune adherence reaction:
   (a) is an example of a reaction that involves complement
   (b) has little application in the clinical laboratory
   (c) can be used for the diagnosis of syphilitic infection
   (d) none of the above
   (Reactions Involving Complement)

7. Antitoxin potency can be measured by:
   (a) precipitation reactions
   (b) flocculation techniques
   (c) *in vivo* tests
   (d) neutralization
   (Neutralization of Toxins and Viruses)

8. Several modifications of the basic immunofluorescent technique exist. These include:
   (a) the double-layer technique
   (b) complement fixation technique
   (c) inhibition technique
   (d) all of the above
   (Fluorescent Antibody Reactions)

9. The utilized enzyme in the ELISA technique:
   (a) should affect tissue structure
   (b) should not affect tissue structure
   (c) may be used in an impure form
   (d) must be stable for storage purposes
   (Enzyme-Linked Immunoassay (ELISA))

10. The titer of a substance:
    (a) refers to the number of antibody molecules per unit volume of the original serum
    (b) cannot be used as an indication of antibody concentration
    (c) can only be used as a measurement of antigen
    (d) is read as the lowest dilution of serum that gives a reaction with antigen
    (Titration)

ANSWER "TRUE" OR "FALSE"

11. The antigen-antibody reaction is reversible.
    (Introduction)

12. The biologic effects of complement activation can be considered as a tertiary manifestation of the antigen-antibody reaction.
    (Types of Immunologic Reaction)

13. In the precipitation reaction, when the reagents are present in optimal proportions, the precipitation line formed will generally be convex to the well containing the reactant of higher molecular weight.
    (Precipitation)

14. Passive agglutination tests cannot be used for the detection of soluble antigen.
    (Agglutination)

15. The complement fixation test can be used in the diagnosis of some parasitic diseases.
    (Reactions Involving Complement)

16. ELISA methods have been used in viral antibody studies.
    (Enzyme-Linked Immunoassay (ELISA))

General References

Bryant, N. J.: An Introduction to Immunohematology, 2nd ed. Philadelphia, W. B. Saunders Company, 1982.

Henry, J. B. (Ed.): Clinical Diagnosis and Management by Laboratory Methods, 17th ed. Philadelphia, W. B. Saunders Company, 1984.

Raphael, S. S. (Ed.): Lynch's Medical Laboratory Technology, 4th ed. Philadelphia, W. B. Saunders Company, 1983.

SIX

SYPHILIS

OBJECTIVES

The student shall know, understand, and be prepared to explain:

1. A brief history of the origin of syphilis
2. The morphology of *Treponema pallidum*
3. The metabolism of *T. pallidum*
4. The syphilis antigens: Wasserman, treponemal
5. The stages of syphilis and their correlation with test results
6. The antibodies in syphilis, specifically:
   a. Development
   b. The production of immunity
7. The treatment of syphilis and its correlation with test results
8. Syphilis and blood transfusion
9. A description of neurosyphilis
10. A description of congenital syphilis
11. The diseases related to syphilis, specifically:
    a. Yaws
    b. Pinta
    c. Bejel
    d. Rabbit syphilis
12. The principles of the laboratory tests for syphilis
13. The methods of syphilis testing, including:
    a. The venereal disease research laboratory slide test with serum and spinal fluid
    b. The fluorescent treponemal antibody absorption test with serum
    c. The dark-field microscopic examination of *T. pallidum*
    d. The rapid plasma reagin card test on serum
    e. The unheated serum reagin test on serum
    f. The *T. pallidum* immobilization test
14. A brief description of the principles of other tests for syphilis

---

Introduction

Two schools of thought exist regarding the origin of syphilis. The first of these, often referred to as the "pre-Columbian theory," states that syphilis was present in Europe prior to the voyage of Columbus but was not recognized as such, was confused with other diseases (*e.g.,* leprosy) or was present in a milder form than is seen today. Hudson (1963) and others believe that the disease probably first appeared in the tropics (Central Africa) as a condition closely resembling the trep-

onematoses of the present day, such as yaws, and was eventually introduced into other parts of the world by travelers and traders. The facts that the treponemes of syphilis and yaws are morphologically indistinguishable, that both respond to the same treatment, and that the same blood tests are reactive in both diseases are points in support of the pre-Columbian theory.

The second school of thought, sometimes referred to as the "Columbian theory," states that syphilis was endemic in Haiti (then called Hispaniola) and was subsequently contracted and carried to Europe by Columbus's crew. In 1494, King Charles VIII of France beseiged Naples, and, shortly after the fall of the city, syphilis became widespread in the army and throughout Italy. The disease was later given its name through a poem "Syphilis sive Morbus Gallicus," written by Fracastorius in 1530, although at the time of the Naples seige, the Italians called it the "French disease," and the French called it the "Italian disease." The English, by contrast, called it the "Spanish disease," and medical literature of the day called it "the great pox" or "the evil pox."

As will be obvious, neither the Columbian theory nor the pre-Columbian theory is entirely satisfactory. The conclusion that a previously endemic disease could so suddenly become epidemic is as difficult to believe as the theory that the disease spread so rapidly from a single port of entry. What is certain is that the disease became the subject of medical literature in the closing years of the fifteenth century, the first mention being in an edict issued by the Diet of Worms on October 7, 1495. In 1497, mercury was being advocated as treatment for the disease by at least two physicians, Widmann and Gilino, and, in 1498, the first major book about syphilis was written by Francisco Lopez de Villalobos.

For centuries, no specific etiology was assigned to syphilis. Many early writers (who were also astrologers) blamed the disease on a malignant alignment of the stars and planets. Later, syphilis, along with certain other diseases, was ascribed to a lack of balance between the humors of the body. The bacteriologic era of medicine, heralded by the work of Pasteur, Koch, Löffler, and others, stimulated a search for the cause of the disease. Numerous bacteria were reported as causal, but the critical experiments resisted confirmation or repetition.

The 5-year period 1905 to 1910 produced, through numerous discoveries, the important contributions to the modern age of syphilis management. In 1905, Schaudinn and Hoffmann of Hamburg discovered that syphilis was caused by a spirochete that they called *Spirochaeta pallida*. The same workers later changed the name to *Treponema pallidum,* but, because the original name had been widely used, both were regarded as correct. A year later, Wassermann, Neisser, and Bruck (1906) described a diagnostic blood test (Wassermann test). As this knowledge developed, so did the methods of treatment. In 1909, Ehrlich of Frankfurt produced "606," or "salvarsan," an organic arsenic preparation that was effective when given intravenously. The term *606* was applied because it was Ehrlich's 606th experiment with drugs of this group. The generic name is *arsphen-amine*. Some years later, Ehrlich produced neoarsphenamine, which was even more effective. Intramuscular injection of bismuth was proposed as treatment by Sazerac and Levaditi in 1921, as a less toxic and more effective substitute for mercury.

With little doubt, the greatest single therapeutic advance in the history of infectious diseases was the discovery of penicillin by Sir Alexander Fleming. Soon after the discovery of the antibiotic (1943), John Mahoney, in New York, reported remarkable results obtained with penicillin in the treatment of four patients with primary syphilis. The healing of lesions was little short of miraculous. Other workers soon confirmed Mahoney's findings, and, within a short period of time, penicillin had completely replaced all other forms of treatment for all phases of the disease. Even now, more than 40 years later, penicillin remains the drug of choice in treatment of the disease.

The prevalence of syphilis is not known with certainty. In the United States, the total number of cases reported each year has declined slightly since the early 1960s, with 33.7 cases per 100,000 population reported in 1976, compared with just over 70 cases per 100,000 population in the mid 1940s. In 1974, almost 40 million people were tested for syphilis, and 1.2 million had positive reactions (Blount and Holmes, 1975). Congenital syphilis has decreased by almost 90 per cent since 1950, and the mortality rate has dropped from about 1 case per 100,000 population in 1967 to just over 0.1 per cent in 1975, although this statistic may be unreliable owing to the fact that in deaths reportedly due to other causes, syphilis may have been a contributing factor.

The incidence of the disease remained relatively steady during the years 1955 to 1958; then it increased from 113,894 cases in 1958 to a peak of 126,245 cases in 1962 and has since declined to 71,761 cases in 1976. In 1977, 9.4 cases per 100,000 population was reported. This increased to 14.6 cases per 100,000 population in 1982, then it decreased to 14.1 cases per 100,000 in 1983. These data can only be regarded as relative, because the vast majority of cases (possibly as high as 70 to 80 per cent) are not reported. A problem that has also recently surfaced in the epidemiology of the disease is the disproportionately high number of cases in homosexual or bisexual males. A study conducted in England, Scotland, and Wales in 1971 revealed that 42 per cent of the males reported to have primary or secondary syphilis were homosexual. A similar study in the United States revealed that 34 per cent of males with syphilis were either homosexual or bisexual, an increase of 10 per cent over the level reported in 1969.

MORPHOLOGY OF *TREPONEMA PALLIDUM*

Treponema pallidum is a member of the order Spirachaetales and the family Treponemataceae. This family contains three genera: Borrelia, Treponema, and Leptospira. The genus Treponema contains four principal species of pathogenic organisms: *T. pallidum* (responsible for human syphilis), *T. pertenue* and *T. carateum* (the etiologic agents for yaws and pinta, respectively), and *T. cuniculi* (responsible for rabbit syphilis).

The morphologic characteristics of *T. pallidum* can be studied microscopically. The usual method used in clinical tests is that of dark-field (or dark-ground) illumination, although both the phase-contrast and the electron microscopes have been used.

T. pallidum is seen microscopically as a close-coiled, thin, regular spiral organism varying in length from 6 to 15 μ and consisting of 8 to 24 coils (Figs. 6–1 and 6–2). The width of the spiral is seldom more than 0.25 μ. Electron microscopic studies have revealed the anatomic structure of the cell, which presents as an axial bundle surrounded by a number of spirally wound filaments, which, when they have become detached from the axial bundle, have been misinterpreted as flagella (Ovčinnikov and Delektorsij, 1966, 1968). There is probably a periplast or capsular structure. Evidence suggests that *T. pallidum* multiplies by transverse fission and that the active phase of this probably occurs about every 30 hours.

In aqueous media, young treponemes spin vigorously around their long axis in an apparently useless type of motion. In more viscous media, however, they achieve sufficient traction to propel themselves. In tissues, they show remarkable flex-

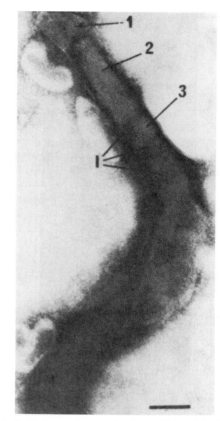

Figure 6–2. Electron micrograph of *T. pallidum* (Nicol's strain). (From Hovind-Hougen, K.: Acta Pathol. Microbiol. (Scand.) 255:1, 1976. Reproduced in Braude, A. I.: Medical Microbiology and Infectious Diseases. Philadelphia, W. B. Saunders Company, 1981, p. 491.)

ibility as they adapt themselves to the intracellular spaces.

METABOLISM OF *TREPONEMA PALLIDUM*

Outside the host, *T. pallidum* is extremely susceptible to a variety of physical and chemical agents that rapidly bring about its destruction. Suspensions of the organism, however, have remained viable and motile for periods up to 15 days when kept at 35°C under anaerobic conditions in medium containing serum albumin, glucose, carbon dioxide, pyruvate, cysteine, glutathione, and serum ultrafiltrate.

The metabolic capabilities of the cultivable treponemes show some variation, although for all of them, nutritional requirements are complex. They require and use glucose (or other fermentable carbohydrate) as a primary energy source, as well as multiple amino acids, purines, and pyrimidines. Many strains also need biocarbonate and one or

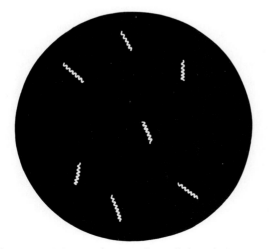

Figure 6–1. Microscopic view of *T. pallidum* (diagrammatic).

more coenzymes. All require at least one exogenously supplied fatty acid; for some oral strains, a short-chain acid is sufficient, but others require one or more acids of 16 to 18 carbon chains.

T. pallidum has not been recovered in blood, serum, or plasma stored at 4°C for more than 48 hours, although organisms may remain alive for up to 5 days in tissue specimens removed from diseased animals. Suspensions of treponemes frozen at −70°C or lower in the presence of glycerol or other cryoprotective agent, however, can be kept viable for years.

ANTIGENS

The Wassermann Antigen

In the original form of the Wassermann test, an extract of liver containing many treponemes from human fetuses with congenital syphilis was used as antigen. The specific ligand involved, however, was later found to be present in alcoholic extracts of normal liver and other mammalian tissues. Subsequently, the ligand was isolated from cardiac muscle and identified as a phospholipid, diphosphatidyl glycerol, which was called *cardiolipin*.

Cardiolipin is a normal constituent of host tissue; therefore, a theory arose that the development of the antibody represented an autoimmune response (a theory supported by the fact that the Wassermann antibody—anticardiolipin—appears in other disorders, *e.g.*, lupus erythematosus). Free cardiolipin, however, is a hapten and must be bound to a suitable carrier to be antigenic. The lipid composition of cultivable treponemes depends to a considerable extent upon the lipids in the growth medium; therefore, it is possible that pathogenic treponemes growing *in vivo* have access to a plentiful supply of this phospholipid, which could be incorporated into the treponeme, the microbial cell being a foreign carrier and the bound cardiolipin serving as the immunogenic determinant.

The Treponemal Antigens

In the treponemes, two classes of antigen have been recognized, those restricted to one or a few species and those shared by many different spirochetes.

The only well-studied treponemal component is a protein that is found in most treponemes, both saprophytic and pathogenic species. This antigen, once widely used in a diagnostic test for syphilis, was first obtained from the Reiter treponeme, a spirochete reputed to be a cultivable, nonvirulent variant of *T. pallidum*. In its purest form, it is a macromolecule associated with RNA. This antigen (or a very similar protein) is present in many indigenous treponemes of the human alimentary tract, and many individuals acquire weak, low-level, "natural" antibodies to it.

THE STAGES OF SYPHILIS (CORRELATION WITH TEST RESULTS)

Syphilis (in humans) is ordinarily transmitted by sexual contact. In the infected male, the offending *T. pallidum* organisms are either present in lesions on the penis or discharged from deeper genitourinary sites along with the seminal fluid. In infected females, the lesions are commonly located in the perineal region or on the labia, vagina wall, or cervix. In approximately 10 per cent of cases, the primary infection is extragenital, usually in or about the mouth.

Primary (or Early) Stage

T. pallidum appears to enter the skin only through small breaks, although, like all other spirochetes, it is capable of passing through intact mucous membranes, after which it is carried by the blood stream to every organ of the body. Multiplication of the organism at the site of entrance results, within as few as 10 and as many as 60 days, in the development of a characteristic primary inflammatory lesion known as a *chancre* (Fig. 6–3).

The chancre usually begins as a papule (a small, circumscribed solid elevation of the skin) and then breaks down to form a superficial ulcer with a clean, firm base. The chancre in males may occur

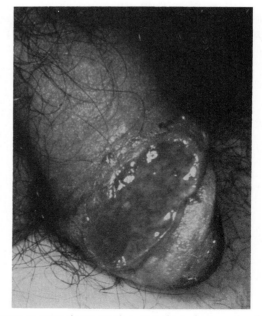

Figure 6–3. Typical primary chancre in the early stage of syphilis.

on any part of the external genitalia, the most common site being the coronal sulcus of the penis. It may also occur inside the urethra (the so-called intrameatal chancre), in which case the only symptom may be scanty serous urethral discharge. In females, the primary chancre may occur on the labium majus or minus, at the fourchette, on the clitoris, near the urethral orifice, on the cervix uteri or (rarely) the vaginal wall, or on the vulva (in which case it can be associated with considerable edema of the labia).

The primary chancre persists for 1 to 5 weeks and then heals spontaneously. During this stage, the serum in 30 per cent of cases becomes serologically active after 1 week; in 90 per cent of cases, it becomes reactive after 3 weeks. Serum tests for syphilis usually give positive results between the first and third weeks after the appearance of the chancre. Less than 10 per cent of cases show a positive reaction by the fifth day. The reagin titer (see later in this chapter) increases rapidly during the first 4 weeks and then remains stationary for approximately 6 months.

Secondary Stage

The secondary stage of syphilis usually occurs from 6 to 8 weeks after the appearance of the primary chancre. In about one third of cases, this systemic secondary stage appears before the chancre disappears and is usually characterized by a generalized rash, which often also involves the mucous membranes (Fig. 6–4).

During the secondary stage, lesions may develop in the eyes, joints, or central nervous system. These secondary lesions, particularly in the mucous membranes, contain large numbers of spirochetes and, when located on exposed surfaces, are highly contagious. As with primary syphilis, these lesions subside spontaneously after 2 to 6 weeks.

In the secondary stage, serologic tests for syphilis are invariably positive.

Note: In some cases (albeit rarely), the primary and secondary stages of syphilis go unnoticed, the first signs and symptoms of the disease being the late (or tertiary) lesions.

The Late Latent Stage

Usually after the second year of infection, syphilis enters the late stage, which is usually noncontagious. The stage begins with a period of latency, in which there are no clinical signs or symptoms of the disease, the only indication of infection being positive serologic tests. This latent stage may last for many years, or even for the rest of the patient's life, with the patient dying from causes unrelated to syphilis.

After an infection has persisted for more than 4 years, it is rarely communicable except between mother and fetus.

Tertiary Stage

The first lesions of the tertiary stage of syphilis are usually seen from 3 to 10 years after the primary stage (or later). The lesions, known as *gummata*, are usually located on the skin, mucous membranes, subcutaneous and submucous tissue, bones, joints, muscles, and ligaments. When gummata are located on the skin or bones, they cause relatively little trouble. Serious manifestations, however, usually result when these lesions are present in the nervous system (causing general

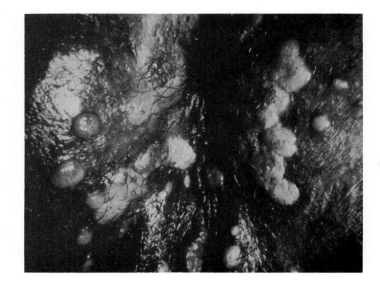

Figure 6–4. Lesions of secondary syphilis (anal area).

paralysis or tabes dorsalis), in the cardiovascular system (causing, in many cases, aortic aneurysm), and in the eyes (where they may cause permanent blindness).

In about one fourth of untreated cases, the tertiary stage is asymptomatic and is recognized only by serologic tests. Note that occasionally the primary and systemic lesions heal so completely that even the serologic tests become nonreactive.

ANTIBODIES IN SYPHILIS

Development

Individuals infected with *T. pallidum* respond immunologically by producing both specific and nonspecific antibodies. The specific antibodies are directed against the pathogenic *T. pallidum*; the nonspecific antibodies are directed against the protein antigen group common to pathogenic spirochetes. The antibody against the group antigen in cases of primary syphilis are fixed with IgG and IgA. Specific anti-treponemal antibodies in early or untreated early latent syphilis are predominantly IgM, although this same immunoglobulin is reported to be present in only 23 per cent of sera from patients with untreated late latent syphilis. This early immune response to infection is rapidly followed by the appearance of IgG antibodies, which soon become predominant. The largest elevations in IgG levels are seen in the secondary stage. Between the secondary and the early latent stage, total IgG does not appear to decrease significantly, but basic IgG does. This suggests a closer relationship of the fluctuations in the number of treponemes with basic IgG levels than with total IgG levels. Nonspecific IgA antibodies increase significantly during the course of untreated syphilis.

Production of Immunity

Immunity to *T. pallidum* develops in the course of syphilis both in rabbits and in humans. Some immunity can be detected in rabbits with experimental syphilis just 3 weeks after infection with the organism. Resistance to reinfection increases to a maximum approximately 3 months after infection. Termination of the disease within the first 3 months by penicillin therapy renders the individual susceptible to reinfection.

Attempts to induce immunity against experimental infection in rabbits by means of *T. pallidum* vaccine have been made by a number of investigators, some reporting failure and others reporting success.

Protective immunity against syphilis can be induced by vaccines containing nonviable *T. palli-*

dum or certain cultivable nonpathogenic treponemata. The need for high-volume dosage and the difficulties in the production of sufficient quantities of *T. pallidum*, however, hamper the general use of vaccines. The comparatively easily cultivable nonpathogenic treponemata would be a preferable source of vaccine, but further study is required to determine the true effectiveness of these preparations in conferring protective immunity.

It is possible that there is no *complete* immunity to *T. pallidum*. Studies have shown that active lesions may be brought under control and animals may be resistant to rechallenge with *T. pallidum*, but the host is not able to rid itself of the infecting organism, which persists in lymph nodes. Human subjects have been found to be resistant to rechallenge with *T. pallidum* during latency, although observations have shown that they have not succeeded in eradicating the infecting organism.

TREATMENT OF SYPHILIS (CORRELATION WITH TEST RESULTS)

If a patient infected with *T. pallidum* is adequately treated before the appearance of the primary chancre, it is probable that the serologic tests will remain nonreactive. If treatment is given before the appearance of reagin (*i.e.,* the seronegative primary stage), the serologic tests also usually give no reaction. After the appearance of reagin (*i.e.,* the seropositive primary stage), the serologic tests usually become nonreactive 6 months after treatment. (Note: Reagin is an anti-cardiolipin antibody, a nonspecific treponemal antibody formed during *T. pallidum* infection. Note that this is not the same as the IgE antibody [the reagin of allergy]; see discussion under IgE in Chapter Two.)

In the secondary stage of the disease, serologic tests usually become nonreactive within 12 to 18 months after treatment. After the secondary stage, however, treatment has variable effects on serologic test results, yet, as a general rule, the sooner treatment is given, the more marked will be the serologic response.

If the patient is treated 10 years or more after the onset of the disease, the serologic tests can be expected to change little, if at all.

In about 10 per cent of cases, patients who receive adequate treatment during the primary or secondary stage of syphilis fail to exhibit a decrease or reversion of serologic test results and show reactive test results indefinitely. These patients are said to be "seroresistant" or "Wassermann-fast." This phenomenon may be due to the continued presence of reagin, indicating a definite immune response or persistent foci of infection. Neurosyphilis is frequently associated with seroresistance in both the early and late stages. In cases of a persistently reactive serologic test, spiral fluid should be examined to determine whether the disease has been controlled.

SYPHILIS AND BLOOD TRANSFUSION

Syphilis may be transmitted by blood transfusion when very fresh blood is used. Blood stored at 4°C for 4 days or more, however, is unlikely to transmit syphilis, because *T. pallidum* is unable to survive under these conditions. In most cases, since the primary routine tests on blood donations take several days to complete, the causative organism is usually dead before transfusion is given. In addition, a serologic test for syphilis is standard procedure for all blood donations; therefore, the disease is rarely a problem.

NEUROSYPHILIS

Neurosyphilis is syphilis of the central nervous system. In all types of neurosyphilis, the essential changes are the same: obliterative endarteritis, usually of the terminal vessels, with associated parenchymatous degeneration, which may or may not be sufficient to produce symptoms.

Neurosyphilis is divided into the following groups, depending upon the type and degree of central nervous system lesions present:

1. Asymptomatic neurosyphilis: The patient is usually seen because of a reactive serologic test for syphilis. There are no signs or symptoms indicative of central nervous system involvement; however, examination of the cerebrospinal fluid, obtained by lumbar or cisternal puncture, reveals an increase in cells and total protein, a positive reagin test, and an abnormal colloidal-gold test.
2. Meningovascular neurosyphilis: There are definite signs and symptoms of nervous system damage, resulting from cerebral vascular occlusion, infarction, and encephalomalacia with focal neurologic signs. The cerebrospinal fluid is always abnormal, with an increase in cells and total protein and a positive reagin test. In this type of neurosyphilis, usually either meningeal involvement or vascular involvement is seen.
3. Parenchymatous neurosyphilis: This type of neurosyphilis presents as paresis (incomplete paralysis) or tabes dorsalis (degeneration of the dorsal columns of the spinal cord and of the sensory nerve trunks, with wasting).
   a. The signs and symptoms of paresis may be myriad, although they are always indicative of widespread parenchymatous damage. Personality changes range from minor to psychotic, and frequently there are focal neu-

rologic signs. Serologic blood tests are reactive, and the cerebrospinal fluid is invariably abnormal.
   b. Tabes dorsalis: The spinal fluid in tabes dorsalis gives abnormal findings in 90 per cent of cases; the serum is reactive in 75 per cent of cases. Signs and symptoms include primarily posterior column degeneration with ataxia (failure of muscular coordination), areflexia (absence of reflexes), paresthesias (abnormal sensations, *e.g.,* burning, prickling), bladder disturbances, impotence and, often, lightning pains. Gastric or abdominal "crises" frequently begin with vomiting (which may result in serious electrolyte imbalance) and severe abdominal pain. Trophic joint changes result from loss or impairment of the sensation of pain; the knee joint is most commonly involved, and severe degeneration is common. Syphilitic optic atrophy is also frequently seen.

The signs and symptoms of paresis and tabes dorsalis frequently coexist in the same patient (so-called taboparesis).

CONGENITAL SYPHILIS

Congenital syphilis is acquired during fetal life from the maternal circulation through the placental passage of *T. pallidum* from the eighteenth week of gestation onward. This is more likely to occur when the mother is suffering from early syphilis, particularly the primary or secondary stage, than when she has late syphilis. Adequate treatment of the mother before the eighteenth week of pregnancy prevents infection of the fetus. Because penicillin will cross the placenta in adequate amounts, treatment of the mother after the eighteenth week of pregnancy will also cure the infected fetus.

The clinical manifestations of congenital syphilis may be divided into early, late, and the stigmata. Ordinarily, the division between the early and late stages of the disease is placed at the second year of life. Many of the lesions of the first 2 years of life are infectious and resemble those of secondary syphilis in the acquired form of the disease. The late lesions, appearing from the third year onward, are mostly of the gummatous type and are noninfectious. The stigmata are the scars or deformities resulting from early or late lesions that have healed.

DISEASES RELATED TO SYPHILIS

Yaws

Treponema pertenue, the organism that causes the tropical disease known as yaws, is virtually indis-

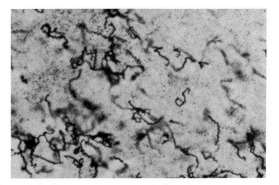

Figure 6–5. *Treponema pertenue* in biopsy specimen. Krajian-Erskine silver impregnation stain. (From Freeman, B. A.: Textbook of Microbiology, 22nd ed. Philadelphia, W. B. Saunders Company, 1985, p. 800.)

tinguishable from *T. pallidum* (Fig. 6–5). In fact, the only difference in the diseases produced by these organisms is the character of the lesions. Both the primary and the secondary lesions of yaws are more persistent than those of syphilis, and, unlike syphilis, scar formation develops at the site of the secondary infection. The lesions are granulomatous or wartlike, with a granular surface similar to that of a raspberry; hence the name *frambesia* (also known as papillomas; Fig. 6–6). The tertiary stage is characterized by nodular or ulcerative necrosis (gummas of skin and subcutaneous tissue), gummas and subperiosteal thickening of the long bones, and plantar hyperkeratosis

(Fig. 6–7). Nasopalatal destructive lesions (gangosa), destruction of joints (particularly the interphalangeal joints), and mobile soft-tissue nodules near the joints (juxta-articular nodes) occur commonly in yaws and are also seen in bejel (discussed later in this chapter). The healed ulcerative lesions leave thin depigmented scars and sometimes severe disfigurement (Fig. 6–8).

In general, yaws is not as grave as syphilis, because it rarely involves the viscera, and congenital yaws is very uncommon. The disease occurs in the tropics, where the combination of high temperature and humidity promotes the persistence of open skin lesions and thus facilitates nonvenereal transmission by direct contact.

Yaws responds dramatically to treatment with penicillin, often requiring only a single long-acting injection.

Pinta

The causative organism of the disease known as pinta is *Treponema carateum*, which, like *T. pertenue*, is morphologically indistinguishable from *T. pallidum* (Fig. 6–9). Pinta is a nonvenereal disease, endemic in Central and South America, that usually occurs in childhood and is contracted through skin contact. Serologic tests are reactive as in cases of syphilis.

The initial lesion in pinta is commonly found on the legs. It starts as a papule but soon forms a circular, scaly patch known as a *pintid*. A papular,

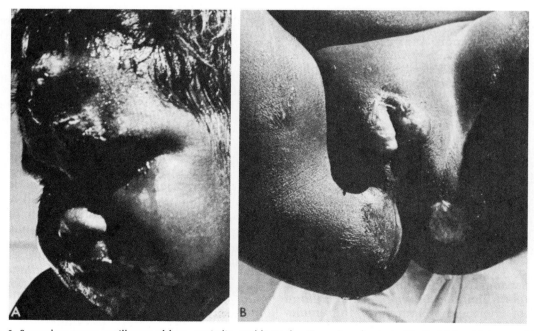

Figure 6–6. Secondary yaws: papillomas of face, genitalia, and buttocks. (From Braude, A. I.: Medical Microbiology and Infectious Diseases. Philadelphia, W. B. Saunders Company, 1981, p. 1616.)

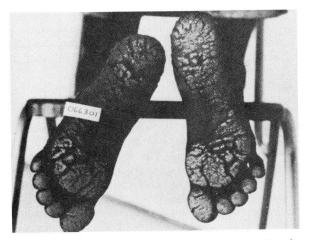

Figure 6–7. Tertiary yaws: plantar hyperkeratosis. (From Braude, A. I.: Medical Microbiology and Infectious Diseases. Philadelphia, W. B. Saunders Company, 1981, p. 1616.)

annular papular, or papulosquamous rash then appears on the limbs and face after an interval of several months. Many years later, lesions of the face, hands, and feet produce atrophy and depigmentation.

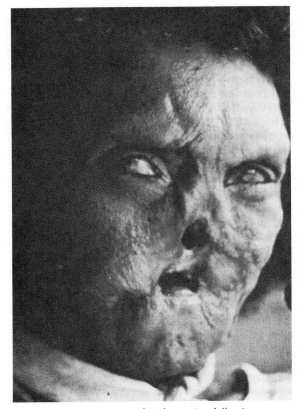

Figure 6–8. Tertiary yaws: facial scarring following gangosa. (From Braude, A. I.: Medial Microbiology and Infectious Diseases. Philadelphia, W. B. Saunders Company, 1981, p. 1618.)

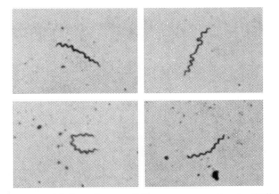

Figure 6–9. Various forms of *Treponema carateum.* Krajian-Erskine silver impregnation stain. (From Freeman, B. A.: Textbook of Microbiology, 22nd ed. Philadelphia, W. B. Saunders Company, 1985, p. 802.)

Pinta is a relatively mild chronic disease, with a good prognosis. Lawton Smith *et al.* (1971) investigated 11 cases of late pinta in Venezuela and found no ocular or neurologic abnormalities except in one patient with pinta and bilateral interstitial keratitis.

Penicillin is effective in treatment, especially in the early stages.

Bejel

Bejel is probably a variety of nonvenereal syphilis. It has been studied by Hudson (1958) and Csonka (1952). Usually no primary lesion is seen. Secondary lesions consist of generalized papular, annular papular, and papulosquamous eruptions. Perineal and genital condylomata and mucous patches are common. After a latency period, tertiary lesions may be observed in subcutaneous tissue, skin, and bones. The nasopharynx and larynx are often involved. The nervous system, cardiovascular system, and other viscera are not involved, however, and there is no evidence of transmission *in utero.*

Differentiation from syphilis is made on clinical grounds. The causative organism (treponeme) is indistinguishable from *T. pallidum* and is sometimes referred to as *T. pallidum II* or *T. pallidum endemicum* to distinguish it from *T. pallidum* of venereal syphilis. Serologic tests for syphilis are positive in cases of bejel.

Penicillin is effective in treatment unless contraindicated by allergy.

Rabbit Syphilis

Rabbit syphilis is a natural venereal infection of rabbits, producing minor lesions of the genitalia. The causative organism is morphologically identical to the spirochete of syphilis and is known as *Treponema cuniculi.* Rabbits with this disease do not give positive Wasserman reactions and do not develop antibodies that immobilize *T. cuniculi*.

SEROLOGIC TESTS FOR SYPHILIS

Principles

Infection of humans with *T. pallidum* provokes in the host a complex antibody response. Serologic tests for syphilis are based on the detection of one or more of these antibodies. No "ideal" single test is available at present, and although more than 200 procedures have been described, only a few are routinely used. Host antibodies are of two known types: (1) non-treponemal antibodies, or reagin, which react with lipid antigens, and (2) treponemal antibodies, which react with *T. pallidum* and closely related strains.

Reagin Tests for Syphilis. In the course of certain diseases, including syphilis, a substance appears in the serum of affected patients that has the properties of an antibody. The substance is known as "reagin," and it possesses the ability to combine with colloidal suspensions of lipoids extracted from animal tissue (most commonly beef heart), which then clump together to form visible masses, a process known as *flocculation*. After combining with reagin, the lipoidal particles have the power to fix complement.

An example of an easily performed reagin test is the VDRL (Venereal Disease Research Laboratory) slide test, which can be used qualitatively and quantitatively for detecting reagin in serum and cerebrospinal fluid (see later in this chapter for test procedure). Other reagin tests include the rapid plasma reagin (RPR) test of Portnoy *et al.* (1957), which uses the incorporation of chlorine chloride to modify the basic VDRL antigen and allows for the testing of plasma without preliminary heating. An extension of this principle is seen in the plasmacrit (PCT) test of Andujar and Mazurek (1959), the unheated serum reagin test described by Portnoy and Carson (1960), the rapid plasma reagin (RPR) (circle) card test (Portnoy, 1963), and the automated reagin test of McGrew *et al.* (1968), developed by the VDRL in 1970. Commercial reagents have been developed and evaluated for other rapid reagin tests that are designed to react at a level comparable to that of the VDRL test (Caputo, 1975; March *et al.*, 1974).

It should be noted that reagin is part of the gamma globulin portion of serum and is probably present in small quantities in all normal sera. These quantities, however, are insufficient to give positive results with standard test procedures.

Treponemal Tests for Syphilis. Nelson (1948) showed that the serum of patients with syphilis contains an antibody that is distinct from reagin

and that, in the presence of complement, inhibits the normal movement of virulent treponemes of syphilis. On the basis of this information, a test was developed by Nelson and Mayer (1949) called the *Treponema pallidum* immobilization (TPI) test. The organisms are extracted from lesions in experimentally infected rabbits and incubated with syphilitic serum and guinea-pig complement. Under these conditions, the organisms lose their motility. If 50 per cent or more treponemes are immobilized, the test is regarded as positive. If fewer than 20 per cent are immobilized, the test is negative. The range 20 to 50 per cent represents an area of "doubtful" result. The TPI test has been accepted as the treponemal test of reference, but it is not useful in assessing therapy, because, once the secondary stage is past, it is likely to remain positive for the rest of the patient's life, regardless of treatment, and it does not distinguish between the treponematoses. It is, however, the test of choice for spinal fluid, especially for detecting neurosyphilis when reagin tests give nonreactive or equivocal results.

Since 1949, efforts have been made to develop simpler techniques for routine laboratory use. Tests using killed *T. pallidum*, such as the *Treponema pallidum* immune adherence (TPIA) test, treponemal agglutination test, and *Treponema pallidum* complement fixation (TPCF) test, have failed to satisfy this goal in terms of simplicity and cost. The so-called Reiter protein complement fixation (RPCF) test is more satisfactory, however. This test uses a protein fraction derived from the cultivable Reiter treponeme, which shares a common group antigen with *T. pallidum* and other treponemes (Wallace and Harris, 1967). The complement fixation test is used with Reiter protein antigen substituted for nonspecific antigen.

Another treponemal test is the fluorescent treponemal antibody test described by Hunter *et al.* (1964). In this technique, a drop of a suspension of dead *T. pallidum* (Nichol's virulent stain) serves as antigen. The suspension is dried and fixed on a slide, and diluted patient's serum is added. If antibody is present, the treponemes become coated with a layer of antibody globulin, detectable by the addition of fluorescein isothiocyanate–labeled antihuman immunoglobulin, which unites with the bound globulin and fluoresces when examined by dark-ground illumination under ultraviolet light.

By this method, an antibody specific for *T. pallidum* and other allied pathogenic treponemes and a group-reactive antibody that reacts with both pathogenic and commensal treponemes are detected. This group antibody, present in most normal sera in low concentrations, becomes increased with syphilis infection. By dilution of the serum in a heated culture filtrate of Reiter treponemes (sorbent), the group antibody is theoretically "blocked," and the specific antibody is then free to unite with the treponemal antigen. This is the basis of the fluorescent treponemal antibody absorption (FTA-ABS) test (Hunter *et al.,* 1964), which has proved extremely sensitive, especially in cases of primary syphilis, and has been shown to have good specificity. False-positive reactions have been noted in patients with balanitis and in those with lupus erythematosus, however. The FTA-ABS test can also be used to detect different immunoglobulin classes by using monospecific conjugates. This is of practical value in the differentiation of neonatal syphilis from passive transfer of maternal antibody, because IgM does not cross the placenta.

The *Treponema pallidum* hemagglutination (TPHA) test (Garner and Clark, 1975) is also extremely sensitive and has the advantage of being easy to perform. The antigen used is a suspension of formolized tanned sheep red cells sensitized with an ultrasonicate of virulent *T. pallidum.* Serum is added to an absorbing diluent to remove cross-reacting antibodies, and sensitized cells are added. Unsensitized cells added to a second tube serve as a control. The tubes are allowed to stand at room temperature. A positive result is revealed by the gradual agglutination of the sensitized cells; the unsensitized cells (control) form a compact button at the bottom of the tube.

The *direct fluorescent antibody* (DFA) test is another useful test for syphilis that has distinct advantages over dark-field examination of chancre fluid for treponemas, in particular, the fact that dried slides can be saved or mailed to a reference laboratory for testing or examination.

NOTES ON SEROLOGIC TESTS FOR SYPHILIS

1. When testing a sample for syphilis, the following should be noted:
   a. More than one screening test should be performed if results are found to be positive to guard against false-positive results.
   b. There is no serologic test that will differentiate syphilis from other treponemal infections (*e.g.,* yaws, bejel).
   c. False-positive results may be the result of:
      i. Human error or contaminated specimens.
      ii. Variations from the normal. (A few patients produce an excess of reagin, giving a positive reagin test, in which case treponemal tests must be performed.)
      iii. Diseases allied to syphilis (*e.g.,* yaws)
      iv. Biologic reactions associated with infections or recent immunizations. These are usually "acute" and last no longer than a few months. "Chronic" false-positive results are seen in cases of leprosy.
2. In the interpretation of serologic tests for syphilis, the following factors should be taken into account:
   a. Geographical area or country of origin. Diseases related to syphilis, whose causative organisms are indistinguishable from *T. pallidum,* can result in misdiagnosis.
   b. Ability of the patient to produce reagin or treponemal antibodies.
   c. Stage of the illness.
   d. Previous antibiotic therapy.
   e. Manner in which serologic tests are performed.
   f. Various conditions that may cause biologic false-positive results (discussed earlier).

Negative Reactions

The technologist should keep in mind that a negative serologic test for syphilis may indicate besides that, in addition to the fact that the patient does not have syphilis, any of the following:

1. The infection is too recent to have produced antibodies that give reactions.
2. The test has been rendered *temporarily* nonreactive by consumption of alcoholic fluids prior to testing.
3. The test is *temporarily* nonreactive because of treatment.
4. The disease is latent or inactive.
5. The patient has not produced protective antibodies because of immunologic tolerance.
6. Inferior technique.

Weakly Reactive Results

Weakly reactive results may be due to:

1. Very early infection.
2. Lessening of the activity of the disease after treatment.
3. Biologic false-positive reaction.
4. Inferior technique.

Positive Results

Positive results usually indicate that the patient has syphilis. The technologist should keep in mind, however, that such results could be due to inferior technique or may be biologic false-positive results.

Control of Serologic Tests for Syphilis

Control sera of graded reactivity should be included each time serologic testing procedures are performed. For the nontreponemal flocculation test with serum and spinal fluid, the antigen suspension should be controlled daily. The results obtained should reproduce the established reactivity pattern; with unacceptable results, testing should be delayed until optimal reactivity has been established. This can be done by preparing another antigen suspension, correcting temperature (room temperature should be 23° to 29°C), adjusting equipment, and so on. For the FTA-ABS test, control sera should be included in each test run. Results should be considered invalid if controls are unacceptable.

Control sera of graded reactivity for nontreponemal and treponemal test procedures are obtainable from commercial sources or may be prepared from individual sera (or pooled sera) after testing. High-titer reactive serum may be used for spinal fluid controls.

Quality control of reagents obtained from commercial sources is also important. Chemicals and distilled water should be of high quality and should always be used according to the manufacturer's directions.

METHOD 1: VENEREAL DISEASE RESEARCH LABORATORY (VDRL) SLIDE TEST WITH SERUM

Materials

1. **Mechanical rotator—adjustable to 180 rpm, circumscribing a circle ¾ inch in diameter on a horizontal plane.**
2. **Slides—2 inch × 3 inch, with 12 paraffin or ceramic rings approximately 14 mm in diameter (Note: If glass slides with ceramic rings are used, the rings must be high enough to prevent spillage when rotated; they must be cleaned so that serum will spread to the inner surfaces of the ceramic rings; they must be discarded if the ceramic rings begin to flake off.)**
3. **Ringmaker to make paraffin rings approximately 14 mm in diameter.**
4. **Slide holder for 2 inch × 3 inch microscope slides.**
5. **18-, 19-, and 23-gauge hypodermic needles**
6. **Syringe—Luer-type, 1 or 2 ml**
7. **30-ml, round, glass-stoppered, narrow-mouthed bottles, approximately 35 mm in diameter, with flat interbottom surfaces. (Note: Bottles with convex interbottom surfaces are unsatisfactory.)**

Reagents

1. **VDRL antigen: Antigen for this test is a colorless, alcoholic solution containing 0.03 per cent cardiolipin, 0.9 per cent cholesterol, and a sufficient amount of purified lecithin to produce standard reactivity (usually 0.21 per cent ± 0.01 per cent). Before being put into use, each lot of antigen must be serologically standardized by comparison with an antigen of known reactivity. Antigen lots, once controlled, are stored in the dark at either refrigerator (6° to 10° C) or room temperature in screw-capped (Vinylite liners) bottles or hermetically sealed glass ampules. At these temperatures, the components of the antigen remain in solution. Formation of a precipitate indicates changes resulting from factors such as evaporation or additive materials contributed by pipets. Such ampules should be discarded.**
2. **1.0 per cent buffered saline solution, prepared by adding 0.5 ml of formaldehyde (neutral, reagent-grade); 0.093 gm Na_2HPO_4 + $12H_2O$; 0.170 gm KH_2PO_4; and 10.0 gm NaCl to 1000 ml of distilled water. This solution yields potentiometer readings of pH 6.0 ± 0.1 and is stored in screw-capped bottles. (Note: When an unexplained change in test reactivity occurs, the pH of the buffered saline should be checked to determine whether this is a contributing factor. Saline with pH outside acceptable range should be discarded).**
3. **0.9 per cent saline, prepared by adding 900 mg of dry sodium chloride (A.C.S.) to each 100 ml of distilled water.**

Preparation of Antigen Suspension

1. **Pipet 0.4 ml of buffered saline to the bottom of a 30-ml round glass- or screw-stopped bottle.**
2. **Add 0.5 ml of antigen directly onto the saline while rotating the bottle on a flat surface gently and continuously. The antigen should be taken from the lower half of a 1.0-ml pipet graduated to the tip, and it should be added drop by drop at a speed that allows 0.5 ml of antigen to be added every 6 seconds. The pipet tip should remain in the upper third of the bottle, and rotation should not be vigorous enough to splash the saline onto the pipet. The proper speed of rotation is achieved when the center of the bottle circumscribes a 2-inch diameter circle approximately three times per second.**
3. **Blow the last drop of antigen from the pipet without allowing the pipet to touch the saline.**
4. **Continue the rotation of the bottle for 10 seconds.**
5. **Add 4.1 ml of buffered saline from a 5.0-ml pipet.**
6. **Place the top on the bottle, and shake from the bottom to the top and back approximately three times a second.**

7. **Antigen suspension is now ready for use and may be kept for 1 day. Each time the suspension is used, it should be mixed gently. Do not mix the suspension by forcing it back and forth through any syringe or pipet; this may cause the breakdown of particles and loss of reactivity.**

Testing Accuracy of Antigen Emulsion Delivery Needles

Because it is of primary importance that the proper amounts of reagents be used, the needles used should be checked daily.

For the slide qualitative test on serum (described later in this chapter), dispense the antigen suspension from a syringe fitted with an 18-gauge needle without bevel that will deliver 60 drops (± 2 drops) of antigen suspension per milliliter when the syringe and needle are held vertically.

For the slide quantitative test on serum (described later in this chapter), two tests are required. The first is performed with a 19-gauge needle without bevel that will deliver 75 drops (± 2 drops) of antigen suspension per milliliter when the syringe and needle are held vertically; the second is performed with a 23-gauge needle (with or without bevel) that will deliver 100 drops (± 2 drops) of *saline* per milliliter when the syringe and needle are held vertically.

Needles that do not meet these specifications should be adjusted and calibrated or discarded.

Preliminary Testing of the Antigen Suspension

1. **Test the control sera of graded reactivity (*i.e.*, reactive, weakly reactive, and nonreactive) using the slide qualitative test (described below).**
2. **Reactions with control sera should reproduce the established reactivity pattern. The nonreactive serum should show complete dispersion of antigen particles. Unsatisfactory antigen suspensions or pools of antigen suspensions should not be used.**

Preparation of Serum for Testing

1. **Heat clear serum obtained from centrifuged, clotted blood in a 56°C water bath for 30 minutes before testing (to destroy complement).**
2. **Examine the serum when it is removed from the water bath, and recentrifuge if it is found to contain particle debris.**
3. **If serum is allowed to remain untested for 4 hours or more after original heating, reheat for 10 minutes at 56°C before testing.**

4. **When tested, the serum must be at room temperature.**

Procedure (VDRL Slide Qualitative Test on Serum)

1. **Pipet 0.05 ml of heated serum into one ring of a paraffin-ringed or ceramic-ringed slide. (Glass slides with concavities, wells, or glass rings are not recommended for this test.)**
2. **Add one drop (1/60 ml) of antigen suspension onto each serum with an 18-gauge needle and syringe.**
3. **Rotate the slides for 4 minutes on a mechanical rotator that describes a ¾ inch–diameter circle when set at 180 rpm.**
4. **Read tests microscopically with a 10× ocular and a 10× objective immediately after rotation.**

Reading and Reporting of Results. At $100\times$ magnification, the antigen particles appear as short rod forms. Aggregation of these particles into large or small clumps is interpreted as degrees of reactivity. Read as follows:

No clumping (or slight roughness)	: Nonreactive
Small clumps	: Weakly reactive
Medium or large clumps	: Reactive

Note: A *prozone reaction* is occasionally encountered. This type of reaction is demonstrated when complete or partial inhibition of reactivity occurs with undiluted serum; maximal reactivity is obtained only with diluted serum. This prozone reaction may be so pronounced that only a weakly reactive (or "rough" nonreactive) result is produced in the qualitative test by a serum that is strongly reactive when diluted. Therefore, it is recommended that any serum producing a weakly reactive (or "rough" nonreactive) result in the qualitative test be retested with the quantitative procedure before a report of the VDRL slide test is released. When a reactive result is obtained on some dilution of a serum that produced only a weakly reactive (or "rough" nonreactive) result before dilution, the test should be reported as reactive, and the qualitative titer should be reported.

Procedure (VDRL Slide Quantitative Test on Serum)

1. **Prepare a 1:8 dilution of the serum under test by adding 0.1 ml of the serum to 0.7 ml of 0.9 per cent saline by using a 0.2-ml pipet graduated in 0.01-ml subdivisions.**

2. Mix thoroughly, and allow the pipet to stand in the dilution tube until all dilutions are prepared (if more than one serum is to be tested).
3. Using this pipet, transfer 0.04 ml, 0.02 ml, and 0.01 ml of the 1:8 serum dilution into the fourth, fifth, and sixth paraffin rings, respectively.
4. Blow out the remaining serum dilution into the dilution tube.
5. With the same pipet, transfer 0.04 ml, 0.02 ml, and 0.01 ml of *undiluted* serum into the first, second, and third paraffin rings, respectively.
6. Add two drops (0.01 ml per drop) of 0.9 per cent saline to the second and fifth rings of each serum with a 23-gauge needle and a syringe.
7. Add three drops (0.01 ml per drop) of 0.9 per cent saline to the third and sixth rings of each serum with a 23-gauge needle and syringe.
8. Rotate the slides gently by hand for about 15 seconds to mix the serum and saline.
9. Add one drop (1/75 ml) of antigen suspension to each ring with a 19-gauge needle and a syringe.
10. Rotate the slide for 4 minutes at 180 rpm.
11. Read the test microscopically immediately after rotation.

Reading and Reporting of Results

1. The result of the reaction between the serum and the antigen is read as either reactive or nonreactive.
2. Definite clumping of the antigen particles is reported as reactive; no clumping or slight roughness of antigen particles is reported as nonreactive.

The highest dilution exhibiting a reaction is considered the "end point." Weakly reactive reactions are not counted as significant in reporting an end point titer; therefore, if a serum shows positive reactions at dilutions of 1:2 and 1:4, weakly reactive reactions at 1:8, and no reaction at higher dilutions, the test is reported as "reactive 1:4." A serum that exhibits a reactive reaction in the undiluted serum *only* is reported as "reactive, undiluted only."

METHOD 2: VENEREAL DISEASE RESEARCH LABORATORY (VDRL) SLIDE TEST WITH SPINAL FLUID

Materials

1. Antigen suspension (prepared as described for the VDRL slide test with serum, see p. 70)
2. 1.0 per cent buffered saline (prepared as described for the VDRL slide test with serum, see p. 70)

3. 10.0 per cent unbuffered saline
4. 0.9 per cent unbuffered saline
5. Slides (agglutination)—1¼ × 3 inches, with 12 concavities, each measuring 16 mm in diameter and 1.75 mm in depth

Preparation of "Sensitized Antigen Suspension"

1. Add one part of 10 per cent saline to one part of VDRL slide test suspension.
2. Mix by gently rotating the bottle or inverting the tube, and allow to stand at least 5 minutes but not more than 2 hours before use.

Testing Accuracy of Antigen Suspension Delivery Needles

For the slide quantitative and qualitative tests on spinal fluid, dispense sensitized antigen suspension from a syringe fitted with a 21- or 22-gauge needle, which will deliver 100 drops (± 2 drops) per milliliter when the syringe and needle are held vertically. Needles not meeting this criterion should be adjusted and calibrated before use or discarded.

Procedure (VDRL Slide Qualitative Test on Spinal Fluid)

Note: Tests should be performed within the temperature range 23° to 29°C, because slide flocculation tests for syphilis are affected by room temperature and lower than room temperature, and test reactivity is decreased.

1. Pipet 0.05 ml of spinal fluid into one concavity of an agglutination slide.
2. Add one drop (0.02 ml) of sensitized antigen suspension to each spinal fluid with a 21- or 22-gauge needle.
3. Rotate slides for 8 minutes on a mechanical rotator at 180 rpm.
4. Read tests microscopically with a low-power objective, at 100× magnification. Record as follows:

Reading Results

Definite clumping or flocculation of antigen particles	: Reactive
Complete dispersion of antigen particles, not agglutination or flocculation	: Nonreactive

Procedure (VDRL Quantitative Test on Spinal Fluid)

Note: Quantitative tests are performed on all spinal fluids found to be reactive in the qualitative test.

1. Prepare spinal fluid dilutions as follows: Pipet 0.2 ml of 0.9 per cent saline into each of five or more tubes. Add 0.2 ml of unheated spinal fluid to tube 1, mix well, and transfer 0.2 ml to tube 2. Continue mixing and transferring 0.2 ml from one tube to the next until the last tube is reached. The dilutions are 1:2, 1:4, 1:8, and so forth.
2. Test each spinal fluid and undiluted spinal fluid as described for the qualitative procedure.
3. Report results in terms of the highest dilution of spinal fluid giving a positive reaction.

METHOD 3: FLUORESCENT TREPONEMAL ANTIBODY ABSORPTION (FTA-ABS) TEST WITH SERUM

Materials

1. Incubator—adjustable for 35° to 37°C
2. Dark-field fluorescent microscope assembly
3. Bibulous paper
4. Diamond-point pencil (optional)
5. Template—used as a guide for cutting circles of 1.0 cm inside diameter on glass slides (optional)
6. Slide board or holder
7. Moist chamber: Place moistened paper inside a convenient cover fitting and slide board
8. Loop—bacteriologic, standard 2-mm, 26-gauge platinum wire loop
9. Oil—immersion, low-fluorescence, nondrying
10. Microscope slides—1 inch × 3 inch, frosted end, approximately 1 mm thick
11. Cover slips—No. 1, 22 mm square
12. Dish—staining, glass or plastic, with removable slide carriers
13. Glass rods—approximately 100 × 4 mm, both ends fire polished

Reagents

1. *Treponema pallidum* antigen: The antigen for this test is a suspension of *T. pallidum* (Nicols strain) extracted from rabbit testicular tissue, containing a minimum of 30 organisms per high dry field. The antigen may be stored at 6° to 10°C or may be processed by lyophilization. Lyophilized antigen is also stored at 6° to 10°C and is reconstituted for use according to directions when needed. Any antigen that becomes bacterially contaminated or does not give the appropriate reactions with control sera must be discarded.
2. FTA-ABS test sorbent: This is a standardized product prepared from cultures of Reiter treponemes. It may be purchased in lyophilized or liquid state and should be stored according to the manufacturer's directions.

3. Fluorescein-labeled antihuman globulin (conjugate): This should be of proven quality for the FTA-ABS test. Each new lot of conjugate should be tested to ensure its dependability with respect to working titer and to verify that it meets the criteria concerning nonspecific staining and standard reactivity. The lyophilized conjugate should be stored at 6° to 10°C. Rehydrated conjugate should be dispensed in not less than 0.3-ml quantities and should be stored at −20°C or lower. For practical purposes, a conjugate with a working titer of 1:400 or higher may be diluted 1:10 with sterile phosphate-buffered saline (containing Merthiolate in a concentration of 1:5000) before storage. When conjugate is thawed for use, it should not be refrozen but should be stored at 6° to 10°C. It may then be used as long as acceptable reactivity is obtained with test controls. If a change in FTA-ABS test reactivity is noted in routine testing, the conjugate should be retitered to determine whether this is the contributing factor.
4. Phosphate-buffered saline (PBS), pH 7.2 ± 0.1: The solution is prepared in the following way:

> To each liter of distilled water add
> NaCl—7.65 gm
> Na_2HPO_4—0.724 gm
> KH_2PO_4—0.21 gm

Several liters may be produced and stored in large Pyrex (or equivalent) or polyethylene bottles. The pH of the solution should be 7.2 ± 0.1. PBS outside this range should be discarded.
5. Tween-80: To prepare PBS containing 2 per cent Tween-80, heat the two reagents in a 56°C water bath. To 98 ml of PBS, add 2 ml of Tween-80 (by measuring from the bottom of the pipet). The 2 per cent Tween-80 solution should be pH 7.0 to 7.2 and should be checked periodically, because the solution may become acid. Store at refrigerator temperature, and discard if a precipitate forms or if the pH moves out of the acceptable range.
6. Mounting medium, consisting of one part PBS, pH 7.2, plus nine parts glycerin (reagent quality).
7. Acetone (A.C.S.).

Preparation of *Treponema pallidum* Antigen Smears

1. Mix the antigen suspension well with a disposable pipet and rubber bulb, drawing the suspension into and expelling it from the pipet at least 10 times to break the treponemal clumps and to ensure an even distribution of treponemes.

To ensure that treponemes are adequately dispersed before making slides for the FTA-ABS test, check by dark-field examination. Additional mixing may be required.

2. Cut two circles of 1 cm inside diameter with a diamond-point pencil on clean slides. Wipe the slides with clean gauze to remove loose glass particles. Slides with pre-etched circles are also satisfactory for this test.

3. Smear one loopful of *T. pallidum* antigen evenly within each circle by using a standard 2-mm, 26-gauge platinum wire loop. Allow to air dry for 15 minutes.

4. Fix the smears in acetone for 10 minutes, and allow them to air dry thoroughly. Not more than 60 slides should be fixed with 200 ml of acetone. Store the acetone-fixed smears at −20°C or lower. Fixed, frozen smears can be used indefinitely provided that satisfactory results are obtained with controls. Antigen smears should not be thawed and refrozen.

Preparation of Sera

Test and control sera should be heated at 56°C for 30 minutes before testing. Previously heated test sera should be reheated for 10 minutes at 56°C on the day of testing.

Note: Bacterial contamination or excessive hemolysis may render specimens unsuitable for testing.

Controls

Control sera from commercial sources should be stored and controlled according to the manufacturer's directions. Include the following controls in each test run:

1. Reactive (4+) control. Reactive serum or a dilution of reactive serum should demonstrate strong (4+) florescence when diluted 1:5 in PBS and only slightly reduced fluorescence when diluted 1:5 in sorbent. Prepare as follows:
   a. Using a 0.2-ml pipet and measuring from the bottom, add 0.05 ml of reactive control serum to a tube containing 0.2 ml of PBS. Mix well—at least eight times.
   b. Using a 0.2-ml pipet and measuring from the bottom, add 0.05 ml of sorbent. Mix well—at least eight times.

2. Minimally reactive (1+) control. Dilutions of reactive serum demonstrating the *minimal* degree of fluorescence reported as "reactive" for use as a reading standard. The reactive (4+) control serum may be used for this control when diluted in PBS according to directions.

3. Nonspecific serum controls. A nonsyphilitic serum known to demonstrate at least 2+ non-

specific reactivity in the FTA test at a dilution of PBS of 1:5 or higher should be used. Prepare as follows:
   a. Using a 0.2-ml pipet and measuring from the bottom, add 0.05 ml of nonspecific control serum to a tube containing 0.2 ml of PBS. Mix well—at least eight times.
   b. Using another 0.2-ml pipet and measuring from the bottom, add 0.05 ml of nonspecific control serum to a tube containing 0.2 ml of sorbent. Mix well—at least eight times.

4. Nonspecific staining controls:
   a. Antigen smear treated with 0.03 ml of PBS.
   b. Antigen smear treated with 0.03 ml of sorbent.

Controls 1, 3, and 4 are included for the purpose of controlling reagents and test conditions. Control 2 (minimally reactive control serum) is included as the reading standard (Table 6–1).

Check Testing of New Lots of Reagents

Each new lot of reagents should be tested in parallel with a standard reagent giving satisfactory results before being placed into routine use.

Procedure

1. Identify the previously prepared slides by numbering the frosted end with a lead pencil (see preparation of *T. pallidum* antigen smears).

2. Number the tubes to correspond with the sera and control sera being tested, and place in racks.

3. Prepare controls—reactive (4+), minimally reactive (1+), and nonspecific control serum dilutions as already described.

4. Pipet 0.2 ml of sorbent into a test tube for each test serum.

5. Using a 0.2-ml pipet and measuring from the bottom, add 0.05 ml of the heated serum into the appropriate tube, and mix at least eight times.

Table 6–1. CONTROL PATTERN ILLUSTRATION

	Reaction*
Reactive control	
a. 1:5 PBS dilution	R4+
b. 1:5 sorbent dilution	R(4+ to 3+)
Minimally reactive (1+) control	R1+
Nonspecific serum controls	
a. 1:5 PBS, dilution	R(2+ to 4+)
b. 1:5 sorbent dilution	N
Nonspecific staining controls	
a. Antigen, PBS, and conjugate	N
b. Antigen, sorbent, and conjugate	N

*R = reactive; N = normal. Test runs in which these control results are not obtained are considered unsatisfactory and should not be reported.

Table 6–2. METHOD OF RECORDING INTENSITY OF FLUORESCENCE

Reading	Intensity of Fluorescence	Report
2+ to 4+	Moderate to strong	Reactive (R)
1+	Equivalent to minimally reactive (1+) control	Reactive (R)
Less than 1+	Weak but definite, less than minimally reactive (1+) control	Borderline (R)
—	None or vaguely visible	Nonreactive (N)

Note: The interval between preparing serum dilutions and placing them on the antigen smears should not exceed 30 minutes.

6. Cover the appropriate antigen smears with 0.03 ml of the reactive (4+), minimally reactive (1+), and nonspecific control dilutions.
7. Cover the appropriate antigen smears with 0.03 ml of the PBS and 0.03 ml of the sorbent for "nonspecific" staining controls a. and b., respectively.
8. Cover the appropriate antigen smears with 0.03 ml of the test serum dilutions.
9. Place in a moist chamber to prevent evaporation.
10. Place the moist chamber in an incubator at 35° to 37°C for 30 minutes.
11. Rinsing procedure: Place the slides in slide carriers and rinse slides with running PBS for about 5 minutes. Then place the slides in a staining dish containing PBS for 5 minutes. Agitate the slides by dipping them in and out of the PBS at least 10 times. Again, place the slides in a staining dish containing *fresh* PBS for 5 minutes, and agitate by dipping them in and out at least 10 times. Rinse the slides in running distilled water for about 5 seconds.
12. Blot the slides *gently* with bibulous paper to remove all water drops. Alternatively, shake off excess water, place the slides on a clean towel, and then dry them with a hair dryer (not hot air).
13. Dilute the conjugate to its working titer in PBS containing 2 per cent Tween-80.
14. Place approximately 0.03 ml of diluted conjugate on each smear. Spread uniformly with a glass rod to cover the entire smear.
15. Repeat steps 9, 10, 11, and 12.
16. Mount the slides immediately by placing a small drop of mounting medium on each smear and applying a cover slip.
17. Examine slides as soon as possible. If a delay is unavoidable, slides may be placed in a darkened room and read within 4 hours.
18. Read microscopically, using a ultraviolet light source and a high-power dry objective. A combination of BG 12 exciting filter, not greater than 3 mm in thickness, and OG1 barrier filter (or their equivalents) has been found to be satisfactory for routine use.
19. Check the nonreactive smears by using illumination from the tungsten light source in order to verify the presence of treponemes.
20. Using the minimally reactive (1+) control slide as the reading standard, record the intensity of fluorescence of the treponemes as shown in Table 6–2.

Note: All specimens with intensity of fluorescence of 1+ or less should be retested. When a specimen initially read as 1+ is retested and subsequently read as 1+ or greater, the test is reported as "reactive." All other test results on retest are reported as "borderline." It is not necessary to retest nonfluorescent (nonreactive) specimens (see Table 6–3).

Borderline Results

A report should accompany each "borderline" result stating that the result cannot be interpreted as "reactive" or "nonreactive." If the result is found the *first* time the specimen is submitted from a particular patient, a new specimen should be requested for retesting. On subsequent occasions, the laboratory should suggest a careful review of the patient's history and findings, because it will be on these criteria that diagnosis will be based.

METHOD 4: DARK-FIELD MICROSCOPY EXAMINATION OF *TREPONEMA PALLIDUM*

Materials

1. Dark-field microscope assembly. This is an ordinary microscope equipped with the following:
   a. Mechanical stage
   b. Dark-field condenser

Table 6–3. THE FTA-ABS REPORTING SCHEME

Test Reading	Repeat	Report*
4+		R
3+		R
2+		R
1+	1+ or greater	R
	1+, less than 1+, or negative	B
Less than 1+	1+, less than 1+, or negative	B
		N

*R = reactive; B = borderline; N = nonreactive.

   c. 10× ocular(s)

   d. Low-power objective (10×)

   e. High dry objective (40 to 45×)

   f. Oil-immersion objective fitted with a funnel stop or equipped with a built-in iris diaphragm to lower the numerical aperture of the objective below that of the condenser

Preferably, the microscope should be *parafocal* (*i.e.*, when objectives are changed, the correct focus is maintained).

  2. Illuminator. Preferably external with iris diaphragm and a 100-watt bulb. Internal microscope base illuminators are satisfactory when connected to a rheostat transformer.

  3. Microscope slides—1 × 3 inches, frosted ends

  4. Cover glass—size No. 1, 22 × 22 mm square

  5. Oil—immersion, nondrying

  6. Lens paper

  7. Lens cleaner

  8. Forceps, cover glass

  9. Applicator sticks

 10. Surgical gloves—rubber or plastic

 11. Gauge—2 × 2 inch square, sterile

 12. Saline—physiologic, sterile

 13. Scalpel

 14. Loop—bacteriologic

 15. Pipet—capillary, disposable sterile

 16. Bulb—rubber, 1- or 2-ml capacity

 17. Speculum—bivalve

 18. Clamp—Kelly or hemostat

 19. Alcohol—70 per cent, or iodine solution

 20. Syringe—1- or 2-ml, sterile

 21. Needles—20- and 23-gauge, sterile

Collection and Submission of Specimens

Careful specimen collection for dark-field examination is especially important, because the objective is to obtain serous fluid that is rich in *T. pallidum* and is as free as possible of red blood cells and tissue debris, which may obscure the treponemes. The lesion should be thoroughly cleansed to remove tissue debris and superficial spirochetal flora, such as the larger *Borrelia*-like organisms and the smaller indigenous treponemes (*e.g.*, *T. genitalis*). When collecting specimens, the technologist should use rubber gloves and take *all necessary precautions to avoid accidental infection*. Remove any scab or crust covering the lesion; cleanse with a gauze pad wet with tap water or physiologic saline. (Note: Do not use antiseptics or soap because of the potential anti-treponemal effect.) Dry the area; abrade the lesion with a dry gauze pad to provoke slight bleeding and exudation of tissue fluid. As oozing occurs, wipe away the first few drops containing red blood cells, and await the appearance of relatively clear serous exudate. If necessary, apply pressure at the base of the lesion or apply a suction cup over the lesion to promote the appearance of tissue fluid. Ideally, the specimen should be obtained from the depths of the lesion rather than from its surface because of the greater likelihood of finding motile treponemes. For direct examination, apply clean cover glasses or slides to the oozing lesion, or use a bacteriologic loop to transfer the fluid from the lesion to glass slides. Flatten the cover glass evenly on the side with the blunt end of an applicator stick to remove air bubbles, and examine immediately. (Note: It may be necessary to examine several slides before treponemes are found.)

Lesions of early syphilis that are not manifest but are suspected necessitate special management. In the female, lesions of the cervix and vaginal vault present special problems for the collection of satisfactory material for dark-field examination. With visualization provided by a bivalve speculum, remove all cervical or vaginal discharge of an interfering nature. Cleanse the lesion with physiologic saline, dry it, and abrade it as before (in this instance, by rubbing with a gauze pad held by a Kelly clamp). As the bleeding stops and serous exudate appears, obtain the material with a bacteriologic loop.

Lesions of the skin, even in the fading stage, merit examination. Materials can be obtained by making a small linear incision, by scraping with a sharp scalpel (or the side of the bevel of a hypodermic syringe by using it as a knife edge), or by injection of a drop or two of sterile saline in the base of the lesion with a small-gauge hypodermic needle and syringe. Mucous membrane lesions (patches) usually present no problem except in the mouth, where other treponemes that are almost identical morphologically to *T. pallidum* and that have the same motility may be present as part of the indigenous flora (*e.g.*, *T. microdentium*).

If it proves impossible to find treponemes after several examinations, a sample from the regional lymph node may be obtained, particularly if the node is palpable. The skin over the node should be sterilized by swabbing with iodine and alcohol or some other suitable agent. Rinse a sterile 20-gauge needle and 2-ml syringe with sterile saline, and allow a few drops of saline to remain in the needle. Hold the node firmly, and insert the needle well into the node. The ability to manipulate the node freely with the needle tip is a good indication that the capsule has been pierced. Leaving the needle in place, carefully detach the syringe, draw a small amount of air (approximately 0.1 ml) into it, and reattach it to the needle. Inject the residual saline into the node, macerate the tissue by gently manipulating the needle in various directions, and aspirate as much material as possible. Discharge the aspirated material on slides for immediate examination. (Note: This procedure should be done by a physician.)

Dark-field examination should be accomplished immediately, either by bringing the patient to the microscope or by bringing the microscope to the patient. Any appreciable delay in examination of the specimen may result in questionable findings because of reduced or complete loss of motility of the treponemes.

Adjustment of the Microscope for Dark-Field Examination

Dark-field illumination is accomplished by blocking out the central rays of light with an opaque stop in the dark-field condenser and reflecting peripheral rays from the side to the upper surface of the microscope side. The only direct rays of light entering the objective are those reflected from the surface of an object in the field. The object appears bright against a dark background.

1. Align the microscope and the illuminator. The external illuminator should be 6 to 20 inches in front of the plane (or flat) side of the microscope mirror.
2. Adjust the iris diaphragm on the front of the illuminator to a diameter of about 20 mm.
3. Using a piece of paper placed across the mirror surface, adjust the illuminator so that the image of the filaments of the light bulb is shown in sharp focus on the center area of the plane side of the mirror. This is done with the focusing knob on the light housing or by moving the housing backward and forward.
4. Remove the paper, and adjust the angle of the mirror to direct the light beam into the bottom of the condenser.
5. Raise the substage containing the condenser to its maximal height. The top of the condenser should be just slightly below the level of the stage. Adjust the height by rotating the top of the condenser clockwise to lower and counterclockwise to raise.
6. Lower the substage slightly, and place 2 or 3 drops of immersion oil on the top of the condenser.

To complete the microscope adjustment and to verify the adjustment before examination of patient material, prepare a suspension of gingival scrapings in a drop of saline on a slide and mount with a cover slip. Proceed as follows:

7. Place the slide on the stage, and center the specimen over the condenser with the mechanical stage.
8. Slowly raise the substage until there is an oil contact between the top of the condenser and the bottom of the slide (with care to avoid trapping air bubbles).
9. Rotate the objective turret to center the 10× objective over the specimen.
10. Bring the specimen into focus by using the coarse adjustment knob.
11. Center the light in the field by adjusting the mirror or by rotating the two centering screws located at the base of the condenser.
12. Focus the condenser by raising or lowering the substage until the smallest diameter of the circular area of intense light is seen.
13. Recheck the centering of the light, and adjust if necessary.
14. Rotate the objective turret, and center the high dry (40 to 45×) objective over the specimen.
15. Using the fine adjustment knob, bring the specimen into focus.
16. Open the iris diaphragm on the light until the entire field is illuminated.

Examination of Specimens

1. Place the slide to be examined under the microscope, and adjust the microscope if necessary.
2. Search the entire specimen methodically for spiral organisms having morphology and motility characteristics of *T. pallidum*.
3. If a suspected organism is seen, center it in the field with the mechanical stage for examination with the oil-immersion objective.
4. Rotate the objective turret halfway so that a *small* drop of immersion oil can be placed on the cover glass.
5. Continue rotation of the turret until the oil-immersion objective is in place over the specimen and in contact with the oil on the cover glass.
6. Examine the organism carefully for identification; focus with the fine adjustment knob only.
7. If organisms are found that have the characteristic morphology and motility of *T. pallidum*, make a positive report. (Note: Do not make the negative report until a careful and exhaustive search of several slides has been made.)

Care should be taken to ensure that the organism seen is, in fact, *T. pallidum*. This can be accomplished only after experience with identification. Practically speaking, *T. pallidum*, as opposed to other spiral organisms, is usually uniform in size, shape, and motility. In contrast, *Borrelia*-like organisms are usually mixed with many other spiral and bacterial types, so that any one preparation will contain spiral forms of various sizes, shapes, and motilities. Experience in this case is the best teacher. In general, though, *T. pallidum* is a thin, tightly wound, rigid, spiral organism exhibiting little flexibility and does not move rapidly from place to place. Any coarsely wound spiral organism exhibiting great flexibility and rapidly moving from place to place, therefore, is *not T. pallidum*.

Interpretation

The demonstration of treponemes with characteristic morphology and motility of *T. pallidum* constitutes a positive diagnosis of syphilis in either the primary, secondary, early congenital, or infectious relapse stages, regardless of the results of serologic testing. In primary syphilis, it may be possible to identify the etiologic agent and to diagnose the disease before the serologic tests become reactive.

Failure to find the organism does not rule out the diagnosis of syphilis. In addition to meaning that the lesion is not syphilitic, negative results of dark-field examination may mean that (1) a sufficient number of organisms were not present to be detected, (2) the patient has received anti-treponemal drugs locally or systemically, (3) the lesion is "fading" or approaching natural resolution or disappearance, or (4) the lesion is one of late syphilis.

When negative results are obtained, the dark-field examination should be repeated on at least three different days, and serologic follow-up should be continued for about 4 months—at weekly intervals for the first month, and every 2 weeks thereafter—before the possibility of syphilis is ruled out.

METHOD 5: RAPID PLASMA REAGIN (RPR) (CIRCLE) CARD TEST ON SERUM

Materials

All equipment and supplies necessary to perform the RPR (circle) Card Test are contained in a kit supplied by Hynson, Westcott and Dunning, Inc., Baltimore, MD, with the exception of controls, the rotating machine and the humidifier cover.

1. The kit contains the following:
   a. RPR Card Test antigen: This cardiolipin is similar to that prepared for the unheated serum reagin test (Method 6). It also contains a suspension of especially prepared charcoal particles, which allows the test to be read macroscopically. The antigen should be stored according to the manufacturer's directions (usually 2° to 8°C), in which case the unopened ampule will have a shelf life of at least 12 months from the date of manufacture. Once the ampule has been opened, it usually remains stable for about 3 months and should not be used after the expiration date on the ampule. Each new lot of antigen suspension should be carefully compared with an antigen suspension of known reactivity before being placed into routine use.
   b. 20-gauge needle without bevel
   c. Plastic dispensing bottle
   d. Plastic-coated cards—each with 10 18-mm circle spots
   e. Dispenstirs—0.05 ml per drop
   f. Capillary pipets—0.05-ml capacity
   g. Rubber bulbs
   h. Stirrers
2. Rotating machine—adjustable or fixed at 100 rpm, circumscribing a ¾ inch diameter circle on a horizontal plane
3. Humidifier cover—any convenient cover containing a moistened pan may be used to cover the cards during rotation
4. Pipets (optional)—these may be used in place of Dispenstirs or capillary pipets
   0.2-ml, graduated in 0.01-ml subdivisions
   0.5-ml, graduated in 0.01-ml subdivisions
   1.0-ml, graduated in 0.01-ml subdivisions

Testing the Accuracy of Delivery Needles

The 20-gauge disposable needle without bevel should be checked each day by placing the needle on a 2-ml syringe or a 1-ml pipet, filling it with antigen suspension, and counting the number of drops delivered in 0.5 ml when the needle is held in a vertical position. The needle is considered satisfactory if 60 drops ± 2 drops are obtained in 1.0 ml. A needle not meeting this specification should be discarded.

Preliminary Testing of Antigen Suspension

1. Attach the needle hub to the tapered fitting on the plastic dispensing bottle. Shake the antigen ampule to resuspend the antigen particles, snap the ampule neck at the break line, and withdraw all the RPR Card Test antigen into the dispensing bottle by suction, collapsing the bottle and using it as a bulb. Shake the dispenser gently before each series of antigen drops is delivered.
2. Test the control sera of graded reactivity each day as described under "procedure" (below). Serum controls can be obtained from the daily test runs or from individual donors.
3. Use only those suspensions that have given the designated reactions with the controls.

Preparation of Serum

1. Centrifuge the blood specimen at room temperature at a force that is sufficient to separate the serum from the cells (generally 1500 to 2000 rpm for 5 minutes).
2. Retain the serum in the original collection tube.
3. Serum is tested without heating but should be at 23° to 29°C at the time of testing.

Procedure

Note: Serum and RPR Card Test antigen suspension should be at 23° to 29°C at the time of testing.

1. Place 0.05 ml of unheated serum on an 18-mm circle of the test card, using a Dispenstir, a 0.05-ml capillary pipet with attached bulb, or a serologic pipet.
2. Spread the serum with the Dispenstir (inverted, using the closed end) or a stirrer (broad end) to fill the entire circle. (Note: Be careful not to scratch the card surface.)
3. Add exactly one drop (1/60 ml) of RPR Card Test antigen suspension to each test area containing serum. Do not stir.
4. Place the card on the rotator, and cover with the humidifier cover.
5. Rotate for 8 minutes at 100 rpm.
6. Read the tests without magnification immediately after rotation. The card may be briefly rotated or tilted by hand if necessary to differentiate nonreactive from minimally reactive results.
7. Report the results as follows:

Small to large clumps:	Reactive (R)
No clumping, or slight roughness:	Nonreactive (N)

Note: Specimens giving any degree of clumping should be subjected to further serologic study, including quantitation.
8. Upon completion of tests, remove the needle, rinse in water, and air dry. Do not wipe the needle; this removes the silicone coating. Recap the dispensing bottle, and store it in the refrigerator.

METHOD 6: UNHEATED SERUM REAGIN (USR) TEST ON SERUM

Materials

1. Centrifuge—angle head, Servall SS-2, type "XL," or equivalent
2. Tachometer
3. Cotton gauze
4. Rotating machine—adjustable to 180 rpm, circumscribing a circle ¾ inch in diameter on a horizontal plane
5. Tubes—stainless steel, 50-ml capacity, without flange
6. Ring maker—to make paraffin rings approximately 14 mm in diameter
7. Slide holder for 2 × 3 inch microscope slides
8. Hypodermic needle–180-gauge, without bevel
9. Syringe—Luer-type, 1- or 2-ml
10. Bottles—30-ml, round, glass-stoppered, narrow-mouth, approximately 35 mm in diameter, with *flat* interbottom surface
11. VDRL antigen
12. VDRL buffered saline
13. Phosphate (0.02M) Merthiolate (0.2 per cent) solution—prepared by dissolving 1.42 gm Na_2HPO_4, 1.36 gm KH_2PO_4, and 1.00 gm Merthiolate in distilled water to a final volume of 500 ml. The pH of the solution should be 6.9. It should be stored in the dark at room temperature and may be used, thus stored, for a period of 3 months.
14. Choline chloride solution (40 per cent)—prepared by dissolving the entire contents of a 250-gm bottle of choline chloride in distilled water to a final volume of 625 ml
15. EDTA (0.1M)—prepared by dissolving 3.72 gm EDTA ([ethylenedinitrilo] tetra-acetic acid disodium salt) to a volume of 100 ml in distilled water. This solution may be used for 1 year.
16. Resuspending solution, prepared as follows:
    EDTA (0.1M) 1.25 ml
    Choline chloride (40 per cent) 2.5 ml
    Phosphate (0.02M) Merthiolate (0.2 per cent) 5.0 ml
    Distilled water 1.25 ml
    (Note: This solution should be prepared each time antigen suspensions are made.)

Preparation of Antigen Suspensions

1. Prepare antigen suspensions as for the VDRL slide tests (see Method 1).
2. Centrifuge measured amounts of the antigen suspension into stainless steel tubes in an angle centrifuge at room temperature at 200 gm for 15 minutes (start timing when centrifuge *reaches* desired speed). From 5 to 30 ml may be centrifuged in a single centrifuge tube.
3. Locate the sediment, and decant supernatant fluid by inverting the tube away from the side containing the sediment. While holding the tube in an inverted position, wipe the inside with cotton gauze without disturbing the sediment.
4. Resuspend with a volume of resuspending solution equal to that of the original volume of antigen suspension that was centrifuged.
5. If more than one centrifuge tube is used, combine all suspensions in a bottle, stopper tightly, and shake gently for a few seconds to obtain an even suspension. This is the completed antigen suspension.
6. Each new lot of antigen suspension should be compared with an antigen suspension of known reactivity before use. Store the antigen suspension at 3° to 10°C, at which it will remain stable for at least 6 months.

Testing Accuracy of Delivery Needles

The 18-gauge needle without bevel should be checked each day by placing it on a syringe, filling it with antigen suspension, and counting the number of drops delivered in 1.0 ml when the needle is held in a vertical position. The needle is considered satisfactory if 45 drops (± 1 drop) are obtained from 1 ml of antigen suspension. A needle that does not meet this specification should be discarded.

Preliminary Testing of Antigen Suspension

Withdraw only sufficient antigen suspension from the stock bottle for 1 day's testing, and return the stock bottle to the refrigerator. The antigen suspension should be kept at room temperature for not less than 30 minutes before it is used.

Test control sera of graded reactivity every day as described under Procedure. Serum controls can be obtained from the daily test runs or from individual donors.

Use only those suspensions that give satisfactory results with controls.

Preparation of Serum

1. Centrifuge the blood specimen at room temperature at a force sufficient to separate the serum from the cellular elements (usually 1500 to 2000 rpm for 5 minutes).
2. Retain the serum in the original collection tube.

Procedure

Note: Serum and USR antigen suspensions should be at 23° to 29°C at the time of testing.

1. Pipet 0.05 ml of unheated serum from the original collection tube into one ring of a paraffin-ringed glass slide.
2. Add one drop (1/45 ml) of antigen suspension onto each serum.
3. Rotate slides on the rotating machine at 180 rpm for 4 minutes.
4. Read tests microscopically with a 10× ocular and a 10× objective immediately after rotation.
5. Report the results as follows:

Medium and large clumps:	Reactive (R)
Small clumps:	Weakly reactive (W)
No clumping, or very slight roughness:	Nonreactive (N)

Note: Specimens giving any degree of clumping should be subjected to further serologic study, including quantitation.

THE *TREPONEMA PALLIDUM* IMMOBILIZATION (TPI) TEST

The TPI test has undergone extensive clinical and laboratory evaluation and has been accepted as the treponemal test of *reference* (*i.e.,* it is the standard test against which all other treponemal tests were evaluated). The test, however, has certain limitations:

1. It requires live treponemes from infected animals and is difficult to perform.
2. It does not distinguish the various treponematoses (*i.e.,* yaws, pinta, bejel).
3. It cannot distinguish between active and latent infection.
4. It cannot be used as an index of therapeutic response.
5. It fails to detect early syphilis.
6. It is ineffective when the patient is on antibiotics.

On the positive side, the test is the one of choice for spinal fluids, especially for detecting neurosyphilis when reagin tests give nonreactive or equivocal results.

Briefly, the test involves the mixing of live, actively motile *T. pallidum* extracted from the testicular chancre of a rabbit and complement. The mixture is incubated in an atmosphere of 5 per cent CO_2 and 95 per cent N_2 and is then observed with a dark-field microscope to determine the proportion of treponemes immobilized relative to the controls. Sera causing immobilization are called TPI positive.

Perhaps the greatest value of the test is in confirming syphilis or ruling out biologic false-positive reactions; yet only a few research laboratories currently perform the test. This is primarily because of the exacting nature of the procedure, the fact that it is not well standardized, and few laboratories desire to maintain "cultures" of live *T. pallidum.*

OTHER TESTS FOR SYPHILIS

The *T. pallidum hemagglutination test* (TPHA, or, when microtechniques are used, the MHA-TP) is a fairly recent addition to syphilis serology. In this test, tanned sheep red cells are coated with antigen from the Nichol's strain of *T. pallidum,* and the serum is absorbed with sorbent similar to that in the FTA-ABS test. A positive reaction is considered to be due to serum antibodies specific for syphilis. The test is simple, rapid, and reproducible and is available in kit form from Ames Division, Miles Laboratories Inc., Elkhart, Indiana. Studies have shown that the MHA-TP test is comparable to the FTA-ABS test in all categories of syphilis except the primary stage, in which the MHA-TP is less reactive than either the FTA-ABS or the VDRL tests. In general, however, the MHA-TP is highly specific and can be considered a satisfactory substitute for the FTA-ABS test. The chief advantages of MHA-TP when compared with FTA-ABS are its simplicity and economy. The reagents and equipment are less expensive, and the procedure technically lends itself to automation. In this regard, it can be used as a highly specific screening test. Furthermore, the reading of the test is less subjective, and quality control is significantly easier.

The **enzyme-linked immunosorbent assay (ELISA)** methodology is also being applied to syphilis serology. In this test, tubes coated inside with *T. pallidum* antigen are incubated with dilute serum from patients. The tubes are washed, and enzyme-labeled antihuman immunoglobulin is added. The amount of enzyme (commonly, alkaline phosphatase) activity is measured by adding substrates to the tube and measuring the reaction product formed. The principles of the ELISA technique are discussed in Chapter Five.

REVIEW QUESTIONS

MULTIPLE CHOICE

Choose the phrase, sentence, or symbol that completes the statement or answers the question. More than one answer may be correct in each case. Answers are given at the end of this book.

1. Which of the following pathogenic organisms is responsible for human syphilis?
   (a) *Treponema parridum*
   (b) *Treponema pallidum*
   (c) *Treponema pertenue*
   (d) *Treponema cuniculi*
   (*Introduction*)

2. The genus Treponema contains:
   (a) two principal species of pathogenic organisms
   (b) three principal species of pathogenic organisms
   (c) four principal species of pathogenic organisms
   (d) five principal species of pathogenic organisms
   (*Morphology of* Treponema pallidum)

3. The length of the *T. pallidum* organism varies from:
   (a) 6–15 microns
   (b) 12–24 microns
   (c) 1–3 microns
   (d) 0.25–0.75 micron
   (*Morphology of* Treponema pallidum)

4. Under anaerobic conditions, *T. pallidum* can be kept viable and motile for periods up to:
   (a) 4 hours at 35°C in appropriate medium
   (b) 1 day at 35°C in appropriate medium
   (c) 72 hours at 35°C in appropriate medium
   (d) 15 hours at 35°C in appropriate medium
   (*Metabolism of* Treponema pallidum)

5. The nutritional requirements of *T. pallidum* include:
   (a) a fermentable carbohydrate
   (b) multiple amino acids
   (c) at least one exogenously supplied fatty acid
   (d) none of the above
   (*Metabolism of* Treponema pallidum)

6. *T. pallidum* has not been recovered from blood, serum, or plasma that has been stored at 4°C for more than:
   (a) 2 hours
   (b) 6 hours
   (c) 24 hours
   (d) 48 hours
   (*Metabolism of* Treponema pallidum)

7. In cases of human syphilis, the primary lesion is extragenital in:
   (a) 1 per cent of cases
   (b) approximately 10 per cent of cases
   (c) approximately 90 per cent of cases
   (d) approximately 50 per cent of cases
   (*The Stages of Syphilis*)

8. During the primary (or early) stage of human syphilis:
   (a) the chancre persists for 1 to 5 weeks, then heals spontaneously
   (b) the serum in 30 per cent of cases becomes serologically active after 1 week
   (c) serum tests for syphilis usually give positive results between the first and third weeks after the appearance of the chancre
   (d) the disease is not communicable
   (*The Stages of Syphilis: Primary (or Early) Stage*)

9. The secondary stage of syphilis:
   (a) occurs from 6 to 8 months after the appearance of the primary chancre
   (b) is usually characterized by a generalized rash
   (c) is characterized by negative serologic tests for syphilis
   (d) in most cases, goes unnoticed
   (*The Stages of Syphilis: Secondary Stage*)

10. The late latent stage of human syphilis:
    (a) usually begins after the second year of infection
    (b) is usually noncontagious
    (c) is highly contagious
    (d) is still contagious between mother and fetus
    (*The Stages of Syphilis: The Late Latent Stage*)

11. The tertiary stage of human syphilis:
    (a) is characterized by lesions known as gummata
    (b) is asymptomatic in 25 per cent of untreated cases
    (c) usually begins 3 to 10 years (or later) after the primary stage
    (d) in a quarter of untreated cases is recognized only by serologic tests
    (The Stages of Syphilis: Tertiary Stage)

12. Specific anti-treponemal antibodies in early or untreated early latent syphilis are predominantly:
    (a) IgG
    (b) IgM
    (c) IgA
    (d) IgE
    (Antibodies in Syphilis)

13. Immunity to *T. pallidum:*
    (a) develops in the course of syphilis both in rabbits and in humans
    (b) can be detected in rabbits with experimental syphilis just 3 weeks after infection with the organism
    (c) can be induced by vaccines containing nonviable *T. pallidum*
    (d) is probably never *complete*
    (Production of Immunity)

14. If treatment is given in a case of syphilis that is in the seropositive primary stage, the serologic tests usually become nonreactive after:
    (a) 1 month
    (b) 6 months
    (c) 5 years
    (d) a considerable amount of time and, in most cases, remain nonreactive for life
    (Treatment of Syphilis)

15. Blood stored at 4°C for 4 days or more:
    (a) is unlikely to transmit syphilis
    (b) is likely to transmit syphilis
    (c) provides an ideal environment for *T. pallidum*
    (d) should always be tested for the presence of *T. pallidum* before transfusion is given
    (Syphilis and Blood Transfusion)

16. Neurosyphilis:
    (a) is syphilis of the central nervous system
    (b) may be asymptomatic
    (c) usually involves obliterative endarteritis
    (d) all of the above
    (Neurosyphilis)

17. Congenital syphilis:
    (a) is acquired through the placental passage of *T. pallidum* from the sixth week of gestation onward
    (b) is more likely to occur when the mother has late syphilis
    (c) cannot be prevented by treatment of the mother after the eighteenth week of gestation
    (d) none of the above
    (Congenital Syphilis)

18. The organism *T. pertenue* causes the tropical disease known as:
    (a) pinta
    (b) yaws
    (c) bejel
    (d) rabbit syphilis
    (Diseases Related to Syphilis)

19. Which of the following are categorized as "reagin tests" for syphilis?
    (a) VDRL slide test
    (b) TPIA test
    (c) RPR (circle) card test
    (d) FTA-ABS test
    (Serologic Tests for Syphilis: Principles)

20. When testing a sample for syphilis:
    (a) more than one screening test should be performed if results are found to be positive
    (b) false-positive results may result from diseases that are related to syphilis present in the individual under test
    (c) the results may be inaccurate due to the fact that the patient has been recently immunized
    (d) the differentiation of syphilis from other treponemal infections is not a problem
    (Notes on Serologic Tests for Syphilis)

21. A negative serologic test for syphilis may indicate:
    (a) that the infection is too recent to have produced antibodies that give reactions
    (b) that the test could be temporarily nonreactive because of the consumption of alcoholic beverage by the patient prior to testing
    (c) that the disease is latent
    (d) that the patient has not produced protective antibodies because of immunologic tolerance
    (Notes on Serologic Tests for Syphilis)

22. When testing a specimen for syphilis, weakly reactive results may be due to:
    (a) very early infection
    (b) lessening of the activity of the disease after treatment
    (c) biologic false-positive reaction
    (d) biologic false-negative reaction
    (Notes on Serologic Tests for Syphilis)

ANSWER "TRUE" OR "FALSE"

23. The causative organism of syphilis was originally called *Spirochaeta pallida.*
    (Introduction)

24. Suspensions of treponemes frozen at $-70°C$ or lower in the presence of glycerol or other cryoprotective agent will remain viable for 7 days.
    (Metabolism of Treponema pallidum)

25. During the secondary stage of syphilis, serologic tests are invariably negative.
    (The Stages of Syphilis: Secondary Stage)

26. Individuals infected with *T. pallidum* respond by

producing both specific and nonspecific antibodies.
(Antibodies in Syphilis)

27. Certain patients with syphilis are seroresistant.
(Treatment of Syphilis)

28. The organism that causes the disease known as pinta is morphologically indistinguishable from *T. pallidum.*
(Diseases Related to Syphilis: Pinta)

29. Penicillin should not be used for the treatment of bejel.
(Diseases Related to Syphilis: Bejel)

30. Rabbits with rabbit syphilis give positive Wassermann reactions and develop antibodies that immobilize *T. cuniculi.*
(Diseases Related to Syphilis: Rabbit Syphilis)

General References

Braude, A. I. (Ed.): Medical Microbiology and Infectious Diseases. Philadelphia, W. B. Saunders Company, 1981.

Finegold, S. M., and Martin, W. J.: Diagnostic Microbiology, 6th ed. St. Louis, The C. V. Mosby Co., 1982.

Freeman, B. A.: Burrows Textbook of Microbiology, 21st ed. Philadelphia, W. B. Saunders Company, 1979.

Raphael, S. S. (Senior Author): Lynch's Medical Laboratory Technology, 4th ed. Philadelphia, W. B. Saunders Company, 1983.

SEVEN

VIRAL HEPATITIS

OBJECTIVES

The student shall know, understand, and be prepared to explain:

1. A brief description of hepatitis
2. The hepatitis viruses
3. Hepatitis A with respect to:
   a. Hepatitis A virus (HVA)
   b. Antibodies to HAV
   c. Serologic tests for HAV
4. Hepatitis B, with respect to:
   a. Hepatitis B virus (HBV)
   b. Markers for HBV
   c. Subtypes of HbsAg
   d. Antibodies to HBAg
   e. Incidence of hepatitis B
   f. Transmission of hepatitis B
   g. Clinical signs and symptoms of hepatitis B
   h. Protection against HBV by antibody
   i. HBV vaccine
5. Non-A, non-B hepatitis, with respect to:
   a. Incidence of non-A, non-B hepatitis
   b. Transmission of non-A, non-B hepatitis
   c. Clinical signs and symptoms of non-A, non-B hepatitis
   d. Serologic tests for non-A, non-B hepatitis
6. The serologic detection of hepatitis markers—principles
7. Practical considerations in hepatitis testing
8. The serologic methods used in hepatitis testing, specifically:
   a. Ouchterlony double diffusion
   b. Counterelectrophoresis
   c. Rheophoresis
   d. Complement fixation
   e. Reversed passive latex agglutination
   f. Reversed passive hemagglutination
   g. Radioimmunoassay
   h. Enzyme-linked immunoassay
9. The serologic detection of anti-HBs
10. The serologic detection of HBcAg and anti-HBc
11. The serologic detection of HBeAg and anti-HBe

Introduction: Hepatitis

Hepatitis is a generic term referring to an inflammation of the liver. The term, however, is more generally used to refer to the clinical, laboratory, and/or histologic effects of liver injury, whether or not inflammation is present.

The vast majority of cases of hepatitis are the result of damage to the liver cells (hepatocytes), caused by viruses, bacteria, fungi, parasites, drugs, toxins, or physical agents such as heat, hyperthermia, radiation and so forth, or by excessive alcohol intake, although some cases are idiopathic—no etiology is identified. Some hepatocytes are affected much more severely than others, and a certain proportion are irreversibly injured. In nonfatal cases, the lost hepatocytes are usually replaced by the regeneration of new cells. The term *fulminant hepatitis* is applied when the number of hepatocytes destroyed is so great that too few remain to maintain basic liver function (*i.e.,* hepatic failure).

The morphologic changes that occur in the liver vary with the cause of hepatitis. Generally, the hepatocytes show nonspecific evidence of injury, with cell swelling (called *ballooning degeneration* when severe) and necrosis—either as eosinophilic bodies (acidophil bodies) or as small cytoplasmic fragments of ruptured hepatocytes.

Because of the many different causes of hepatitis, wherever possible, the term should be qualified with an etiologic modifier (*e.g.,* viral hepatitis, alcoholic hepatitis, radiation hepatitis). This chapter will be confined to the study of viral hepatitis.

The Hepatitis Viruses

Although many viruses may cause hepatitis, the terms *viral hepatitis* and *acute viral hepatitis* are generally used only to refer to cases caused by specific hepatotropic viruses. These include hepatitis A virus, hepatitis B virus, non-A, non-B hepatitis (NANB—*i.e.,* hepatitis viruses other than A and B. The NANB viral hepatitis is caused by a number of different viruses [*e.g.,* CMV, EBV]). All three of these viruses produce acute inflammation of the liver, characterized clinically by fever, nausea, vomiting, and jaundice. The characteristic differences of hepatitis A, B, and non-A, non-B viruses are given in Table 7–1.

Two classic epidemiologic patterns of transmission of viral hepatitis were recognized early and formed the basis for the classification of the disease into two major clinical types. So-called *infectious hepatitis* is the more common variety, which often involves many people and a short incubation period (caused by the type A virus). *Serum hepatitis,* which is caused by the type B virus or the non-A, non-B virus, usually follows blood transfusions or needle wounds and has a longer incubation period.

HEPATITIS A

Hepatitis A (infectious hepatitis) is the type seen in most epidemic outbreaks of hepatitis in the normal population. The disease is transmitted by a fecal-oral route and is therefore more common in countries with low standards of living, where it affects the population at a younger age. Outbreaks

Table 7–1. CHARACTERISTICS OF HEPATITIS VIRUSES

Characteristic	A Virus	B Virus	Non-A, Non-B Virus
Epidemiology	Endemic and epidemic, water-borne and food-borne epidemics	Endemic	Endemic
Transmission	Fecal-oral	Direct inoculation ? venereal	Direct inoculation ? other
Incubation period (weeks)	2–7	4–26	2–8
Disease	Acute	Acute and chronic	Acute and chronic
Size of virus	27 nm	42 nm (27 nm core)	?
Coat protein	No	Yes	?
Nucleic acid	RNA	Circular DNA (mainly double-stranded; molecular weight about 2.1 $\times 10^6$)	?
DNA polymerase	−	+	?
Cell culture system	+	−	−
Animal infection	Marmosets, chimpanzees	Chimpanzees	Chimpanzees
Chronic carrier	−	+	+
Vaccine	−	+	?
Passive immunity with immunoglobulin	+	+	? +

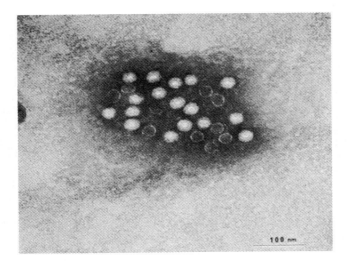

Figure 7–1. Electron micrograph of HAV particles extracted from HAV-infected marmoset liver showing electron dense cores (× 328,600). (From Braude, A. I.: Medical Microbiology and Infectious Diseases. Philadelphia, W. B. Saunders Company, 1981, p. 628.)

also show a seasonal pattern (*e.g.*, when children return to school and interact with one another).

Hepatitis A Virus (HAV)

The virus causing hepatitis A is a nonenveloped, icosahedral, single-stranded RNA particle that belongs to the family Picornaviridae. It has been isolated from the stool of acutely ill patients by Feinstone *et al.* (1973). Electron microscopic observations with positive staining of the particles showed that many have a dense core that is presumably composed of nucleoprotein (Fig. 7–1). This picornavirus localizes primarily in the cytoplasm of the liver, where it multiplies easily. Unlike hepatitis B virus, it does not produce a coat protein (see later discussion) and is not detectable in serum. It is stable in ether and to a pH of 3.0. Its properties resemble those of an enterovirus. Three major polypeptides are associated with the RNA.

HAV has not been grown in tissue culture; however, Dienhardt *et al.* (1967) did attempt to transmit the virus to marmosets (small monkeys found in the tropical forests of the Americas)—studies that eventually led to the isolation of strain CR326 of HAV through serial passage in marmosets. HAV has also been purified fom human and chimpanzee stool extracts, from infected marmoset and chimpanzee livers, and from bile of infected chimpanzees (Deinstag *et al.*, 1975).

Antibodies to HAV (Immunity)

At the onset of clinically apparent hepatitis A, antibodies to HAV appear in the plasma. Initially, the antibody is IgM (anti-HAV IgM), which is subsequently replaced by IgG that persists for years, probably for life (Fig. 7–2). This antibody will aggregate highly purified HAV (Fig. 7–3).

At the present time, there is no vaccine for hepatitis A infection. Passive protection with immunoglobulin, however, appears to both prevent and ameliorate the disease.

Serologic Tests for HAV

Until quite recently, hepatitis A infection was diagnosed after hepatitis B infection had been ruled out by appropriate laboratory tests—therefore by assumption. The recognition that non-A, non-B hepatitis is more common than originally thought, however, has made this assumption less reliable. The HAV antigen (HAAg) has been identified in feces (and occasionally in serum) by rather complex electron microscopic and radioimmunoassay methods—tests that are not readily adapted to the clinical laboratory. Recently, serologic tests have been devised that use antigen extracts from infected marmoset livers or infectious human feces. These include a complement fixation test (modified) and an immune adherence hemagglutination assay (IAHA), both of which have been used to demonstrate antibody titer responses to

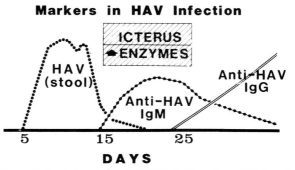

Figure 7–2. Markers in acute HAV infection. (From Pittiglio, D. H. (Ed.): Modern Blood Banking and Transfusion Practices. Philadelphia, F. A. Davis Co., 1983, p. 388.)

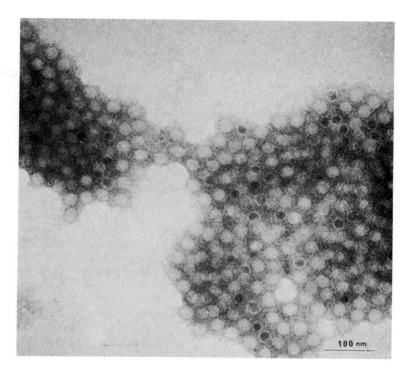

Figure 7–3. Highly purified HAV from pre-acute phase chimpanzee stool aggregated by anti-HAV (× 256,300). (From Braude, A. I.: Medical Microbiology and Infectious Diseases. Philadelphia, W. B. Saunders Company, 1981, p. 629.)

hepatitis A by comparing sera that are obtained 2 or 3 weeks apart. The IAHA is based on the principle that human red cells of group O are aggregated in the specific antigen–antibody–complement reaction (Miller, 1975) and shows particular promise for clinical application.

HEPATITIS B

Formerly known as serum hepatitis and post-transfusion hepatitis, hepatitis B commonly follows parenteral exposure to an infected individual, although other modes of transmission are known to occur (see later discussion). The incubation period is 4 to 26 weeks (*i.e.*, 1 to 6 months). In Western Europe and North America, cases of hepatitis B usually appear singly, whereas in Asia, large segments of the population have been found to be infected. In some cases, infection even seems to be acquired.

An important advance in the control of the spread of hepatitis B resulted from the discovery, in serum, of an antigen associated with the disease. This antigen was first recognized in the serum of an Australian aborigine and was given the provisional name *Australia antigen*. At first, the antigen appeared to be associated with acute leukemia (Blumberg *et al.*, 1965), yet it was not long before this was realized not to be so, and the association with hepatitis was confirmed (Prince, 1968; Blumberg *et al.*, 1968). Australia antigen is now known

to be unassembled viral coat (see later discussion) or "surface" antigen and is termed *HBsAg*.

Hepatitis B Virus (HBV)

HBV is a hepatotropic virus that is microbiologically unrelated to HAV. It is a double-stranded DNA particle, which exists in three forms:

1. A spherical (disc) particle, 22 nm in diameter
2. A filamentous form, 22 nm wide by 50 to 250 nm long
3. A Dane particle, 42 nm in diameter, which represents the virion, consisting of a 27-nm nucleocapsid DNA-containing core, surrounded by an outer lipoprotein coat (Figs. 7–4 and 7–5).

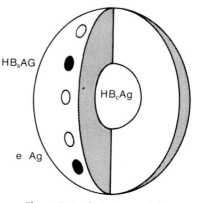

Figure 7–4. The Dane particle.

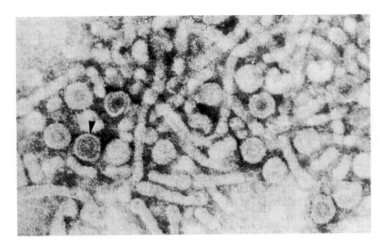

Figure 7–5. Electron micrograph of particulate Australia antigen (HBsAg) showing discs, filaments, and Dane particles (arrow) (× 250,000). (From Braude, A. I.: Medical Microbiology and Infectious Diseases. Philadelphia, W. B. Saunders Company, 1981, p. 630.)

The predominant form seen in the blood of patients with hepatitis B is the spherical particle (1); the filamentous form (2) is slightly less common; and the Dane particle (3) is the least common. It was suggested that the larger particles represented the complete virion and that the other morphologic forms were excess coat protein. This suggestion was given experimental foundation when the internal component of the Dane particle was released by treating the particles with 0.5 per cent Tween-80 (polysorbate) in phosphate buffered saline (Almeida *et al.,* 1971). In addition, the filamentous forms could be converted to the spherical (disc) forms by exposure to mildly acidic buffers.

Markers for Hepatitis B Virus

HBsAg. The outer lipoprotein coat (or envelope) of hepatitis B virus is known as *hepatitis B surface antigen (HBsAg).* It is 22 nm in diameter and is found in the body fluids of patients with hepatitis B viral infection. It is produced in the cytoplasm of infected hepatocytes.

HBcAg. The core of the HBV is known as *hepatitis B core antigen (HBcAg).* It is 27 nm in diameter and is located in the nuclei of hepatocytes in patients with HBV infection.

HBeAg. A soluble antigen, called *e antigen (HBeAg)* is also found in the sera of patients with HBV infection. The antigen appears during acute infection and then usually disappears, but it can be carried chronically in patients with chronic hepatitis B antigenemia and chronic hepatitis. The exact nature of the e antigen is unknown. Three antigenic subtypes, known as HBe_1Ag, HBe_2Ag, and HBe_3Ag, are recognized. The presence of e antigen appears to be associated with the presence of Dane particles. The persistence of the antigen usually indicates chronic hepatitis and may be a marker for infectivity of HBsAg-positive blood.

HBδAg. A new HBsAg-associated delta antigen has been demonstrated by immunofluorescence in the nuclei of hepatocytes from certain patients with HBV infection. The presence and persistence of anti-delta seems to be associated with chronic HBV infection and the development of progressive liver damage.

Subtypes of HBsAg

HBsAg contains a common immunologic determinant, a, and several major subdeterminants that are specified by the viral genome (LeBouvier, 1971). The subdeterminants can be detected by the presence of spurs in immunodiffusion tests with various antisera. Eight distinct categories and two of mixed subtype have been recognized (Table 7–2). In addition, several minor antigenic subtypes have been described.

The major subtypes consist of various combinations of the subdeterminants d/y and w/r, which appear to constitute two groups, composed of d/y on the other hand and w1, w2, w3, w4, and r on the other. The two mixed subtypes (adwr and adyr) are extremely rare and may be due to phenotypic or genotypic mixing of immunologic mark-

Table 7–2. MAJOR AND MINOR SUBTYPES OF HEPATITIS B SURFACE ANTIGEN

Major Subtypes	Minor Subtypes
ayw1	q
ayw2	x
ayw3	f
ayw4	t
ayr	j
adw2	n
adw4	g
adr	
adwy	
adyr	

ers during simultaneous infection associated with more than one subtype of HBsAg. Of the minor subtypes, "g" has been found with w2.

Antigenic subtypes ayw2 and ayw3 appear to be more common in Africa and the Middle East, whereas subdeterminant r appears to predominate in the Far East and is very common in Japan. The antigenic subtype adw2 is common in the United States.

HBsAg of adw and ayw subtypes appears to differ in both biophysical and biochemical characteristics.

Subtype-specific antibodies are determined by studying inhibition of the antibody reactions with different known HBsAg subtypes in the same passive hemagglutination or radioimmunoassay techniques used in anti-HBs detection (see later discussion).

Antibodies to HBAg

Subsequent to infection with HBV, antibodies to HBcAg (anti-HBc) usually appear (often at the same time that enzyme elevations are first seen). Antibody to the surface antigen (anti-HBs) usually appears later, sometimes being delayed by 6 to 12 months after the acute episode and often coinciding with the disappearance of circulating HBsAg.

Both human and animal studies indicate that anti-HBc tends to decrease gradually and may become undetectable after 1 or 2 years, although high titers are found in carriers, and, during the recovery phase of acute hepatitis B, anti-HBc may be present in the absence of HBsAg and anti-Hbs. (Donations of blood taken at this time can cause post-transfusion hepatitis [Hoofnagle *et al.*, 1978]). Anti-HBs lasts much longer and may persist throughout life. This antibody bestows immunity to further infection with HBV. As mentioned, HBeAg is present during the incubation period of acute hepatitis B, and anti-HBe develops either during recovery or with the onset of overt liver disease. The presence of the antibody is considered to be a good prognostic sign (Fig. 7–6).

Incidence of Hepatitis B

Hepatitis B has now assumed major public health importance in a number of situations, the incidence varying from one geographic area to another. In the United States, 0.5 to 0.9 per cent of adults are potentially infectious carriers of the virus, and 8 to 12 per cent of adults are antibody-positive. These rates increase to significantly higher levels among certain "high-risk" groups, such as health care workers (who are repeatedly exposed to blood or blood products), patients (and staff) in hemodialysis units, immunosuppressed patients, institutionalized groups (*e.g.*, prisoners, military recruits), illicit drug users, homosexual males, and individuals from areas in which the virus is endemic (Table 7–3).

HBV infection varies from an inapparent or unrecognized course to a rapidly fatal, fulminant course. Many cases are probably asymptomatic and, as such, are mistaken for a mild influenza attack. For this reason, many individuals who have no history of hepatitis present with serologic evidence of prior exposure to HBV (and HAV; Table 7–4).

Transmission of Hepatitis B

Although parenteral infection is considered to be the most important mode of transmission of hepatitis B, infections can be acquired by casual contact with infected blood or serum, whereby inoculation may occur through often trivial or even unnoticed breaks in the skin or mucous membranes. The minimum infective dose of plasma from a carrier was estimated to be 1×10^{-6} ml (Murray, 1955). Drake *et al.* (1952) found that 4

Figure 7–6. Markers in acute HBV infection. (From Pittiglio, D. H. (Ed.): Modern Blood Banking and Transfusion Practices. Philadelphia, F. A. Davis Co., 1983, p. 387.)

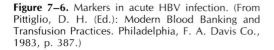
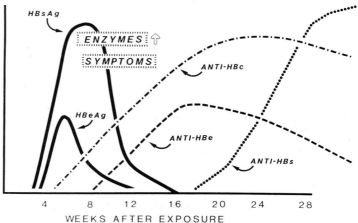

Table 7–3. HEPATITIS MARKERS IN HIGH-INCIDENCE GROUPS

Marker	Positive (%)		
	Southeast Asian Immigrants (483)*	Male Homosexuals (1077)*	Renal Dialysis Patients (163)*
Anti-HAV			—
IgG	90.2	35.6	—
IgM	1.0	—	
HBsAg	20.3†	4.5	71.7‡
Anti-HBs and Anti-HBc	46.8	50.4	—
Anti-HBs	2.9	—	—
Anti-HBc	1.4	5.1	—
HAV and/or HBV	94.6	67.9	—

*Number tested
†50% HBeAg positive, 50% anti-HBe positive, and 100% anti-HBc positive
‡71.8% HBeAg positive and 100% anti-HBc positive
From Pittiglio, D. H. (Ed.): Modern Blood Banking and Transfusion Practices. Philadelphia, F. A. Davis Co., 1983, p. 389.

$\times$ 10^{-5} ml of plasma given by subcutaneous injection could transmit the disease.

Apart from the transfusion of blood or blood products (which still appear to be the most dangerous source of infection), recognized modes of transmission of hepatitis B include the use of common needles and syringes among drug addicts, failure to sterilize dental equipment and tattooing needles, the sharing of razors and toothbrushes, and sexual contact (particularly among male homosexuals). Arthropod spread (mosquitos, bedbugs) is suspected in some tropical areas, although this, like fecal-oral routes, remains uncertain.

Susceptibility to the disease is not confined to any age group; maternal transmission to the fetus or newborn has been reported and often leads to chronic infection of the infant.

The many different modes of transmission of hepatitis B is almost certainly due to the fact that almost all body secretions (*e.g.*, saliva, semen, urine, sweat, colostrum) have been shown to contain the viral surface antigen.

Clinical Signs and Symptoms of Hepatitis B

Individuals exposed to HBV through accidental needle puncture or transfusion do not usually show the expected initial symptoms (weakness, fatigue, nausea, and jaundice) until about 10 to 16 weeks after exposure. In some individuals, however, pain in the joints and/or rash or urticaria may occur several weeks before the illness is recognized as hepatitis.

The acute phase of the illness is also of variable length but in most cases has a duration of only a few weeks. The vast majority of individuals who develop acute hepatitis recover completely and develop immunity. About 10 per cent, however, do not develop immunity and may become chronic carriers or develop chronic active or chronic persistent hepatitis. The reason that this small minority become chronic carriers is not known, although it may be associated with their immunologic status at the time of exposure. (Note: The clinical signs

Table 7–4. VIRAL HEPATITIS MARKERS IN BLOOD DONORS WITH AND WITHOUT A HISTORY OF PRIOR EXPOSURE

	Percentage Positive for One or Several Markers				
	HBsAg	Anti-HBc	Anti-HBc/HBs	Anti-HBc/HBs/HAV	Anti-HAV
Random donors (529)*	0	0.2	4.0	3.5	19.1
Health care personnel (donors) (569)	0	0.002	4.3	0.005	7.7
Donors rejected for hepatitis history (203)	0	0	5.1	1.0	27.6

*Number tested
From Pittiglio, D. H. (Ed.): Modern Blood Banking and Transfusion Practices. Philadelphia, F. A. Davis Co., 1983, p. 390.

and symptoms of HAV infection are almost identical to those seen in acute HBV disease.)

Protection Against HBV by Antibody

The administration of immunoglobulin prepared from subjects with relatively potent anti-HBs was found to reduce the risk of hepatitis in individuals accidentally exposed to HBV (Grady and Lee, 1975), whether through inoculation, ingestion orally, or when blood or blood products are splashed onto mucous membranes. In these cases, hepatitis B immunoglobulin with a high titer of anti-HBs should be given in a dose of approximately 5 ml (for adults) as soon as possible after exposure (WHO, 1977).

Standard immunoglobulin is usually of little value in prophylaxis due to a low titer of anti-HBs (Seeff *et al.*, 1977).

HBV Vaccine

The clinical value of a vaccine against HBV infection was demonstrated by Szumness *et al.* (1980). The vaccine used was prepared from the plasma of chronic carriers of HBsAg; 20 nm spherical particles were purified from the plasma and then treated with formalin to kill any residual live virus. This material was shown to produce anti-HBs in 96 per cent of vaccinated individuals after two injections given 1 month apart. In a high-risk population (male homosexuals), the incidence of both clinical and subclinical HBV infection was significantly less in the vaccinated group (1.4 to 3.4 per cent) than in the control group (18 to 27 per cent). The side effects from the vaccine are minimal, and the vaccine is probably effective in preventing infection even after exposure to HBV. It should be noted that the vaccine is not intended for use in transfusion practice, because most cases of post-transfusion hepatitis are caused by non-A, non-B virus.

The licensing of the HBV vaccine was announced by the FDA in 1981, and the *Journal of the American Medical Association* (June, 1984) stated that the vaccine is safe and recommended for health care personnel worldwide.

Recent work by researchers at Merck, Sharpe and Dohme Research Laboratories, West Point, PA (reported in the American Association of Blood Banks New Briefs, July, 1984) has resulted in the development of a version of the vaccine made by a recombinant strain of the yeast *Saccharomyces cerevisiae*. This preparation was found to have positive effects on human volunteers. Thirty-seven healthy, low-risk adults were tested, each receiving 10 μg of HBsAg at 0, 1, and 6 months. Antibody to HBsAg was found to be present in 27 to 40 per cent of the vaccinees by 1 month and in 80 to 100 per cent by 3 months. Following the third dose at 6 months, large boosts of titer were noted. The formed antibody was found to be specific for the "a" determinant of HBsAg. There were no serious reactions to the vaccination—the only common complaint being transient soreness at the site of injection. The researchers pointed out that this may be the first use in man of a vaccine prepared by recombinant DNA technology.

The three-dose program is believed to offer immunity for about 5 years, when a booster dose would become necessary. The fear of contracting acquired immune deficiency syndrome (AIDS; see page 44) from these inoculations has been shown to be groundless according to James Maynard, M.D., Ph.D., chief of the Hepatitis Branch of the Centers for Disease Control and director of the World Health Organization Collaborating Center for Reference and Research on Viral Hepatitis.

Many new types of vaccines are currently under investigation, including those made with yeast using a synthetic protein and other recombinant DNA techniques. It is hoped that this research will yield a resonably priced, steady supply of source material and freedom from the biologic hazards associated with donor serum.

NON–A, NON–B HEPATITIS

Until recently, viral hepatitis that could not be associated with hepatitis B, cytomegalovirus, or Epstein-Barr virus infection was presumed to be due to hepatitis A. The development of specific diagnostic methods for all these other agents has shown this to be an erroneous assumption. Because it could be proved that in some cases, hepatitis was not caused by HAV or HBV, the rather clumsy term *non-A, non-B hepatitis* was suggested. Although some texts use the term *hepatitis C*, this is not strictly correct, because there is evidence suggesting that there is more than one kind of non-A, non-B virus; in fact, a heterogeneous group of viruses may be involved.

Incidence of Non–A, Non–B Hepatitis

Non-A, non-B hepatitis has been shown to be quite common. In the United States, between 89 and 100 per cent of cases of post-transfusion hepatitis may be related to this agent.

Anicteric cases of post-transfusion hepatitis are more common than icteric cases. For example, Seeff *et al.* (1977) reported a study in the United States in which 2204 patients were followed and in which post-transfusion hepatitis was diagnosed in 241 patients. The disease was found to be icteric in less than one fifth of these patients. In 14 prospective studies reviewed by Blum and Vyas (1982), the overall frequency of hepatitis in patients receiving blood tested as HBsAg negative (from volunteer donors) varied from 4 to 13 per cent.

The incidence of non-A, non-B hepatitis in patients who have received blood transfusions is directly related to the level of alanine aminotransferase (ALT) in the relevant blood donors (Aach et al., 1981). Although non-A, non-B hepatitis does develop in some patients who have received only blood from donors with normal ALT levels, it can be deduced that at least 21 per cent of cases of transfusion-associated hepatitis might be prevented by excluding donors with ALT levels above 44 IU (Holland et al., 1981).

Non-A, non-B hepatitis is seen in populations of low socioeconomic status and is associated with a chronic carrier state (Alter, 1980). The minimum carrier rate in volunteer blood donors in the United States has been estimated to be 1.6 per cent, and, in commercial (paid) donors, it has been estimated to be 5.4 per cent (Blum and Vyas, 1982).

Although non-A, non-B hepatitis is usually associated with transfusion, sporadic cases have also been documented without known exposure to blood or blood products.

Transmission of Non–A, Non–B Hepatitis

The mode of transmission of non-A, non-B hepatitis is sometimes similar to that of hepatitis B. Although its association with transfusion is clear, its prevalence among populations of low socioeconomic status suggests transmission by close person-to-person contact.

Experimental transmission of non-A, non-B hepatitis has shown that it can be transmitted from human to human and from human to chimpanzee (Tabor et al., 1978).

Clinical Signs and Symptoms of Non–A, Non–B Hepatitis

The majority of patients with non-A, non-B hepatitis have minimal clinical manifestations, and few patients require hospitalization. The incubation period varies from 6 to 10 weeks, with a peak of about 8 weeks (Alter, 1980). Up to 60 per cent of cases reveal abnormal ALT levels for more than a year; if a liver biopsy is taken, most cases show histologic evidence of a significant chronic liver disease, and about 10 per cent show features of cirrhosis (Alter, 1980). The tendency for serum hepatic enzyme levels to fluctuate markedly over

a relatively short period of time is a striking feature of non-A, non-B hepatitis. Although the disease differs in many respects from hepatitis B, there is considerable overlap, and the two forms cannot be differentiated on clinical grounds alone.

Serologic Tests

A variety of test systems have been described with respect to non-A, non-B hepatitis, yet none have been universally accepted as markers of the infection. The diagnosis of non-A, non-B hepatitis is therefore currently made by ruling out other known causes of hepatitis by appropriate serologic tests.

THE SEROLOGIC DETECTION OF HEPATITIS MARKERS
Serologic Detection of Anti–HAV

The serologic tests that have been described to identify anti-HAV include complement fixation, immune adherence hemagglutination, and radioimmunoassay. Of these, only radioimmunoassay is available commercially, and it is the most commonly used technique for this purpose.

The radioimmunoassay test for anti-HAV (HAVAB, Abbott Laboratories) uses a solid phase (bead) that is coated with an anti-HAV-HAV complex. The bead is incubated with a mixture of patient's serum and ^{125}I-labeled anti-HAV. The anti-HAV in the patient's serum competes with the known labeled antibody for the available binding sites, resulting in a decrease in counts per minute (cpm). A 50 per cent or greater reduction in the counts when compared with the negative control cpm indicates that the unknown contains anti-HAV.

One of several methods available to identify IgM–anti-HAV involves the use of staphylococcal protein A (Newman DC or Cowen strain) to absorb IgG from diluted serum prior to testing. Other methods, including column chromatography and labeled anti-IgM have also been used. The radioimmunoassay technique for detecting IgM–anti-HAV (HAVAB-M, Abbott Laboratories) involves the incubation of patient's serum with an anti-IgM–coated solid phase. Purified HAV particles are added to the bound IgM fraction of the patient's serum. These will bind to IgM having anti-HAV specificity. ^{125}I-labeled anti-HAV is added after incubation and washing (to remove unbound protein), and an increase in cpm of the test when compared with the negative control indicates the presence of IgM–anti-HAV in the test sample.

Serologic Detection of HBsAg

The most frequently used serologic tests for the detection of HBsAg include:

1. Ouchterlony double diffusion (agar gel diffusion)
2. Counterelectrophoresis
3. Rheophoresis
4. Complement fixation
5. Reversed passive latex agglutination
6. Reversed passive hemagglutination
7. Radioimmunoassay
8. Enzyme-linked immunosorbent assay (ELISA)

These tests may be grouped into first generation, second generation, and third generation, according to sensitivity—third generation being the most sensitive and therefore preferred in most clinical situations. In this connection, Ouchterlony double diffusion (agar gel diffusion) is regarded as a first generation test; radioimmunoassay, reversed passive hemagglutination, enzyme-linked immunosorbent assay (ELISA), and reversed passive latex agglutination are regarded as third generation; and the remainder, counterelectrophoresis, rheophoresis, and complement fixation are regarded as second generation (Table 7–5).

Sources of antisera for the detection of HBsAg are:

1. Human, including multiply-transfused patients, patients giving an anamnestic response following transfusions of blood and blood products, volunteers stimulated with noninfectious HBsAg-positive material, and sporadic sources (*i.e.,* not associated with blood and blood sources).
2. Animals hyperimmunized with purified HBsAg
3. Laboratory animals (guinea pigs, rabbits, mice, monkeys, chimpanzees)
4. Domestic animals (horses, sheep, goats)

It should be noted that although HBsAg has been found to be present for as long as a year in the serum of carriers, it has also been reported that most patients with clinical or serum enzyme patterns consistent with a diagnosis of serum hepatitis do not retain HBsAg for more than 3 months after the acute phase of the disease.

PRACTICAL CONSIDERATIONS IN HEPATITIS TESTING

In practice, tests for HBV and HBsAg are performed to:

1. Identify blood donors who are infected with HBV and who might, therefore, transmit the infection to recipients.
2. Establish the etiology of clinical cases of hepatitis.

To this end, any method that optimally demonstrates the presence of HBsAg in serum or plasma is satisfactory. Third generation tests, naturally, are the methods of choice for both of these applications.

In cases of clinical hepatitis in which HBsAg is *not* detected, sensitive methods for the detection of anti-Hbs or anti-HBc (see later discussion) are useful, although tests for anti-HBc may be of limited usefulness in many situations (see Serologic Detection of HBcAg and anti-HBc, later in this chapter). Anti-HBs detection by less sensitive methods is useful for identifying donors whose plasma contains high anti-HBs titer and is therefore suitable for the production of HBIG (hepatitis B immune globulin) and potent antisera for *in vitro* diagnostic methods. When evaluating the safety and effectiveness of passive and active immunization with experimental HBIG preparations and vaccines, however, third generation methods are preferable.

Suggested Rules for Practical Testing

In testing for hepatitis B surface antigen and antibody (and all other hepatitis-related viruses, antigens, and/or antibodies), extreme caution should be exercised by the technologist to guard against the spread of infection. To this end, the following rules should be followed when handling any biologic specimens known to contain or suspected of containing the viruses.

General Rules

1. Smoking, eating, and drinking should not be permitted in laboratory areas. Food must not be stored in the same refrigerator as blood or blood products.
2. The technologist should avoid all contact between the fingers and the mouth, including the licking of labels, pencils, fingers, and so on.

Table 7–5. TESTS AVAILABLE FOR HBsAG DETECTION

Third Generation
Radioimmunoassay
Reversed passive hemagglutination
Enzyme-linked immunosorbent assay (ELISA)
Reversed passive latex agglutination

Second Generation
Counterelectrophoresis
Rheophoresis
Complement fixation

First Generation
Ouchterlony double diffusion (agar gel diffusion)

3. Mouth pipetting should be expressly forbidden.
4. Technologists should not wipe their hands on lab coats or gowns.
5. Technologists must wash in a hand basin (not a laboratory sink) after handling a specimen. A strong antiseptic solution should be used for this purpose (*e.g.,* povidone-iodine [Betadine; Proviodine]).
6. In each laboratory, a safety officer should be appointed to supervise work and to educate staff.

Clothing

1. A plastic apron should be worn in the laboratory, and it should be cleaned with weak hypochlorite and then water after each use.
2. Plastic gloves should be worn, and these should be discarded into a plastic bag to be incinerated after use. Gloves should be changed every 2 hours.
3. A clean gown that can be autoclaved after use should be worn.
4. If there is danger of production of an aerosol (*e.g.,* in shaking and gassing of samples), safety spectacles or a visor should be worn.
5. Opening of specimens and all pipetting should be performed in a fume hood.
6. The hands should be washed well with povidone-iodine after gloves are removed.

Work Areas

1. Before and after each use, work benches must be cleaned with strong hypochlorite solution (10,000 ppm available chlorine)
2. A freshly prepared bottle of prepared hypochlorite, a disposal jar with hypochlorite swabs, and a plastic disposable bag should be on hand at all times for wiping up any spills.
3. The hypochlorite solution should be checked several times a day with starch iodide paper (paper turns blue if solution is active).
4. All paper work should be done in a separate, clean area.

Specimens

1. Specimens from patients suspected of having serum hepatitis should arrive at the laboratory in a plastic bag with proper identification as a "high-risk" specimen attached to the outside of the bag.
2. Any leaking specimen should be discarded unopened.

3. Open the container *carefully* after covering the cork with gauze squares.
4. Pipetting should be done with a rubber teat or other device, and the sample should be expelled *gently* down the wall of the receiving vessel.
5. Pipets should be completely immersed in hypochlorite immediately after use and then autoclaved before washing.
6. If it is necessary to centrifuge the specimen, do so in a tightly capped tube. If the tube breaks in the centrifuge, any removable contaminated parts should be autoclaved or immersed in 2 per cent activated glutaraldehyde (Cidex), and the rest of the centrifuge should be swabbed with Cidex and left for 1 hour. (Note: Hypochlorite corrodes centrifuges.)

Accidents

1. If the eyes or mouth is contaminated, wash the area well with tap water.
2. Pricks or cuts incurred while processing the specimen or pre-existing skin lesions that become contaminated with samples for examination should be washed at once with hypochlorite solution, followed by water. Any such accidents should be recorded and reported.

OUCHTERLONY DOUBLE DIFFUSION (AGAR GEL DIFFUSION)

Ouchterlony double diffusion (or agar gel diffusion) was the first method used in establishing the relationship of HBsAg to type B hepatitis. The technique has the following advantages:

1. It demonstrates specificity by the formation of lines of identity between HBsAg in test samples and in positive control sera.
2. It distinguishes the subtypes of HBsAg by lines of partial identity or spur formation.
3. It is the simplest method available for HBsAg (and anti-HBs) detection in that no special equipment is required.
4. A number of different well configurations and agar and buffer combinations have given satisfactory results.

The disadvantages of the technique are:

1. It is less sensitive than other techniques.
2. It requires 24 to 72 hours for optimal results.
3. Optimal test conditions are somewhat dependent upon the antiserum used.

Ouchterlony double diffusion can provide a convenient method for the identification of very potent antisera because of its relative insensitivity.

METHOD 1: OUCHTERLONY DOUBLE DIFFUSION (AGAR GEL DIFFUSION)

Materials

1. Buffers—phosphate-buffered saline at pH 7.4. (Good results have also been reported with tris-EDTA or Veronal. The pH of the buffer should be between 7.2 and 8.2.)
2. Gels—agarose. Different types of agar (Noble agar, ionagar, and agarose) can be used, but agarose gives the most reproducible results. Agarose concentrations between 0.6 and 2.0 per cent work well; 1.1 per cent is generally most convenient. Dilute in buffer (1).
3. Plates—3¼- × 4¼-inch lantern slides. (Microscope slides or Petri dishes work equally well.) The plates can be prepared and stored provided that they are precoated with a thin film of 2 per cent Noble agar, which is applied when the plates are warm and subsequently dried in a 50° to 60°C chamber for 30 minutes. Prepunched plates are available from several commercial firms, but they are expensive, and freshness cannot be ensured.

Method

1. Pipet 15 ml of a 1.1 per cent agarose solution onto a lantern slide, giving a gel of about 1.5 mm thickness.
2. After the gel has hardened, punch a seven-hole pattern on the agarose-coated plate with a metal punch. Wells of 2 to 3 mm diameter and from 3 to 4 mm apart give satisfactory results, although they can be as large as 5 mm in diameter and 6 to 7 mm apart.
3. The wells are filled with a Pasteur (or capillary) pipet: a separate pipet is used for each serum sample. Serum known to contain HBsAg is placed in the upper and lower wells. Anti-HBs is placed in the central well; this allows for the observation of lines of identity or nonidentity between the control precipitins produced by sera under test, which are placed in the four adjacent wells (Fig. 7–7).
4. Incubate the slide in a moist chamber for 24 to 72 hours.

Interpretation

Ideally, plates should be read in a darkened room. The appearance of a white precipitation line (read against a dark background) indicates the presence of HBsAg.

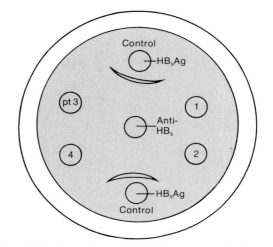

Figure 7–7. Ouchterlony double diffusion (agar gel diffusion).

COUNTERELECTROPHORESIS

The technique of counterelectrophoresis (CEP) is based on the fact that HBsAg and its antibody, anti-HBs, have differing electrophoretic mobilities in an electrical field. Thus, a slide covered with a thin layer of agarose containing a series of punched *opposing* wells, when placed in an electrical field with antigen and antibody properly oriented in opposite wells, allows the fast migration of antibody and antigen *toward* each other and results in a visible precipitate between the wells where the antigen and antibody meet (Fig. 7–8).

The advantages of this technique in comparison with Ouchterlony double diffusion are twofold:

1. It is possible to obtain a positive reaction in 30 to 90 minutes with CEP, as opposed to 24 to 72 hours with Ouchterlony double diffusion.
2. The reagents are moving in one direction rather than diffusing radially from the wells, so there is a greater degree of sensitivity.

METHOD 2: COUNTERELECTROPHORESIS
(Alter *et al.*, 1971; Das *et al.*, 1971; Dreesman *et al.*, 1972; Gocke and Howe, 1970)

Note: A number of CEP reagents and kits are available from commercial sources.

Materials

Many variations of this technique exist with respect to reagents, concentrations, and so on. All of the many variations have been reported to give satisfactory results.

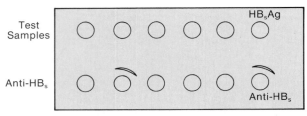

Figure 7–8. Counterelectrophoresis.

1. **Buffer—barbital buffer (0.05 M, pH 8.6)**
2. **Gels—17 ml of agarose (1 per cent concentration) diluted in buffer (1)**
3. **Plates—3¼- × 4-inch lantern slides**

Method

1. **Pipet 16 ml of 1 per cent agarose solution onto 3¼- × 4-inch lantern slides to have a gel of uniform thickness.**
2. **After the agar has cooled and hardened, cut two parallel rows of 15 wells, 3 mm in diameter and 7 mm apart, edge to edge, in the agar with a metal punch.**
3. **Fill the wells in one row with the sera under test; fill the other set of wells with anti-HBs of adequate potency to form a precipitin reaction in agar gel diffusion (see Fig. 7–8).**
4. **Connect the slides to the barbital buffer in an electrophoresis cell by wicks of chromatographic paper, with the wells containing anti-HBs proximal to the anode and the wells containing test sera proximal to the cathode.**
5. **Electrophoresis is carried out for 2 hours at 15 mA constant current per slide.**
6. **An HBsAg-positive control serum should be included on each slide.**

Interpretation

Slides may be examined for immunoprecipitin reaction 1 to 24 hours after completion of electrophoresis. The presence of a white precipitation line (read against a dark background) indicates the presence of HBsAg.

RHEOPHORESIS

The technique known as *rheophoresis* uses the same principle as Ouchterlony double diffusion. In this technique, however, samples containing HBsAg are forced to migrate toward the anti-HBs by evaporation (see Fig. 7–9).

Comparison tests with Ouchterlony double diffusion, counterelectrophoresis, and complement fixation performed by Zambazian and Holper (1972) indicate that rheophoresis has sensitivity similar to that of counterelectrophoresis and complement fixation and is more sensitive than the

Ouchterlony double diffusion technique. In addition, rheophoresis was found to be particularly convenient for determining HBsAg subtypes with appropriate sub-type–specific antisera.

METHOD 3: RHEOPHORESIS
(Jambazian and Holper, 1972)

Materials

1. **Buffer—0.01 M tris buffer, pH 7.6**
2. **Gel—1.25 ml 0.8 per cent agarose**
3. **Plate—Ouchterlony double diffusion dish (a molded plastic cup, 3 cm in diameter and approximately 6 mm deep, will serve the purpose.)**

Method

1. **Fit a gel diffusion dish with a cylindrical Teflon ring (3 cm outside diameter, 2.5 cm inside diameter, and 0.55 cm in length).**
2. **Pour melted agarose (1.25 ml, 0.8 per cent, pH 7.6) into the dish, and allow it to solidify.**
3. **Cut a pattern of six peripheral wells (5 mm in diameter) and a central well (3 mm in diameter) in the agar with a center-to-center distance of 7 mm (Fig. 7–9).**
4. **Carefully remove the Teflon ring, leaving a circular moat around the periphery of the dish.**
5. **Fill the moat with 0.01 M tris buffer, pH 7.6.**
6. **Fill two opposing peripheral wells with serum containing HBsAg to serve as a control. Fill the remaining peripheral wells with test samples.**
7. **Fill the central well with anti-HBs.**
8. **One minute after adding anti-HBs, cover the central well with a 3-mm plastic cover to prevent evaporation.**
9. **Place a 3-cm² plastic cover with a central hole (0.8 cm in diameter) over the entire plate with**

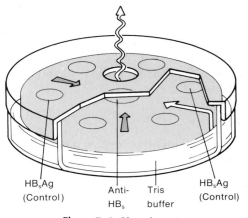

HBsAg   Anti-   Tris   HBsAg
(Control)   HBs   buffer   (Control)

Figure 7–9. Rheophoresis.

the center of the plastic cover located directly over the antibody well.
10. Incubate the plate at 37°C, and read after 8 to 16 hours' incubation (16 to 24 hours if incubation is at 28° to 32°C).

Interpretation

The presence of a white precipitate line (read against a dark background) indicates the presence of HBsAg.

COMPLEMENT FIXATION

Complement fixation techniques are, in general, more sensitive than double diffusion or counterelectrophoresis for measuring HBsAg or anti-Hbs but are less sensitive than hemagglutination or radioimmunoassay techniques for measuring anti-HBs. Both quantitative and qualitative complement fixation tests can be completed within 2 hours; involve simple, easily obtainable equipment; are easy to perform with standardized reagents; and can be automated. The major advantage of this test is that it allows for the detection of antibodies in the patient's serum by their complement-fixing properties.

The test has the following disadvantages:

1. The necessity for standardizing reagents.
2. The need to test more than one dilution of serum, especially when testing for HBsAg, to avoid prozoning.
3. The possibility of nonspecific anti-complementary reactions in certain sera.

All recognized subtypes of HBsAg can be detected by this technique with high-titer, multispecific complement–fixing antibody. It should be noted, however, that there are many examples of "hyperimmune" anti-HBs that do not fix complement, even though they are excellent precipitins.

The most common complement fixation technique used in HBsAg and anti-HBs detection is the microtiter technique.

METHOD 4: THE MICROTITER COMPLEMENT FIXATION TECHNIQUE

Note: The microtiter complement fixation method described here is as described by Barker, Peterson, and Murray (1970), which is patterned after the technique originally described by Sever (1962).

Method

1. Heat serum for testing to 56°C for 30 minutes.
2. Prepare a series of twofold dilutions in Veronal buffered saline supplemented with calcium and magnesium. Dilutions should start at 1:5, using microtiter plates.
3. Add 0.025 ml of complement, 1.7 to 2 U, and 0.025 ml of antibody, 2 to 4 U, to each dilution, and allow to incubate for 16 to 20 hours at 4°C. Note: In practice, overnight fixation at 4°C is commonly used, but short fixation at 37°C for 1 hour allows for completion of the test within 2 hours. Tests by Schmidt and Lennette (1971) revealed that although the shorter test tended to give slightly lower antigen titers, its sensitivity was comparable to that of the overnight test.
4. Add 0.025 ml of 1 per cent suspension of hemolysin-sensitized sheep red blood cells.
5. Incubate for 30 minutes at 35°C, shaking the plates to keep the cells in suspension.
6. Read microscopically.

Interpretation

The end point is the highest serum dilution at which 3 to 4 plus fixation of complement occurs.

REVERSED PASSIVE LATEX AGGLUTINATION

The reversed passive latex agglutination test is the most rapid and the most simple first generation test for HBsAg. The test is, in principle, the agglutination of latex particles coated with anti-HBs by HBsAg in test samples. Because false-positive results are frequently seen, confirmation of this reaction (and all other agglutination reactions) by another method of equal or greater sensitivity is essential.

METHOD 5: REVERSED PASSIVE LATEX AGGLUTINATION
(Fritz and Rivers, 1972; Hirata *et al.*, 1973; Leach and Ruck, 1971; Malin and Edwards, 1972)

Note: Goat polystyrene–latex particles with a gamma globulin fraction containing rabbit anti-HBs are obtainable from commercial sources.

Method

1. Using a small rod, mix one drop of serum under test with one drop of the latex suspension on a black plastic or glass slide.
2. Set up a control in parallel, using serum known to possess HBsAg.
3. Tilt the slide by hand or with an appropriate mechanical shaker for 5 minutes at room temperature.

Interpretation

Agglutination of the particles becomes apparent not later than 5 minutes after mixing when HBsAg is present in the serum under test.

Note: **Perform a confirmatory test to guard against false positives, if necessary.**

REVERSED PASSIVE HEMAGGLUTINATION

Agglutination of red cells coated with anti-HBs (reversed passive hemagglutination) provides a rapid, sensitive, and simple method for detecting HBsAg.

The same caution given for reversed passive latex agglutination applies here, in that false-positive results are frequently seen; another method is essential before results are finally interpreted.

Reversed passive hemagglutination is based on the principle that antibody globulins are readily bound to the surface of red blood cells that have been treated with tannic acid. Highly purified antibody (from horse serum) is attached to tanned turkey erythrocytes to yield a "sensitized" cell suspension that will agglutinate in the presence of HBsAg.

METHOD 6: REVERSED PASSIVE HEMAGGLUTINATION
(Chrystie *et al.*, 1974; Hopkins and Das, 1973; Juji and Yokochi, 1969)

Materials

1. **Test cells—1 per cent suspension of formalinized tanned turkey erythrocytes coated with purified horse anti-HBs dispersed in phosphate-buffered saline (pH 7.2, 0.15 M containing 5 per cent sucrose, 1.5 per cent normal rabbit serum, and 0.1 per cent sodium azide). This preparation is available from commercial sources.**
2. **Control cells—formalinized, tanned turkey erythrocytes coated with normal horse globulin.**
3. **Buffer—sterile 0.15 M phosphate–buffered saline, pH 7.2, containing normal horse serum, normal human serum, and 0.1 per cent sodium azide.**

These reagents can be stored at 4°C. Cells from commercial sources should be reconstituted 15 minutes before use with the manufacturer's recommended volume of sterile distilled water. Once reconstituted, the cells will keep for 1 day at 4°C.
4. **Titration plates—U-bottom, disposable.**

Method

1. **Prepare two dilutions of each test serum by placing three drops of diluent in the first row** of wells of a U-bottom, disposable titration plate and one drop in the second row of wells, using a disposable 0.025-ml dropper. Using a 0.025-ml microtiter loop, take up 0.025 ml of the patient's serum and mix with the diluent in the first well, giving a 1:4 dilution. Transfer the diluter to the second well, giving a 1:8 dilution. Rinse the diluter in strong bleach (Javex), and follow with two distilled water rinses. Repeat for each test serum.
2. **Set up positive and negative controls using 1 ml of heat-inactivated, diluted HBsAg-positive human serum as a positive control and 1 ml of normal human serum as a negative control.**
3. **To each of the 1:8 dilutions, add one drop (0.025-ml dropper) of the test cells.**
4. **Mix the contents of the wells by gently shaking the plates. Cover with a plastic sealer, and allow to settle at room temperature.**
5. **Read after 30 to 60 minutes.**

Interpretation

Positive Reaction. Cells may be partially or completely agglutinated to form a carpet at the bottom of the well (Fig. 7–10).

Negative Reaction. Cells fall to the base of the U and form a tight ring or button in the center of the well (Fig. 7–10).

Weak Positive Reaction. Incomplete agglutination with a central carpet of agglutinated cells surrounded by a definite ring pattern is seen. The ring is of larger diameter than that of a negative pattern and can usually be distinguished by its slightly crenelated edge (Fig. 7–10).

Note: Perform a confirmatory test to guard against false-positive reactions.

RADIOIMMUNOASSAY

Radioimmunoassays are the most sensitive methods for the detection of HBsAg and anti-HBs. The two most widely used techniques are the solid-phase radioimmunoassay and the double-antibody or radioimmunoprecipitation (RIP) tests. The solid

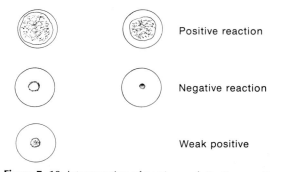

Figure 7–10. Interpretation of passive agglutination results.

phase radioimmunoassay system for HBsAg detection uses the "sandwich" principle; test samples are added to plastic tubes or beads coated with anti-HBs. In the radioimmunoprecipitation technique for HBsAg, known quantities of anti-HBs and ^{125}I-labeled HBsAg are incubated with antibody against gamma globulin, and antigen-antibody complexes are precipitated.

Radioimmunoassay methods are more sensitive than hemagglutination methods and much more sensitive than second generation methods (e.g., counterelectrophoresis) for the detection of HBsAg and anti-HBs.

METHOD 7: RADIOIMMUNOASSAY
(Aach et al., 1971, 1973; Oberby et al., 1973)

The technique described here is that intended for use with the Austria 11-125 kit provided by Abbott Laboratories, North Chicago, Illinois.

Materials

The kit contains:

1. Beads—coated with hepatitis B surface antigen (guinea pig)
2. Vials (10 ml each) of anti-HBs ^{125}I (human)—approximately 7 microcuries per vial; preservative—0.1 per cent sodium azide
3. Vial (5 ml) of negative control (nonreactive for HBsAg); preservative—0.1 per cent sodium azide
4. Vial (3 ml) of positive control (positive for HBsAg); preservative—0.1 per cent sodium azide
5. Four reaction trays (20 wells each), 8 sealers, and 80 tube identification inserts
6. Counting tubes (8 cartons, 20 tubes each) properly positioned for transfer of beads from reaction trays

Additional materials needed (not provided with the kit):

1. Precision pipets or similar equivalent to deliver 0.2 ml
2. Device for delivery of rinse solution such as Cornwall syringe, Filamatic, or equivalent
3. An aspiration device for washing coated beads, such as a cannula or aspirator tip, and a vacuum source and trap for retaining the aspirate
4. A well-type gamma scintillation detector capable of efficiently counting ^{125}I
5. Gently circulating water bath, capable of maintaining temperature at 45°C ± 1°C
6. Austria confirmatory neutralization test kit (Note: All Austria 11-125 reactive samples must

be confirmed with the test procedure provided with this kit.)

Collection and Preparation of Samples

1. **Only serum and recalcified plasmas can be tested. Collect blood specimens, and separate the serum from the sample. Plasma can be tested only after conversion to serum.**
2. **If specimens are to be stored, they should be refrigerated at 2° to 8°C or frozen. If specimens are to be shipped, they should be frozen.**

Procedure

Seven negative and three positive controls should be assayed with each run of unknowns. Ensure that reaction trays containing controls and reaction trays of unknowns are subjected to the same process and incubation times. Use a clean pipet or disposable tip for each transfer to avoid cross-contamination.

1. **Adjust the temperature of the water bath to 45°C.**
2. **Remove the cap from the clear plastic tube that contains antibody-coated beads. Hold the bead dispenser directly over the top of the reaction tray incubation well, and push down with the index finger to release one bead into a well for each sample to be tested.**
3. **Using precision pipets, add 0.2 ml of serum and positive and negative controls to the bottom of their respective wells. Ensure that the antibody-coated bead is completely surrounded by serum. Tap the reaction tray to release any air bubbles that may be trapped in the serum sample.**
4. **Apply a cover sealer to each tray, and incubate the trays in the 45°C water bath for 2 hours.**
5. **At the end of 2 hours, remove the trays from the water bath. Remove the cover sealer and discard. Using a semiautomated aspiration and rinsing system, aspirate the serum; rinse each well and bead with a total of 5 ml of distilled or deionized water. Repeat this wash procedure one additional time. Note: A manual system of washing the wells and beads may also be used. Using disposable pipets or cannulas and a Cornwall syringe delivery system, or equivalent, and a vacuum source, rinse each well and bead with extreme care not to overflow the reaction well but ensuring that the bead is totally immersed throughout the wash procedure. Place the pipet or cannula, attached to the vacuum source, into the bottom of the well next to the bead, and simultaneously add slowly, with the Cornwall syringe, 5 ml of distilled or deionized water.**

6. With precision pipets, add 0.2 ml of ^{125}I-labeled anti-HBs (human) to the bottom of each reaction well. Ensure that the antibody-coated bead is surrounded by the labeled antibody solution. Tap the tray to release any air bubbles that may be trapped in the solution.

7. Apply a new cover sealer to each tray, and incubate the trays in the 45°C water bath for 1 hour.

8. At the end of 1 hour, remove the trays from the water bath. Remove the cover sealer, aspirate the antibody solution from each well, and rinse the well and antibody-coated bead it contains with a total of 5 ml of distilled or deionized water, as in step 5.

9. Transfer the beads from the reaction wells to properly identified counting tubes; align the inverted rack of oriented counting tubes over the reaction tray, press the tubes tightly over the wells, and then invert the tray and tubes together so that beads fall into properly labeled tubes.

10. Place the counting tubes in a suitable well-type gamma scintillation counter, and determine the count rate. The position of the bead at the bottom of the counting tube is not important. Although it is not critical that the counting be done immediately, it should be performed as soon as practicable. All control samples and unknowns must be counted together.

Interpretation

The presence or absence of HBsAg is determined by relating net counts per minute of the unknown sample to net counts per minute of the negative control mean times the factor 2.1. Unknown samples whose net count rate is higher than the mean cutoff value established with the negative control are to be considered positive with respect to HBsAg.

The mean value for the positive control samples should be at least five times the negative control mean. If not, the technique may be suspect, and the run should be repeated.

Note: For gamma counters that do not automatically subtract machine backgrounds, the gross counts may be used if the cutoff value for the negative control is calculated as described below.

Calculation of the Negative Control Mean. An example of the calculation of the negative control mean is given in Table 7–6.

Elimination of Aberrant Values. Discard those individual values in the negative control samples that fall outside the range of 0.5 to 1.5 times the mean.

Table 7–6. AN EXAMPLE OF THE CALCULATION OF THE NEGATIVE CONTROL MEAN

Negative Control Sample Number	Net Count Rate Per Minute
1	380
2	400
3	410
4	375
5	350
6	390
7	400
	Total 2705

$$\frac{\text{Total net cpm}}{7} = \frac{2705}{7} = \text{net cpm (mean)}$$

Example (from Table 7–6)

$0.5 \times 386 = 193$ and $1.5 \times 386 = 579$
Range = 193 cpm to 579 cpm

Note: In this example, no negative control sample is rejected as aberrant. The negative control mean therefore need not be revised. Typically, all negative control values should fall within the range of 0.5 to 1.5 times the control mean. If more than one value is consistently found to be outside this range, technical problems should be suspected.

Calculation of the Cutoff Value (from Table 7–6)

1. Multiply the net negative control mean, 386 cpm, by the factor 2.1.
2. The calculated cutoff value is then 811 cpm.
3. Unknowns whose net count rate is higher than the cutoff value should be considered positive with respect to HBsAg.

Note: Many gamma counters have no capacity for automatically subtracting background. In this case, as an alternative to subtracting instrument background manually from each sample, uncorrected sample counts per minute can be compared with a cutoff modified as follows:

(Negative control mean − Background) × 2.1 + Background = Cutoff

Example (from Table 7–6)

Gross negative control mean = 436 cpm
Instrument background = 50 cpm
Cutoff = (436 − 50) × 2.1 + 50 = 861

Samples with gross count rates greater than 861 are to be considered reactive with respect to HBsAg.

Calculation of Positive Control to Negative Control Ratio (from Table 7–6)

1. **Divide the positive control mean value by the negative control mean value after correcting for background:**

$$\frac{\text{Net positive control mean}}{\text{Net negative control mean}} = \text{P/N ratio}$$

2. **This ratio should be at least 5; otherwise, the technique may be suspect, and the run should be repeated.**

Using the figures in Table 7–6:

Net positive control mean value = 5906 cpm
Net negative control mean value = 386 cpm
P/N ratio = 5906 ÷ 386 = 15.3

Technique is acceptable, and data may be considered valid.

Limitations of the Procedure

Nonrepeatable Positives. Some positive results may test nonreactive on repeat. This phenomenon is highly dependent upon the technique used in running the test. The most common sources of such nonrepeatable positives are:

1. **Inadequate rinsing of the bead.**
2. **Cross-contamination of nonreactive samples caused by transfer of residual droplets of high-titer, antigen-containing sera on the pipetting device.**

Nonspecific False Positives. The nonspecific false positives resulting from cross-reactions with guinea pig serum are essentially eliminated by using ^{125}I-labeled anti-HBs of human origin; however, all sensitive immune systems have a potential for false positives, and before notifying a patient or donor that he or she may be a carrier of HBsAg, positive results must be confirmed as follows:

1. *Repeatability.* **Further testing of the sample in question will verify whether it is repeatedly positive. In making an evaluation of data, consideration should be given to the actual test values obtained. The value 2.1 times the negative control mean is used as the cutoff for single determinations. This value has been selected in order to decrease the total number of nonrepeatable positives.**

   If repeat testing shows the sample to be less than 2.1 times the negative control mean, the original result may be classified as a nonrepeatable positive. If repeats are above the cutoff value, the sample should be presumed reactive for HBsAg. Such results are contingent on determination of the specificity of the repeatable positives.

2. *Specificity.* **Specificity analysis must be performed prior to informing a donor that he or she is a HBsAg carrier. A suitable method must be used for confirmation of screening procedure on all reactive specimens. A repeatable reactive specimen, confirmed by neutralization with human antiserum, must be considered HBsAg-positive.**

ENZYME-LINKED IMMUNOASSAY

The enzyme-linked immunosorbent assay (ELISA) technique is based on the same principle as the radioimmunoassay technique, but an enzyme label rather than a radiolabel is used as an indicator. In this technique, after incubation and washing to remove unbound label, a chromogenic substrate is added. Degradation of the substrate by bound enzyme produces a color change and an optical density increase that is proportional to the HBsAg concentration in the unknown sample.

Serologic Detection of Anti–HBs

Serologic testing for anti-HBs is usually not helpful in diagnosis, because the antibody often appears weeks to months after antigenemia has subsided. Testing, however, is useful in determining past infection and possible immunity in individuals who may have been exposed to infection or in those who are likely to work in situations where exposure risks are high. In these cases, anti-HBs can be easily detected by passive hemagglutination of antigen-sensitized red blood cells or by radioimmunoassay.

Serologic Detection of HBcAg and Anti–HBc

Hepatitis B core antigen and antibody are detectable by several serologic procedures with varying degrees of sensitivity, notably complement fixation, counterelectrophoresis, immune adherence hemagglutination, and radioimmunoassay.

Serologic tests for anti-HBc have proved valuable for seroepidemiologic studies and diagnosis of HBV infection, whereas tests for HBcAg are seldom used in the diagnosis of type B hepatitis. Lack of availability of reagents for both HBcAg and anti-HBc has to some extent limited their use for anti-HBc in research laboratories.

HBcAg has been purified from the following sources:

1. The liver of immunosuppressed chimpanzees experimentally infected with HBV. The HBcAg in these cases is purified by differential centrifugation and isopyknic banding in cesium chloride.
2. Plasma of chronic carriers of HBcAg, which contains large numbers of Dane particles.

In the latter technique, the Dane particles are purified by isopyknic and rate zonal centrifugation procedures. The HBsAg is removed by treatment with a nonionic detergent. The free cores are then purified by isopyknic banding in cesium chloride. Two populations of cores have been detected by such means:

1. "Heavy" cores, with a density of about 1.37 gm per cubic centimeter and a high specific DNA polymerase activity. These cores serve as a source of antigen for radioimmunoprecipitation tests for anti-HBc.
2. "Light" cores, with a density of about 1.30 to 1.32 gm per cubic centimeter and deficient in DNA polymerase activity. These cores have been used successfully as a source of antigen for complement fixation and immune adherence hemagglutination tests for anti-HBc.

Of the tests available, complement fixation is probably the most widely used for anti-HBc detection; although it is insufficiently sensitive to diagnose many inapparent or subclinical infections, almost all patients with chronic infection (clinical or subclinical) have anti-HBc detectable by complement fixation. The source of antigen for complement fixation tests is chimpanzee liver. The test is performed in the same way as complement fixation tests for anti-HBs (see earlier in this chapter) yet has the disadvantage of requiring a large quantity of antigen compared with other tests for anti-HBc. Counterelectrophoresis is as sensitive as complement fixation for anti-HBc and provides results in 2 hours. Again, relatively large quantities of HBcAg purified from chimpanzee liver are required. The test procedure is the same as that for HBsAg (see earlier in this chapter).

A more satisfactory test is the immune adherence hemagglutination (IAHA) technique, which, according to Tsuda et al. (1975) is about 10 times as sensitive as complement fixation and counterelectrophoresis for detecting anti-HBc. Relatively small quantities of HBcAg are required and therefore can be obtained from Dane particle-rich plasma as well as from liver.

The most sensitive tests for HBcAg and anti-HBc, however, are radioimmunoassays. The antigen source is high-density Dane particle cores purified from HBsAg-positive plasma. The tests are said to be 300 times more sensitive than complement fixation or counterelectrophoresis in anti-HBc detection.

Serologic Detection of HBeAg and Anti–HBe

Tests for HBeAg and anti-HBe are not generally used in a routine setting, because although there may be prognostic implications of such detection, the utilized tests (immunoprecipitation, such as the Ouchterlony double diffusion method) have not been proved to be sufficiently sensitive in this respect.

REVIEW QUESTIONS

MULTIPLE CHOICE

Choose the phrase, sentence, or symbol that completes the statement or answers the question. More than one answer may be correct in each case. Answers are given at the end of this book.

1. Hepatitis is the result of damage to hepatocytes, which may be caused by:
   (a) viruses
   (b) drugs
   (c) heat
   (d) excessive alcohol intake
   (Introduction: Hepatitis)

2. Infectious hepatitis:
   (a) is caused by hepatitis A virus
   (b) is caused by hepatitis B virus
   (c) is caused by hepatitis non-A, non-B virus
   (d) usually results from needle punctures or needle wounds
   (The Hepatitis Viruses)

3. Hepatitis A:
   (a) is also known as *serum hepatitis*
   (b) is transmitted by a fecal-oral route
   (c) is more common in countries with low standards of living
   (d) is the type seen in most epidemic outbreaks of hepatitis in the normal population
   (Hepatitis A)

4. The hepatitis A virus:
   (a) produces a coat protein
   (b) is detectable in the serum of patients with hepatitis A

(c) is stable in ether

(d) is stable to a pH of 3.0

(Hepatitis A Virus (HAV))

5. Anti-HAV:
   (a) appears in the plasma at the onset of clinically apparent hepatitis A
   (b) initially occurs as IgM
   (c) initially occurs as IgG
   (d) persists in the circulation until the symptoms of the disease are no longer apparent
   (Antibodies to HAV (Immunity))

6. Hepatitis B:
   (a) is also known as *post-transfusion hepatitis*
   (b) commonly follows parenteral exposure to HBV
   (c) has an incubation period of 2 to 4 weeks
   (d) has an incubation period of 1 to 6 months
   (Hepatitis B)

7. The hepatitis B virus:
   (a) exists in three forms
   (b) is microbiologically related to hepatitis A virus
   (c) is a double-stranded DNA particle
   (d) none of the above
   (Hepatitis B Virus (HBV))

8. The outer lipoprotein coat (or envelope) of hepatitis B virus is known as:
   (a) HBsAg
   (b) HBcAg
   (c) HBeAg
   (d) HBδAg
   (Markers for Hepatitis B Virus)

9. The number of antigenic subtypes that have been recognized for HBeAg is:
   (a) one
   (b) two
   (c) three
   (d) none
   (Markers for Hepatitis B Virus)

10. The two mixed subtypes of HBeAg, adwr and adyr, are:
    (a) extremely common in Japan
    (b) extremely rare
    (c) may be due to phenotypic or genotypic mixing of immunologic markers during simultaneous infection associated with more than one subtype of HBsAg
    (d) none of the above
    (Subtypes of HBsAg)

11. Antibodies to HBsAg:
    (a) occur at the onset of clinically apparent hepatitis B
    (b) often appear in coincidence with the disappearance of circulating HBsAg
    (c) bestow immunity to further infection with hepatitis B virus
    (d) may persist throughout life
    (Antibodies to HBAg)

12. Which of the following individuals may be considered "high-risk" groups with respect to hepatitis B infection?

(a) patients in hemodialysis units

(b) homosexual males

(c) immunosuppressed patients

(d) illicit drug users

(Incidence of Hepatitis B)

13. Hepatitis B may be transmitted through:
    (a) transfusion of blood or blood products
    (b) unsterilized dental equipment
    (c) sexual contact
    (d) all of the above
    (Transmission of Hepatitis B)

14. Viral surface antigen has been found in:
    (a) saliva
    (b) semen
    (c) sweat
    (d) colostrum
    (Transmission of Hepatitis B)

15. An HBV vaccine made by a recombinant strain of the yeast *Saccharomyces cerevisiae*:
    (a) has been found to have positive effects on human volunteers
    (b) causes the production of antibody in recipients after a three-dose program
    (c) produces an antibody in recipients that is specific for the "a" determinant of HBsAg
    (d) has several serious side effects
    (HBV Vaccine)

16. The transmission of non-A, non-B hepatitis is:
    (a) associated with transfusion of blood or blood products
    (b) similar to that of hepatitis B
    (c) believed to be through close person-to-person contact
    (d) not possible between humans and chimpanzees
    (Transmission of Non-A, Non-B Hepatitis)

17. Which of the following is/are third generation tests for HBsAg?
    (a) Ouchterlony double diffusion
    (b) enzyme-linked immunoassay
    (c) counterelectrophoresis
    (d) complement fixation
    (Serologic Detection of HBsAg)

18. Sources of antisera for the detection of HBsAg include:
    (a) horses
    (b) mice
    (c) multiply-transfused human patients
    (d) goats
    (Serologic Detection of HBsAg)

19. In practical testing of HBsAg:
    (a) mouth pipetting is acceptable under certain circumstances
    (b) pipetting should be performed in a fume hood
    (c) leaking specimens should be carefully cleaned before use
    (d) specimens should be centrifuged in a tightly capped tube
    (Practical Considerations)

20. The most sensitive method for the detection of HBsAg is:
    (a) complement fixation
    (b) Ouchterlony double diffusion
    (c) radioimmunoassay
    (d) rheophoresis
    (Serologic Detection of HBsAg)

21. HBcAg has been purified from:
    (a) latex particles
    (b) the liver of immunosuppressed chimpanzees experimentally infected with HBV
    (c) cesium chloride
    (d) the plasma of chickens
    (Serologic Detection of HBcAg and Anti-HBc)

22. "Heavy" cores:
    (a) have a high specific DNA polymerase activity
    (b) are deficient in DNA polymerase activity
    (c) are successfully used as a source of antigen for complement fixation tests
    (d) have a density of 1.30 gm per cubic centimeter
    (Serologic Detection of HBcAg and Anti-HBc)

ANSWER "TRUE" OR "FALSE"

23. The term *hepatitis* refers to inflammation of the liver.
    (Introduction: Hepatitis)

24. Hepatitis A is transmitted by a fecal-oral route.
    (Hepatitis A)

25. IgG–anti-HAV will aggregate highly purified HAV.
    (Antibodies to HAV (Immunity))

26. HBcAg was originally known as *Australia antigen*.
    (Hepatitis B)

27. Of the three forms of HBV, the Dane particle is the most common form seen in patients with hepatitis B.
    (Hepatitis B Virus (HBV))

28. HBeAg is a soluble antigen.
    (Markers for Hepatitis B Virus)

29. Three subtypes of HBsAg have been recognized.
    (Subtypes of HBsAg)

30. Post-transfusion hepatitis is usually related to the non-A, non-B virus, although sporadic cases have been documented without known exposure to blood or blood products.
    (Incidence of Non-A, Non-B Hepatitis)

General References

Braude, A. I. (Ed.): Medical Microbiology and Infectious Diseases. Philadelphia, W. B. Saunders Company, 1981.

Bryant, N. J.: An Introduction to Immunohematology, 2nd ed. Philadelphia, W. B. Saunders Company, 1982.

Finegold, S. M., and Martin, W. J.: Bailey and Scott's Diagnostic Microbiology, 6th ed. St. Louis, The C. V. Mosby Co., 1982.

Freeman, B. A.: Burrows Textbook of Microbiology, 21st ed. Philadelphia, W. B. Saunders Company, 1979.

Henry, J. B. (Ed.): Clinical Diagnosis and Management by Laboratory Methods, 17th ed. Philadelphia, W. B. Saunders Company, 1984.

Mollison, P. L.: Blood Transfusion in Clinical Medicine, 7th ed. Oxford, Blackwell Scientific Publications, 1983.

Pittiglio, D. H.: Modern Blood Banking and Transfusion Practices. Philadelphia, F. A. Davis Co., 1983.

Raphael, S. S.: Lynch's Medical Laboratory Technology, 4th ed. Philadelphia, W. B. Saunders Company, 1983.

EIGHT

C-REACTIVE PROTEIN

OBJECTIVES

The student shall know, understand, and be prepared to explain:
1. The characteristics of C-reactive protein
2. The properties of C-reactive protein
3. Current and potential uses of C-reactive protein determination
4. The laboratory tests for C-reactive protein, principally:
   a. The latex-fixation test for the qualitative and quantitative determination of CRP in serum
   b. The microprecipitation test for CRP

Introduction

C-reactive protein (CRP) is a trace constituent of serum that was originally defined by its calcium-dependent precipitation with the C-polysaccharide of pneumococcus (Tillet and Francis, 1930). The protein was originally thought to be an antibody to C-polysaccharide and specific for patients with pneumococcal infections, but later studies dispelled this contention, and the relative *nonspecificity* of CRP is now well recognized.

The outstanding characteristic of the CRP is that it appears in the sera of individuals in response to a variety of inflammatory conditions and tissue necrosis and disappears when the inflammatory condition has subsided. It is consistently found in cases of bacterial infection (particularly the colon-typhoid group) (Dawson, 1957), active rheumatic fever (Anderson and McCarthy, 1950), and many malignant diseases, and it is commonly found in cases of active rheumatoid arthritis, viral infection, and tuberculosis. In addition, CRP has been detected in the sera of patients following surgical operations (Crockson, *et al.*, 1966) and blood transfusions, as well as in bullous fluid aspirated from patients with thermal burns, pemphigus vulgaris, and other bullous lesions. The protein usually appears rapidly after the onset of disease (14 to 26 hours) and may increase in concentration by as much as 1000 times its normal amount; thus, it is a useful clinical indicator of disease states (Hayashi and LoGrippo, 1972; Table 8–1).

During the 1940s and 1950s, laboratory testing for CRP was widely used as an aid to diagnosis of a variety of inflammatory conditions; however, certain problems with the test subsequently came to be realized, namely:

1. The nonspecificity of the test, which was considered to be a major problem in its clinical interpretation.
2. The quantitative nature of the original assay procedure, which made it impossible to establish any correlation between the positivity of the test and the severity of a clinical disease.

In addition to these problems, new tests were being developed for monitoring acute-phase reactions, the most popular of which was the erythrocyte sedimentation rate (ESR).

For these reasons, the CRP test gradually lost

Table 8–1. PRESENCE OF C–REACTIVE PROTEIN IN DISEASE

Normally Present	Occasionally Present	Absent
Active rheumatic fever	Pericarditis	Skin diseases
Acute myocardial infarction	Rheumatoid arthritis	URI (upper respiratory infections)
Carcinoma	Pyelitis	Renal disease
Streptococcal infections	Nephritis	Localized infections
Pneumonia	Tuberculosis	

its popularity and by the mid-1970s was being performed by very few laboratories.

The potential role of CRP in the clinical laboratory and as a mediator or modulator of the immune response has recently been restimulated due to studies on the purification of the CRP molecule, the preparation of an antisera specific for it, and the development of sensitive, specific, rapid, and quantitative techniques for its measurement in serum. This resurgence of interest is also stimulated by the fact that a molecule that is produced in such large amounts during the acute inflammatory response must have biologic significance, even if such significance is as yet unrealized.

PROPERTIES OF C-REACTIVE PROTEIN

Human CRP is a homogeneous molecule (MW 120,000) with a sedimentation coefficient of 6.5 and an electrophoretic mobility in the gamma region (Volanakis, *et al.,* 1978) that consists of five probably identical, noncovalently bound subunits of approximately 21,500 to 23,500 daltons each, linked in the form of a cyclic pentamer. It is made up of 100 per cent peptide and has an amino acid composition similar to that of immunoglobulin (IgG). In addition, CRP shares with immunoglobulin the ability to initiate certain functions of potential significance to host defense and inflammation, including precipitation (Tillet and Francis, 1930; Abernethy and Francis, 1937), agglutination (Gal and Miltenyi, 1955), opsonization (Kindermark, 1971), capsular swelling (Lofstrom, 1944), and complement activation (Kaplan and Volanakis, 1974; Siegel *et al.,* 1974). C-reactive protein also combines with T-lymphocytes and inhibits certain of their functions (Mortensen *et al.,* 1975), and it inhibits the aggregation of platelets induced by aggregated human gamma globulin and thrombin (Fidel and Gewurz, 1975). CRP differs from immunoglobulin in antigeneity (McLeod and Avery, 1941), tertiary structure, homogeneity (Gotschlich and Edelman, 1965), stimuli required for formation and release, and binding specificities (for which CRP, in certain reactivities, requires calcium) (Gotschlich and Edelman, 1967), and in that it is produced entirely by hepatocytes or liver parenchymal cells (Kushmer and Feldmann, 1978).

In a physical sense, CRP is thermolabile, being destroyed by heating at 70°C for 30 minutes, and does not cross the human placenta.

The elevation of CRP in a patient above the normal (*i.e.,* 0.5 mg/dl) indicates tissue damage or inflammation or both, with great reliability. If these evaluations are monitored sequentially, they can provide an excellent means of assessing disease activity and of guiding therapy.

CURRENT AND POTENTIAL USES OF CRP DETERMINATION

The serum levels of alpha-1-antitrypsin, haptoglobin, ceruloplasmin, alpha-1-acid glycoprotein, and CRP increase during active inflammation or tissue injury. Serum CRP levels, however, increase within 4 to 6 hours after an acute tissue injury, whereas the serum levels of all the other acute phase reactants increase from 12 to 24 hours after the injury. CRP, therefore, is an earlier and more reliable indicator of clinical disease and its severity than the other reactants.

Studies by Fisher *et al.* (1976) have shown that the CRP test can also be useful as a means of evaluating the postoperative clinical course of a patient as opposed to the traditional parameters used for this purpose (*e.g.,* body temperature, white blood count, erythrocyte sedimentation rate), which are often unreliable. In general, serum CRP levels in uncomplicated surgical cases increase within 4 to 6 hours, reach peak value (usually 25 to 35 mg/dl) between 48 and 72 hours postoperatively, then begin to decrease after the third postoperative day, and reach normal values between the fifth and the twelfth postoperative days. In using CRP levels in this regard, it is important to run tests in series rather than at single, isolated points in the clinical course; it is also important that the preoperative CRP levels be determined. Further, the CRP levels must be determined quantitatively in order to be clinically meaningful and useful.

CRP determinations have also been found to be useful in evaluating the clinical course of bacterial and viral infections, rheumatic diseases, myocardial infarction, burn injuries, and renal transplantation.

Bacterial and Viral Infections. In the differential diagnosis of infectious diseases, CRP was reported by McCarthy *et al.* (1978) to be useful in distinguishing bacterial from viral infections. Studies of sequential determinations of CRP in acute childhood pyelonephritis (Jodal and Hanson, 1976) showed that levels of the protein decreased promptly following successful treatment yet continued to rise or remained ineffective when drug therapy was ineffective. Pepys *et al.* (1977), in studying inflammatory bowel disease, reported that CRP was useful in distinguishing Crohn's disease or transmural colitis from chronic ulcerative colitis—a distinction that is not always possible on clinical and histopathologic grounds.

Rheumatic Diseases. CRP measurements can reflect the activity of various rheumatic diseases. In cases of rheumatoid arthritis, for example, CRP has been shown to be a more reliable indicator of disease activity than the ESR, because the ESR reflects certain blood changes that are not necessarily altered in inflammation (*e.g.,* immunoglobulin and cholesterol concentrations, anemia, the size and shape of erythrocytes), whereas CRP does not (Walsh *et al.,* 1979).

Myocardial Infarction. A sharp increase in the serum CRP level accompanies myocardial infarction (especially in the acute phase), and this increase usually parallels the size of the infarct (Smith *et al.,* 1977). CRP quantitation, therefore, can be useful in differentiating acute infarction from angina. Serious complications are indicated by continued increase (or subsequent increase) of the CRP level.

Burn Injuries. Daniels *et al.* (1974), in studying the serum protein profiles in thermal burns, showed that an increase in CRP levels correlated with the severity of the burn.

Renal Transplantation. Sandoval (1981) observed a sudden increase in the serum CRP level that correlated with the onset of homograft rejection, thereby suggesting the potential of using CRP testing in monitoring patients with kidney transplants.

CRP testing has also proved useful in cases of systemic lupus erythematosus.

DISCUSSION

Although little is known about the precise function of CRP, it is possible that the interactions of this protein with various lymphocyte and monocyte subpopulation may constitute the function of "paving the way" for subsequent, more specific immune response. The finding that CRP has a particularly strong affinity for monocytes bearing Fc receptors may be significant in this respect, although the true nature of this interaction remains yet to be elucidated.

LABORATORY TESTS FOR CRP

CRP protein determination is now considered to be of greater practical significance than all other indices of inflammation in assessing inflammatory diseases. For example, CRP is present at all times when the ESR is abnormally elevated, and, whereas ESR determinations may provide "borderline" results and may, in some cases, remain elevated in the absence of inflammation (*e.g.,* in anemia due to a decrease in number of erythrocytes, in pregnancy due to an increase in fibrinogen, and in nephrosis due to loss of albumin and relative increase in globulin), CRP does not have a variable range between normal and abnormal and is not influenced by anemia or serum protein alteration.

Serologic tests for CRP use the patient's serum and either purified pneumococcal C-polysaccharide or anti-CRP serum obtained from rabbits immunized with purified CRP, the latter being preferred.

The tests that have been devised for CRP can be divided into different categories, depending upon the type of procedure involved:

1. *Agglutination:* Agglutination tests for CRP are performed using latex particles coated with antibodies to human CRP, which interact with the patient's serum either on a microscope slide or in a test tube. This test, known as the latex-fixation test, is by far the most popular of the CRP tests and is claimed to be the most sensitive (Fishel, 1967). (The technique is given later in this chapter.)

2. *Complement fixation:* Complement fixation tests for CRP are not generally suitable for use in a routine clinical laboratory and, therefore, are considered to be of historic and academic interest only.

3. *Fluorescent antibody:* Fluorescent antibody tests are useful in studying the binding of CRP to lymphocytes and their subpopulations and are used primarily as research tools for localizing CRP in tissues.

4. *Precipitation:* Precipitation tests for CRP can be done either in the fluid phase (by a capillary or a tube method) or in the solid gel phase (by the Ouchterlony, Oudin, or Mancini methods). In addition, CRP gel tests involving electrophoresis or electroimmunodiffusion have been described. In 1976, Deaton and Maxwell described the use of laser nephelometry in the measurement of CRP (and other serum proteins). This technique is sensitive, rapid, and reproducible and makes it possible to reliably perform CRP determinations on a large number of samples. In brief, the procedure involves the measurement of the light (from a laser-light source) that is scattered by insoluble immune complexes in a liquid medium containing polyethylene glycol. The patient's serum sample and standards are incubated for 2 hours at room temperature with a specific anti-CRP antiserum diluted in polyethylene glycol containing a buffer (pH 7.4). With the use of a nephelometer, the laser beam is passed from the source through the sample and control solutions (which contain the insoluble CRP immune complexes). The forward-scatter light is measured, within the range of the standard sera, with a photomultiplier tube. The concentration of CRP is proportional to the amount of forward-scatter light, which is displayed by the instrument. (Note: In order to subtract nonspecific background-scatter light, which is related to the patient's serum or the reagents or both, it is necessary to run appropriate blank samples in parallel with the test. In some cases (*e.g.,* when using specimens that

have been frozen and thawed), levels of background-scatter light can be extremely high; this represents the only inconvenience of this technique.)

5. *Radioimmunoassay:* An extremely sensitive radioimmunoassay has been described that is capable of detecting levels of CRP in the nanogram range. For most routine studies of CRP, however, this degree of sensitivity is unnecessary.

METHOD 1: THE LATEX–FIXATION TEST FOR THE QUALITATIVE AND QUANTITATIVE DETERMINATION OF C–REACTIVE PROTEIN IN SERUM
(Asher and Shigekawa)

The test procedure given here is that for the CR-TEST provided in a kit by Hyland Laboratories, Deerfield, Illinois. Test kits for CRP are also provided by Difco Laboratories, Detroit, Michigan; Baltimore Biological Laboratory, Cockeysville, Maryland; and others.

Materials

The kit contains:

1. **CR-TEST Latex–Anti-C-Reactive Protein Reagent (5 ml) containing polystyrene-latex particles complexed with goat, horse, and sheep antihuman CRP globulin. Sodium azide—0.1 per cent (w/v) is present as a preservative.**
2. **CR-TEST Positive Control Serum (human; 1.2 ml). Sodium azide—0.1 per cent (w/v) is present as a preservative.**
3. **CR-TEST Negative Control Serum (human; 1.2 ml). Sodium azide—0.1 per cent (w/v) is present as a preservative.**
The above reagents are stored in the dark between 2° and 8°C.
4. **Glycine-Saline Buffer Diluent (100 ml). This, too, should be stored between 2° and 8°C and should be discarded if it becomes contaminated or cloudy.**
5. **Glass slide with ovals**
6. **Capillary pipets with two rubber bulbs**

Additional materials required:

1. **Water baths (37° to 45°C and 56°C)**
2. **Applicator sticks (or toothpicks)**
3. **Test tubes (12 × 75 mm) and test tube rack**
4. **Serologic pipets**
5. **An adequate light source**
6. **Stopwatch**

Procedure (Qualitative)

1. **Inactivate the test serum at 56°C for 30 minutes. (Note: Use fresh, uncontaminated patient's**
serum. If the test cannot be performed immediately, store serum between 2° and 8°C for no longer than 72 hours after collection. If the analysis is delayed for more than 72 hours, freeze the serum sample. Thaw rapidly when needed in a 37° to 45°C water bath.)
2. **Allow all reagents, controls, and specimens to come to room temperature.**
3. **Prepare 1:5 and 1:50 dilutions of the test specimen. The 1:5 dilution is made by adding 0.1 ml of specimen to 0.4 ml of glycine-saline buffer diluent. The 1:50 dilution is prepared by adding 0.1 ml of the 1:5 dilution to 0.9 ml of the glycine-saline buffer diluent.**
4. **Place the serum specimens and controls on the glass slide as follows:**
   a. **Serum specimen—ovals 1 and 2: Using the same capillary pipet, place one drop of the 1:50 dilution near one end of oval 2 of the slide and then one drop of the 1:5 dilution near one end of oval 1.**
   b. **Negative control—oval 4: Using the dropper cap, place one drop of negative control serum (without further dilution or inactivation) near one end of oval 4 of the divided slide.**
   c. **Positive control—oval 5: Using the dropper cap, place one drop of the positive control serum (without inactivation), which must be diluted 1:5 with the glycine-saline buffer diluent, near one end of oval 5 of the divided slide.**
5. **Mix the latex–anti-CRP reagent by gently inverting the vial. Using the dropper cap, add one drop of this reagent to the opposite ends of ovals 1, 2, 4, and 5.**
6. **Mix the contents of each oval with separate applicator sticks, and spread within the entire area of the oval.**
7. **When the contents of the last oval have been mixed, start the stopwatch. Simultaneously rock and rotate the slide manually for 4 minutes. At the end of 4 minutes, immediately examine the slide with reflected light for macroscopic agglutination. (Note: Reaction time is critical.)**

Interpretation. CR-TEST is an antigen-antibody reaction that is most marked when the reactants are in optimal concentrations. Prozones may be encountered that are avoided by dilution of the serum. In such cases, agglutination will occur with the diluted serum, and a weaker or negative reaction will occur with the undiluted serum. Visible agglutination in either or both diluted and undiluted serums indicates the presence of CRP. Serum that does not contain CRP will give a smooth suspension with no visible agglutination in either diluted or undiluted serum. (See Table 8–2.)

Table 8–2. INTERPRETATION OF TESTS FOR
C–REACTIVE PROTEIN

Undiluted Serum	Diluted Serum	Interpretation
0 to 2+	2+ to 4+	Strongly positive
3+ to 4+		Positive
1+ to 2+	0 to 2+	Weakly positive
	Negative	
Negative	Negative	Negative

Procedure (Quantitative)

1. Allow all reagents, controls, and specimens to come to room temperature.
2. Prepare doubling dilutions beginning at 1:8 of previously inactivated positive patient specimens in glycine-saline buffer diluent. Serum specimens are tested at dilutions of 1:8, 1:16, 1:32, 1:64, and 1:128.
3. Using a capillary pipet, transfer one drop of each specimen dilution to one end of successive ovals on the slide. The same capillary pipet may be used for the series of dilutions if transfer is started with the greatest dilution.
4. Set up a dilution control on the slide by adding one drop of latex–anti-C-reactive protein reagent to one drop of glycine-saline buffer diluent in the remaining oval on the slide.
5. Add one drop of latex–anti-CRP reagent to each drop of specimen dilution.
6. Using a wooden applicator stick and starting with the dilution control and then the greatest specimen dilution, mix the contents of each oval and spread within the entire area of the oval.
7. When the last oval has been mixed, start the stopwatch. Simultaneously, rock and rotate the slide manually for 4 minutes. At the end of 4 minutes, immediately examine the slide with reflected light for macroscopic agglutination.

Controls: The dilution control should form a smooth or slightly granular suspension. If clumping is observed in this oval, the test is invalid and must be repeated.

In addition to the dilution control, the positive control serum and the negative control serum should be checked in separate ovals as a check on the reactivity of the test reagent. The positive control should react at a 1:8 dilution in the glycine-saline buffer diluent.

Interpretation. The titer of the serum is the reciprocal of the highest dilution that exhibits definite agglutination (*i.e.*, more granular than the dilution control).

Notes on the Latex-Fixation Test

When the CRP content of the specimen is markedly elevated, a prozone effect may result in a false-negative reaction with undiluted serum. For this reason, a 1:50 dilution has been included in the rapid slide test.

In order to observe the increase or decrease of CRP protein levels, all positive specimens should be routinely tested with the quantitative titration test described.

Patients with a high titer of rheumatoid factors may give positive results on the CR-TEST.

METHOD 2: MICROPRECIPITATION TEST FOR C-REACTIVE PROTEIN
(Anderson and McCarthy, 1950)

Materials

1. CRP precipitin serum (supplied by Hyland Laboratories, Deerfield, Illinois)
2. Capillary tubes
3. Modeling clay (plasticine) in modeling clay rack

Procedure

1. Use only serum specimens that are clear and free of particulate matter.
2. Dip a capillary tube into the CRP precipitin serum, and allow the fluid to fill approximately one third of the tube.
3. Wipe off the outside of the capillary tube with clean tissue.
4. Draw up an equal volume of the serum under test.
5. Carefully invert the capillary tube several times to effect mixing.
6. Tilt the capillary tube to move the serum column toward one end of the tube, and place the fingertip over the end of the capillary while inserting the tube upright into a modeling clay rack. This procedure will create an air space to hold the serum column above the clay base.
7. Allow the tube to stand at room temperature for 10 to 12 hours. The result may be reported qualitatively or semiquantitatively. In quantitation, report the height (in millimeters) of the precipitate column as the degree of positivity (*e.g.*, 3 mm of precipitate is reported as a 3+ reaction).
8. Alternatively, the tube can be incubated at 37°C for 2 hours. A preliminary result may be reported at this time. If a semiquantitative result is required, the tube is then placed in a refrigerator overnight before the final reading is made.

REVIEW QUESTIONS

MULTIPLE CHOICE

Choose the phrase, sentence, or symbol that completes the statement or answers the question. More than one answer may be correct in each case. Answers are given at the end of this book.

1. CRP:
    (a) is a trace constituent of serum
    (b) was originally defined by its potassium-dependent precipitation with the C-polysaccharide of pneumococcus
    (c) was originally thought to be an antibody to C-polysaccharide
    (d) is a nonspecific protein
    (Introduction)

2. CRP is consistently found in cases of:
    (a) bacterial infection
    (b) active rheumatic fever
    (c) active rheumatoid arthritis
    (d) viral infection
    (Introduction)

3. After the onset of disease, CRP usually appears in the serum within:
    (a) 1 to 3 hours
    (b) 14 to 26 hours
    (c) 3 to 5 weeks
    (d) 1 to 6 months
    (Introduction)

4. Human CRP:
    (a) is a beta globulin
    (b) is made up of 100 per cent peptide
    (c) has an amino acid composition similar to that of IgG
    (d) is not involved in the initiation of complement activation
    (Properties of CRP)

5. CRP has the ability to initiate:
    (a) precipitation
    (b) agglutination
    (c) opsonization
    (d) capsular swelling
    (Properties of CRP)

6. CRP:
    (a) crosses the human placenta
    (b) does not cross the human placenta
    (c) is thermostable
    (d) is thermolabile
    (Properties of CRP)

7. The elevation of CRP above the normal indicates:
    (a) the termination of disease processes
    (b) tissue damage
    (c) inflammation
    (d) none of the above
    (Properties of CRP)

8. CRP:
    (a) is present at all times when the ESR is elevated
    (b) is absent when the ESR is normal
    (c) has a variable range between normal and abnormal
    (d) is influenced by anemia or serum protein alteration
    (Laboratory Tests for CRP)

9. Tests for CRP include:
    (a) precipitation tests
    (b) the latex-fixation test
    (c) the slide agglutination test
    (d) all of the above
    (Laboratory Tests for CRP)

10. The molecular weight of CRP is:
    (a) 120,000 to 140,000
    (b) 250,000 to 300,000
    (c) 500,000 to 800,000
    (d) 60,000 to 80,000
    (Properties of CRP)

ANSWER "TRUE" OR "FALSE"

11. CRP is retained at high levels for many years after conditions of inflammation have subsided.
    (Introduction)

12. CRP has been detected in the sera of patients following surgical operations.
    (Introduction)

13. After the onset of disease, CRP may increase in concentration by as much as 5000 times its normal amount.
    (Introduction)

14. The monitoring of CRP elevations in sequence is of no value in assessing disease activity.
    (Properties of CRP)

15. The latex-fixation test for CRP is considered to be more sensitive than other techniques.
    (Laboratory Tests for CRP)

General References

Alba's Medical Technology, 9th ed. Berkeley Scientific Publications, Anaheim, California, 1980.

Bennington, J. L.: Saunders Dictionary and Encyclopedia of Laboratory Medicine and Technology. Philadelphia, W. B. Saunders Company, 1984.

Braude, A. I. (Ed.): Medical Microbiology and Infectious Diseases. Philadelphia, W. B. Saunders Company, 1981.

Finegold, S. M., and Martin, W. J.: Bailey and Scott's Diagnostic Microbiology, 6th ed. St. Louis, The C. V. Mosby Co., 1982.

Raphael, S. S. (Ed.): Lynch's Medical Laboratory Technology. Philadelphia, W. B. Saunders Company, 1983.

Widmann, F. K.: Clinical Interpretation of Laboratory Tests, 9th ed. Philadelphia, F. A. Davis Co., 1983.

NINE

STREPTOLYSIN O

OBJECTIVES

The student shall know, understand, and be prepared to explain:
1. The characteristics of streptolysin O
2. The properties of streptolysin O
3. The significance of the antistreptolysin O reaction
4. The serologic tests for antistreptolysin O
5. The method of antistreptolysin O titration

Introduction

Streptolysin O (SLO) is a bacterial toxin produced by virtually all strains of *Streptococcus pyogenes*. It is one of two extra-cellular hemolysins (or cytolysins), the other being *streptolysin S* (SLS). SLO is released during infection as indicated by antibody production to it. The toxin is a protein with a molecular weight of approximately 70,000 which, in its reduced state, brings about the lysis of red and white blood cells.

PROPERTIES OF STREPTOLYSIN O

Streptolysin O is so called because of its oxygen lability and is quite distinct from SLS (see later discussion). It is hemolytically inactive in the oxidized form and is characteristic of a group of cytolytic toxins known as the *oxygen-labile toxins* (Bernheimer, 1974), which are produced by several different gram-positive bacteria and possess a number of common properties—they are activated by sulfhydryl (SH) compounds, they appear to be antigenically related, and their biologic activity is completely inhibited by low concentrations (1.0 µg per milliliter) of cholesterol and certain related sterols.

Hemolysis of erythrocytes occurs within minutes after the addition of SLO, and toxic effects of SLO have been demonstrated on several types of mammalian cells in culture (Cinader, 1973). SLO is also cardiotoxic. It may cause interstitial myocarditis in experimental animals and systolic arrest of per-

fused mammalian hearts. Its cardiotoxicity is probably caused by inducing the release from atria of acetylcholine, which poisons ventricles. The first, the (f) site, contains two cystine residues and is responsible for the attachment of the molecule to the red blood cells; the second site, the (t) site, is concerned with the final hemolytic event.

It is evident that membrane cholesterol is the binding site of SLO, because only those cells that contain cholesterol in their membranes are susceptible to the toxin. In addition, SLO is inactivated only by the membrane lipid fraction that contains cholesterol; the addition of exogenous cholesterol to SLO inhibits toxic action, and treatment of erythrocyte membranes with alfalfa saponin or filipin inhibits the absorption of SLO (Shany *et al.,* 1974). These agents are known to bind to cholesterol in the membrane. The actual *mechanism* that results in cell lysis remains to be explained, however.

SIGNIFICANCE OF THE ANTISTREPTOLYSIN O REACTION

Streptolysin O is antigenic, eliciting the formation of antibodies that effectively neutralize its hemolytic action. A high proportion of patients with streptococcal infections show an antibody response during convalescence; therefore, the measurement of serum antistreptolysin O (ASO) has become a valuable and reliable indicator of streptococcal infection (particularly in cases of rheumatic fever and glomerulonephritis).

COMPARISON WITH STREPTOLYSIN S

Unlike SLO, SLS is an oxygen-stable nonantigenic peptide with a molecular weight of about 2800. Whereas SLO is synthesized only by growing streptococci, SLS is synthesized by both growing and resting cells and is found on the surface of washed streptococcal cells as a cell-bound hemolysin. The peptide, however, is loosely bound and can be released into the surrounding medium by a variety of carrier molecules (*e.g.,* serum albumin, alpha-lipoproteins, yeast RNA, and nonionic detergents such as tweens and tritons). Upon release by the carriers, the hemolysin becomes recognized as SLS. Extracellular SLS, therefore, is a complex between a nonspecific carrier molecule and the specific hemolytic peptide. The peptide can be transferred among the various carriers and finally to the surface of mammalian cells. After the interaction with membrane phospholipids, the hemolytic peptide is inactivated. SLS is inhibited by lecithin and beta-lipoproteins, but, unlike SLO, it is not inhibited by cholesterol. Further, red cells treated with SLO show distinct lesions similar to those caused by complement, yet red cells similarly treated with SLS show no such lesions. SLS, when injected intravenously, causes necrosis of the liver and kidney tubules and massive intracellular hemolysis. When injected intra-articularly, it can induce a chronic arthritis.

TESTS FOR ANTISTREPTOLYSIN O

The most widely used test for SLO is the neutralization test used to detect ASO in serum. This test is based on the fact that ASO can be specifically fixed to SLO *in vitro*, where it will neutralize its hemolytic activity. The test, therefore, by doubling dilution, estimates the amount of antibody that can, in the presence of a constant dose of SLO, completely inhibit hemolysis of a given number of red cells.

In the interpretation of ASO titers, many variables, including age, the severity of the infection, previous exposure to streptococcal infection, and the individual's ability to respond immunologically to the toxin, must be taken into account, because no set "normal" titer has been established. Most healthy adults (99 per cent) have ASO titers of 125 Todd units (or less). (The original ASO test procedure was developed by Todd, whose name is still used to express the levels of antibody titer. One Todd unit is that amount of antibody that completely neutralizes two and one half minimal hemolytic doses of SLO.) Children, however, show fluctuating ASO titers from 5 to 125 Todd units. The usual titer normally decreases after 50 years of age, probably owing to a weakened immunologic response.

A rise in ASO titer of at least 30 per cent over the previous level is usually regarded as reliable. In cases of rheumatic fever and glomerulonephritis, a marked increase in ASO titer is often seen during the symptom-free period preceding an attack of the illness. ASO titers in acute cases of rheumatic fever are usually between 300 and 1500 Todd units and are usually maintained at high levels for a period of 6 months from the onset of disease. Drugs commonly used in the treatment of patients with rheumatic fever (*e.g.,* sodium salicylate, aureum salts, and aminophenazone with phenylbutazone [Irgapyrin]) do not affect the production of SLO *in vivo*, but antibiotics (*e.g.,* penicillin, Aureomycin), hormones, and cortisone inhibit the production of the toxin.

Increased ASO titers have been found in a large number of diseases (*e.g.,* scarlet fever, cholera minor, tuberculous diseases, pneumococcal pneumonia, gonorrhea), although they are rarely above 500 Todd units unless the patient has had a recent streptococcal infection. Very low titers are observed in all stages of the nephrotic syndrome, possibly as a result of a defect in formation or increased destruction of antibody protein or loss of antibody protein in the urine.

A single high ASO titer is of little value to the clinician, because a small number of healthy individuals have high titers. Significance should only be attached to changes in ASO titers determined by serial titration.

In addition to the ASO titration, a particle agglutination test has been described, which is generally less frequently used. This test involves coated particles (*e.g.,* latex, treated erythrocytes, or certain bacteria) that are then mixed with diluted test serum on a slide. If the particles agglutinate, ASO can be regarded as present. It is possible to use erythrocytes as particles, because the SLO is in the oxidized state and, therefore, is nonhemolytic. The main advantage of this test when compared with the ASO O titration is that lipoproteins, oxidized SLO, or bacterial growth products do not give false-positive results.

The streptozyme test is a particle agglutination test in which erythrocytes are coated with a crude mixture of streptococcal antigens. It is good for screening but has limited value as a quantitative test.

METHOD 1: ANTISTREPTOLYSIN O TITRATION

Antistreptolysin O titration allows the quantitative analysis of the antibody, based on an internation-

Serum Dilutions	1:10		1:100						1:500				Red Cell Control	SLO Control
Tube	1	2	3	4	5	6	7	8	9	10	11	12	13	14
Add serum dilution, ml	0.8	0.2	1.0	0.8	0.6	0.4	0.3	1.0	0.8	0.6	0.4	0.2	0	0
Add buffer solution, ml Shake gently to mix	0.2	0.8	0	0.2	0.4	0.6	0.7	0	0.2	0.4	0.6	0.8	1.5	1.0
Add streptolysin O, ml Shake gently to mix. Incubate at 37°C for 15 minutes	0.5	0.5	0.5	0.5	0.5	0.5	0.5	0.5	0.5	0.5	0.5	0.5	0	0.5
Add 5 per cent red cell suspension, ml	0.5	0.5	0.5	0.5	0.5	0.5	0.5	0.5	0.5	0.5	0.5	0.5	0.5	0.5
Shake gently to mix. Incubate at 37°C for 45 minutes, shaking tubes after first 15 minutes. Following incubation, centrifuge tubes for 1 minute at 1500 rpm														
Todd unit value	12	50	100	125	166	250	333	500	625	833	1250	2500		

ally recognized unit system (Todd, 1932). The system defines a minimal hemolytic dose of SLO as that amount of toxin that will completely hemolyze 0.5 ml of a 5 per cent suspension of rabbit red blood cells, measured in Todd units.

Materials

1. Saline—0.85 per cent
2. Streptolysin O buffer—This is commercially available from a number of supply houses. It is prepared as follows:
   7.4 gm sodium chloride
   3.17 gm potassium phosphate
   1.81 gm sodium phosphate
   Add to 1000 ml of distilled water. The final pH should be between 6.5 and 6.7. The buffer may be stored at 4° C for up to 1 week.
3. Streptolysin O—This is available in dehydrated form from commercial supply houses and should be rehydrated just prior to use. Once rehydrated, the solution should not be subjected to vigorous shaking, and it must be used within 1 hour or discarded, because the active reagent is subject to inactivation by oxidation.
4. Red blood cells—A 5 per cent suspension of fresh (not more than 1 week old) human red blood cells (group O) are most commonly used in this test, although rabbit red blood cells are equally as sensitive to SLO. The cells must be washed three times in diluent, and the buffy coat (white blood cells) must be removed. The final centrifugation should be at 1500 rpm for 10 minutes, following which the packed red cells may be measured to achieve a 5 per cent suspension. Prepare the final suspension in SLO buffer.
5. Test tubes—12 × 100 mm are commonly used (round bottom).

Procedure

1. Prepare dilutions of fresh or inactivated serum as follows, using SLO buffer as the diluent:
   1:10—0.5 ml of serum + 4.5 ml buffer
   1:100—1.0 ml of 1:10 serum dilution + 9.0 ml buffer
   1:500—2.0 ml of 1:100 serum dilution + 8.0 ml buffer
   The first two serum dilutions are usually sufficient for preliminary titrations.
2. Set up the test according to the protocol given in the table on page 113.

Interpretation

The ASO titer expressed in Todd units is the reciprocal of the serum dilution that completely neutralizes the SLO. For example, a serum showing no hemolysis in tubes 1 through 4, a trace of hemolysis in tube 5, and marked to complete hemolysis in the remaining tubes is reported as containing 125 Todd units.

Before reporting results, always ensure that the controls give the expected results.

REVIEW QUESTIONS

MULTIPLE CHOICE

Choose the phrase, sentence, or symbol that completes the statement or answers the question. More than one answer may be correct in each case. Answers are given at the end of this book.

1. Streptolysin O:
   (a) is a bacterial toxin produced by virtually all strains of *Streptococcus pyogenes*
   (b) is a viral toxin
   (c) is released during infection
   (d) is not antigenic
   (Introduction)

2. Streptolysin O:
   (a) in a reduced state brings about the lysis of red and white blood cells
   (b) in a reduced state brings about the lysis of red cells only
   (c) is so called because of its oxygen lability
   (d) is the same as streptolysin S
   (Introduction, Properties of Streptolysin O)

3. The molecular weight of streptolysin O is:
   (a) about 5000
   (b) about 70,000
   (c) about 250,000
   (d) about 300,000
   (Introduction)

4. The oxygen-labile toxins:
   (a) are activated by sulfhydryl compounds
   (b) are not related antigenically to one another
   (c) are inactivated by sulfhydryl compounds
   (d) are inhibited in their biologic activity by low concentrations of cholesterol
   (Properties of Streptolysin O)

5. Streptolysin O:
   (a) possesses two active sites
   (b) possesses three active sites
   (c) possesses four active sites
   (d) possesses six active sites
   (Properties of Streptolysin O)

6. Streptolysin S:
   (a) is an oxygen-labile toxin
   (b) is nonantigenic

STREPTOLYSIN O **115**

(c) has a molecular weight similar to that of streptolysin O
(d) is synthesized only by growing streptococci
(Comparison with Streptolysin S)

7. In the interpretation of antistreptolysin O titers, which of the following variables must be taken into account:
(a) the age of the patient
(b) previous exposure to streptococcal infection
(c) the individual's ability to respond immunologically to the toxin
(d) all of the above
(Tests for Antistreptolysin O)

8. The ASO titer in children is:
(a) usually high
(b) usually below 5 Todd units
(c) usually between 5 and 125 Todd units
(d) usually between 300 and 500 Todd units
(Tests for Antistreptolysin O)

9. The production of streptolysin O *in vivo* is inhibited by:
(a) sodium salicylate
(b) penicillin
(c) aureum salts
(d) cortisone
(Tests for Antistreptolysin O)

10. The particle agglutination test for streptolysin O:
(a) is more frequently used than the antistreptolysin O titration
(b) involves particles coated with latex, treated erythrocytes, or certain bacteria
(c) is unreliable because of the probability of false-positive results
(d) is a useful quantitative test
(Tests for Antistreptolysin O)

ANSWER "TRUE" OR "FALSE"

11. Streptolysin O is quite distinct from streptolysin S.
(Properties of Streptolysin O)

12. Streptolysin O is cardiotoxic.
(Properties of Streptolysin O)

13. Streptolysin O is inactivated by the membrane lipid fraction of cells that lack cholesterol.
(Properties of Streptolysin O)

14. Red cells treated with streptolysin O show distinct lesions similar to those caused by complement.
(Comparison with Streptolysin S)

15. Increased ASO titers have been found in cases of scarlet fever, where the level is usually more than 1000 Todd units.
(Tests for Antistreptolysin O)

General References

Alba's Medical Technology, 9th ed. Anaheim, CA, Berkeley Scientific Publications, 1980.
Bennington, J. L. (Ed.): Saunder's Dictionary and Encyclopedia of Laboratory Medicine and Technology. Philadelphia, W. B. Saunders Company, 1984.
Braude, A. I. (Ed.): Medical Microbiology and Infectious Diseases. Philadelphia, W. B. Saunders Company, 1981.
Finegold, S. M., and Martin, W. J.: Bailey and Scott's Diagnostic Microbiology, 6th ed. St. Louis, The C. V. Mosby Co., 1982.

TEN

COLD AGGLUTININS: STREPTOCOCCUS MG

OBJECTIVES

The student shall know, understand, and be prepared to explain:

1. The characteristics of cold agglutinins
2. Cold agglutinin syndrome
3. Cold agglutinins in *Mycoplasma pneumoniae* infection and infectious mononucleosis
4. Cold agglutinins in other disease states
5. Tests for cold agglutinins, specifically:
   a. Rapid screen for cold agglutinins
   b. Titration of cold agglutinins
6. The characteristics of streptococcus MG
7. The tests for streptococcus MG, specifically:
   a. The streptococcus MG agglutination test

COLD AGGLUTININS

Introduction

Cold agglutinins were initially demonstrated by Landsteiner (1903) through the observation that agglutination would occur when the serum of an animal was mixed with its own red cells at a temperature near 0°C. It was later shown that this phenomenon also applied to most human subjects (Landsteiner and Levine, 1926). The significance of these cold agglutinins with respect to human disease, however, was not fully appreciated until many years later.

At a shallow but convenient level, cold agglutinins can be divided into two groups: those that are "harmless," having anti-I, anti-H or (rarely) anti-Pr specificity and present in all normal sera; and those that are "harmful," the so-called pathologic cold autoagglutinins, which have anti-I, anti-i, and (rarely) other specificities and are found in cases of chronic cold hemagglutinin disease (also known as cold agglutinin syndrome) and transiently following mycoplasmal infection.

A detailed study of cold agglutinins is unnecessary for the serologist (although the interested reader is referred to the excellent texts by Mollison [1983] and Petz and Garratty [1980] for more detailed information [see General References at the end of this chapter]); therefore, this discussion will be confined to those areas that involve the serology laboratory. Cold agglutinins with respect to autoimmune hemolytic anemia are discussed in Chapter Twelve.

Characteristics

By definition, cold agglutinins are antibodies that react best with red blood cells at temperatures *below* 37°C. The reaction strength is often greatest at temperatures of 0° to 4°C. At temperatures of 25° to 30°C, these reactions are generally not manifest, although the thermal maximum is dependent upon the concentration and binding affinity of the cold agglutinin. Those cold agglutinins that are active only to a temperature of 10° to 15°C are regarded as harmless, whereas those that are active *in vitro* up to a temperature of 30°C or more are generally associated with such harmful effects as blocking of small vessels on exposure to cold, due to red cell agglutination and the production of hemolytic anemia. Between these two extremes are many examples of cold agglutinins that are active up to a temperature of 25°C and that are found in association with disease.

The agglutination observed with cold agglutinins can be eliminated by warming and may be reversed to the original agglutinated state by recooling the specimen. The antibody agglutinates all adult human red blood cells, regardless of group, although some variation in reaction strength is often observed. In addition, the agglutinating serum reacts with the erythrocytes of many unrelated species. They may be absorbed to exhaustion by erythrocytes in the cold but are unaffected by absorption at 37°C. They may be stored in the cold with only slight diminution of potency.

Cold Agglutinin Syndrome

Cold agglutinin syndrome is a condition in which there is a high titer of cold agglutinins causing intravascular agglutination when the blood is cooled in peripheral parts of the body exposed to the cold, which may cause mild hemolytic anemia as a result of complement fixation. The condition is reversible by rewarming the exposed parts of the body.

The syndrome occurs in two distinct clinical settings:

1. In the elderly, chronic cold agglutinin syndrome usually has a gradual onset and chronic course. The agglutinins usually contain monoclonal kappa light chains. This condition may also be due to the presence of a lymphoma in some individuals.
2. Postinfectious cold agglutinin syndrome, which commonly follows infection with *Mycoplasma pneumoniae* or infectious mononucleosis.

Those affected with cold agglutinin syndrome, in addition to a high titer of cold agglutinins, are also found to have large amounts of C3d, resulting in a positive direct antiglobulin test.

Cold Agglutinins in *Mycoplasma pneumoniae* Infection and Infectious Mononucleosis

Cold agglutinins are found in approximately 55 per cent of patients with *M. pneumoniae* pneumonia. In such cases, subclinical hemolysis is common, and, in a few patients, there is an episode of hemolytic anemia (Tanowitz *et al.*, 1978).

Generally, cold agglutinin syndrome in *M. pneumoniae* infections occurs in the second or third week after the onset of the disease. The onset of hemolysis is usually rapid and abnormal IgM cold agglutinins, which characteristically have anti-I

specificity, increase in titer, reaching a peak at day 12 to day 15, then rapidly decreasing after day 20. In some cases, the patient may already have recovered from the respiratory infection, then he becomes ill again. Increasing pallor and jaundice occur, and splenomegaly is generally present. In a few cases, acrocyanosis and hemoglobinuria are seen (Pirofsky, 1969), and, in rare cases, gangrene may result from exposure to the cold. The hemolytic anemia, if this occurs, proceeds at an alarming rate and may be fatal (Dacie, 1962; Tanowitz *et al.*, 1978). The disorder may be more pronounced in cases of glucose-6-phosphate dehydrogenase (G-6-PD) deficiency and sickle-cell disease (Tanowitz *et al.*, 1978).

The involvement of cold agglutinins in *M. pneumoniae* infections has been the subject of several investigations. The fact that the antibody has anti-I specificity suggests the possibility of the presence of I-like antigen in the *M. pneumoniae* organism and a cross-reactive response (Janney *et al.*, 1978). This is supported by the fact that, whereas intact *M. pneumoniae* do not inhibit anti-I, lipopolysaccharide prepared from these organisms does. Furthermore, the cold agglutinins produced in rabbits following an injection of *M. pneumoniae* will inhibit these organisms (Costea *et al.*, 1972).

In *M. pneumoniae* pneumonia, there is a positive correlation between the frequency of cold agglutinins and the severity of the disease, the extent of pulmonary involvement and the duration of the illness. Extremely high titers are sometimes found in cases of hemolytic anemia. A fourfold rise in titer is significant of acute involvement. Antibiotic therapy may interfere with the development of cold agglutinins.

In infectious mononucleosis, cold agglutinins of anti-I specificity are frequently present as a transient phenomenon (Jenkins *et al.*, 1965; Rosenfield *et al.*, 1965). Worlledge and Dacie (1969), in reviewing published cases, concluded that anti-i is present in about 50 per cent of patients with the disease: 14 of 30 sera from afflicted individuals agglutinated cord red cells (which possess the highest concentration of the i antigen) to a titer of 16 or more, whereas normal sera agglutinated the same cells only to a titer of 4 at 4°C. The antibody in patients with infectious mononucleosis is normally detectable *in vitro* up to a temperature of about 24°C, although in patients who developed a hemolytic syndrome (less than 1 per cent), the antibody was found to be active *in vitro* up to a temperature of at least 28°C.

Goldberg and Barnett (1967), in investigating a case of hemolytic anemia complicating infectious mononucleosis, found that the agglutinin involved was an IgG-IgM complex. The autoantibody (presumably anti-i) was found to be IgG, and the IgM was an anti-IgG antibody. Both antibodies reacted more strongly at 4°C, and the separated IgG was found *not* to be an agglutinin, although it sensitized red cells to agglutination by anti-IgG. Capra *et al.* (1969) suggested that these findings represented the rule in infectious mononucleosis with hemolytic anemia, although subsequent investigations have cast doubt on this conclusion (Chaplin, 1980). Many examples of IgM anti-i infectious mononucleosis have been reported (*e.g.*, Troxel *et al.*, 1966; Wollheim and Williams, 1966).

Infectious mononucleosis is further discussed in Chapter Eleven.

Cold Agglutinins in Other Disease States

In the early literature on cold agglutinin syndrome, an association with several pathogenic states was reported, although the significance of the relationship, in most cases, is questionable. Included in this group are trypanosomiasis, relapsing fever, cirrhosis, malaria, septicemia, pernicious anemia, and various forms of carcinoma (Pirofsky, 1969). The production of high-titer cold agglutinins has also been found (by the same author) to occur during influenza virus infection, occasionally involving an episode of hemolytic anemia.

Tests for Cold Agglutinins

In the serology laboratory, tests for cold agglutinins are most commonly requested in cases of suspected primary atypical pneumonia, where rapid screening tests have proved useful. If strongly positive reactions or reactions that increase in strength as the temperature decreases are observed, titration of the antibody is recommended. Tests should be performed regularly, because an increase in titer through the duration of the illness is of greater diagnostic significance than a positive result on a single specimen.

The fact that cold agglutinins are absorbed by erythrocytes in the cold is of major importance in the determination of cold agglutinins. If specimens are stored and/or transported in the cold, most cold agglutinins of significance will attach themselves to the red blood cells and will therefore be absent from the serum when testing is performed. For this reason, specimens should be collected at 37°C and transported to the laboratory submerged in water at 37°C. If this is not possible, specimens should be warmed to 37°C for 30 minutes before the serum is separated from the cells. Centrifugation is not recommended, but if it is unavoidable, refrigerated centrifuges must not be used.

METHOD 1: RAPID SCREEN FOR COLD AGGLUTININS

Method

1. **Place the specimen in a water bath at 37°C as soon as it arrives in the laboratory.**
2. **Separate the serum from the clot when the clot has retracted completely.**
3. **Using a Pasteur pipet, transfer the serum into a labeled tube and centrifuge at 3400 rpm for 2 minutes.**
4. **Prepare a 5 per cent suspension of the patient's cells.**
5. **Set up two test tubes in a test tube rack.**
6. **Place two drops of the patient's serum in each tube. To each tube consecutively, add:**
   a. **one drop of the patient's red cells**
   b. **one drop of group O cord red cells**
7. **Incubate the serum-cell mixture at 20°C for 1 hour.**
8. **Read and record results.**
9. **Incubate the same tubes in a water bath at 15°C for 1 hour.**
10. **Read and record results.**

Interpretation

If agglutination is observed at 15°C and 20°C, proceed with the titration technique as described in Method 2.

If agglutination is observed at 15°C but disappears as the tube is warmed to 20°C or higher, record as negative.

METHOD 2: TITRATION OF COLD AGGLUTININS

Method

1. **Set out 10 tubes in a test tube rack.**
2. **Place 1.5 ml of diluent (physiologic saline) in tube 1 and 1.0 ml of diluent (physiologic saline) in tubes 2 through 10.**
3. **Add 0.5 ml of the patient's serum to tube 1, mix and transfer 1.0 ml to tube 2, mix and transfer 1.0 ml to tube 3, and so on, through tube 9. Tube 10 will serve as a cell control. By this method, dilutions will be 1:4 to 1:1024.**
4. **Add 0.1 ml of the patient's own red cells (2 per cent suspension) to each tube.**
5. **Mix the contents by vigorous shaking of the test tube rack, and place racks at 4°C overnight.**
6. **Remove the tubes from the refrigerator and read immediately.**

Interpretation

The titer of cold agglutinins is read as the reciprocal of the highest dilution exhibiting any agglu-

tination (1+ agglutination is usually taken as the weakest when read macroscopically). After reading, place the tubes at 37°C for 2 hours and reread. If the titer was due to cold agglutinins, the erythrocytes will be dispersed and no agglutination will be seen.

Note: As for the rapid screen, specimens for titration of cold agglutinins must be kept at 37°C at all times until the serum and cells are separated.

STREPTOCOCCUS MG

Streptococcus MG is a nonhemolytic, gram-positive coccus that is isolated from the throats of patients with primary atypical pneumonia. During convalescence, patients with this disease often develop antibodies to streptococcus MG, which are specific and react with the capsular polysaccharide of the organism.

Forty-four per cent of patients with primary atypical pneumonia demonstrate positive streptococcus MG reactions. Agglutinins occur in more than 75 per cent of patients with severe attacks of the disease of long duration; only 20 per cent of patients with mild attacks of short duration develop agglutinins.

Streptococcus MG agglutinins occur in normal serum at low titers (1:10). A titer of 40 or greater in a single specimen is considered to be suggestive of primary atypical pneumonia, but a fourfold rise in titer of antibodies to streptococcus MG during convalescence is of greater diagnostic significance than a single positive result. These agglutinins are usually detectable approximately 2 to 3 weeks after onset of the disease.

Antibodies to streptococcus MG are distinct from cold agglutinins, many individuals showing one but not the other reaction. The agglutinins to streptococcus MG are found in only about 4 per cent of patients with other diseases where they have no value as a diagnostic aid, the titers varying considerably yet never being extremely high.

Tests for Streptococcus MG

The most common test for the detection of streptococcus MG is the streptococcus MG agglutination test. Specimens for this test may be allowed to clot in the refrigerator, because antibodies to streptococcus MG are not absorbed by red blood cells as are cold agglutinins. The serum should be separated from the red cells and stored at 4°C. Excellent commercial antigens for streptococcus MG are available from Difco Laboratories, Detroit, Michigan and from Baltimore Biological Laboratories, Cockeysville, Maryland.

It should be noted that, although the streptococcus MG agglutination test is helpful in the diagnosis of primary atypical pneumonia, the coccus itself is not the etiologic agent of the disease.

METHOD 1: THE STREPTOCOCCUS MG AGGLUTINATION TEST

Method

1. **Set up 10 tubes in a test tube rack.**
2. **Add 0.2 ml of diluent (physiologic saline) to each tube.**
3. **Add 0.2 ml of the patient's serum to tube 1. Mix and transfer 0.2 ml to tube 2. Continue mixing and transferring, and discard 0.2 ml from tube 9. Tube 10 will then serve as an antigen control.**
4. **Add 0.2 ml of antigen suspension to each tube. The final dilutions are 1:4 through 1:1024.**
5. **Shake the rack, and incubate at room temperature or 37°C for 18 hours.**
6. **Read and record results.**

Interpretation

The highest dilution showing definite agglutination (1+) is taken as the end point. The titer is expressed as the reciprocal of this dilution (e.g., if the agglutination end point occurs at 1:128, the titer is 128). Note that low titers (i.e., less than 20) are not considered significant.

REVIEW QUESTIONS

MULTIPLE CHOICE

Choose the phrase, sentence, or symbol that completes the statement or answers the question. More than one answer may be correct in each case. Answers are given at the end of this book.

1. The term *cold agglutinins:*
   (a) refers to antibodies that react best with red blood cells at temperatures below 37°C
   (b) refers to antibodies that react best with red blood cells at temperatures above 37°C
   (c) refers to antibodies that have a thermal range between 25° and 30°C
   (d) refers to antibodies that most often react best at 0° to 4°C
   (Characteristics)

2. The thermal maximum of cold agglutinins is:
   (a) 0°C
   (b) 4°C
   (c) 10°C
   (d) dependent upon the concentration and binding affinity of the cold agglutinin
   (Characteristics)

3. The agglutination observed with cold agglutinins:
   (a) can be eliminated by warming the specimen
   (b) is reversible with changes in temperature
   (c) cannot be eliminated by warming the specimen
   (d) can be eliminated by cooling the specimen below 0°C
   (Characteristics)

4. Cold agglutinins:
   (a) agglutinate all adult human red blood cells regardless of group
   (b) agglutinate red cells of group O only
   (c) exhibit varying reaction strength from one sample to another
   (d) can be absorbed to exhaustion by erythrocytes at 37°C
   (Characteristics)

5. Chronic cold agglutinin syndrome in the elderly:
   (a) usually has a gradual onset and a chronic course
   (b) produces agglutinins in the patient that usually contain polyclonal kappa light chains
   (c) may be due to the presence of a lymphoma in some individuals
   (d) produces agglutinins in the patient that usually contain monoclonal lambda chains
   (Cold Agglutinin Syndrome)

6. Those individuals affected with cold agglutinin syndrome:
   (a) have a high titer of cold agglutinins
   (b) have large amounts of C3d on their cells
   (c) have a positive direct antiglobulin test
   (d) usually have a negative direct antiglobulin test
   (Cold Agglutinin Syndrome)

7. In *Mycoplasma pneumoniae* infection:
   (a) all patients have high titers of cold agglutinins
   (b) about 55 per cent of patients have abnormal cold agglutinins that have anti-I specificity
   (c) hemolytic anemia is the result in the vast majority of patients
   (d) there is a positive correlation between the frequency of cold agglutinins and the severity of the disease
   (Cold Agglutinins in Mycoplasma pneumoniae *Infection and Infectious Mononucleosis)*

8. In infectious mononucleosis:
   (a) cold agglutinins of anti-I specificity are frequently present
   (b) cold agglutinins of anti-i specificity are frequently present and thereafter persist throughout life
   (c) a hemolytic syndrome may develop in fewer than 1 per cent of cases
   (d) the cold agglutinin formed will react with cord red blood cells to a temperature of about 24°C
   (Cold Agglutinins in Mycoplasma pneumoniae *Infections and Infectious Mononucleosis)*

9. Streptococcus MG:
   (a) is a nonhemolytic, gram-positive coccus
   (b) is a nonhemolytic, gram-negative coccus
   (c) is isolated from the throats of patients with primary atypical pneumonia
   (d) often stimulates the production of antibodies in patients with primary atypical pneumonia
   (Streptococcus MG)

10. Agglutinins to streptococcus MG:
    (a) are found in 44 per cent of patients with primary atypical pneumonia
    (b) occur in normal serum at high titers (1:40 or greater)
    (c) are the same as cold agglutinins
    (d) are found in high titers in patients with a number of diseases
    (Streptococcus MG)

ANSWER "TRUE" OR "FALSE"

11. Cold agglutinins that are active only to a temperature of 10° to 15°C are regarded as harmless.
    (Characteristics)

12. Cold agglutinins will react with the erythrocytes of many unrelated species.
    (Characteristics)

13. Cold agglutinins are found in approximately 90 per cent of patients with *Mycoplasma pneumoniae* infection.
    (Cold Agglutinins in Mycoplasma pneumoniae *Infection and Infectious Mononucleosis)*

14. Antibiotic therapy has no effect on the development of cold agglutinins.
    (Cold Agglutinins in Mycoplasma pneumoniae *Infection and Infectious Mononucleosis)*

15. Anti-i is present in all normal sera to a titer of 16.
    (Cold Agglutinins in Mycoplasma pneumoniae *Infection and Infectious Mononucleosis)*

16. Specimens for cold agglutinin testing should be collected at 37°C and, if possible, transported to the laboratory submerged in water at 37°C.
    (Tests for Cold Agglutinins)

17. Streptococcus MG is the etiologic agent of primary atypical pneumonia.
    (Tests for Streptococcus MG)

18. Antistreptococcus MG antibodies react with the capsular polysaccharide of streptococcus MG.
    (Streptococcus MG)

General References

Alba's Medical Technology, 9th ed. Anaheim, CA, Berkeley Scientific Publications, 1980.

Bennington, J. L. (Ed.): Saunders Dictionary and Encyclopedia of Laboratory Medicine and Technology. Philadelphia, W. B. Saunders Company, 1984.

Finegold, S. M., and Martin, W. J.: Bailey and Scott's Diagnostic Microbiology, 6th ed. St. Louis, The C. V. Mosby Co., 1982.

Mollison, P. L.: Blood Transfusion in Clinical Medicine, 7th ed. Oxford, Blackwell Scientific Publications, 1983.

Petz, L. D., and Garratty, G.: Acquired Immune Hemolytic Anemias. New York, Churchill Livingstone, 1980.

Raphael, S. S. (Ed.): Lynch's Medical Laboratory Technology, 4th ed. Philadelphia, W. B. Saunders Company, 1983.

Widmann, F. K.: Clinical Interpretation of Laboratory Tests, 9th ed. Philadelphia, F. A. Davis Co., 1983.

ELEVEN

INFECTIOUS MONONUCLEOSIS

OBJECTIVES

The student shall know, understand, and be prepared to explain:

1. The Epstein-Barr virus
2. The characteristics of the disease
3. A general outline of heterophil antibodies
4. The role of heterophil antibodies in infectious mononucleosis
5. The serologic tests for infectious mononucleosis, including:
   a. The Paul-Bunnell test
   b. The Davidsohn differential test
   c. Rapid differential slide tests (spot tests)

Introduction

Infectious mononucleosis is a self-limiting disease caused by the Epstein-Barr virus (EBV). The disease may be confused with similar but more serious diseases such as diphtheria, pharyngitis, Vincent's angina, lymphadenitis with scarlet fever, hepatitis, or pertussis (whooping cough). The most effective method of diagosis (currently) is serologic.

THE EPSTEIN–BARR VIRUS

The Epstein-Barr virus is an enveloped, double-stranded DNA virus that belongs to the family Herpetoviridae. It is ubiquitous and may be transmitted through saliva and blood transfusions, and possibly by mosquitos. Eighty to 90 per cent of healthy adults have antibody to EBV. Infectious mononucleosis results from primary infection with EBV, after which neutralizing antibodies develop and lifelong immunity protects against further exogenous reinfections. Once infected, however, an individual remains a lifelong carrier of the virus. EBV has been known to survive in peripheral blood lymphocytes for years without producing disease.

Several different diseases are associated with EBV, notably Burkitt's lymphoma and nasopharyngeal carcinoma. EBV has several different antigens that may be used to relate different diseases to EBV infections. The viral capsid antigens (VAC) are found in all persons affected by acute phase infectious mononucleosis. The antibody to VAC achieves maximum strength during the second week of the disease, then gradually decreases in strength, remaining at a low level throughout life. The so-called early antigens are also found in cases of infectious mononucleosis, but they disappear early after recovery. Both of these antigens can be detected by immunofluorescence techniques.

CHARACTERISTICS

Infectious mononucleosis is an acute infectious disease of the reticuloendothelial system. Clinically, the disease presents as fever, malaise, lethargy, sore throat with exudate, enlarged lymph nodes in the neck, mild hepatitis, enlarged spleen, and (sometimes) blotchy skin rash. The disease usually lasts about 2 weeks, although convalescence may take months. Characteristic of infectious mononucleosis are enlarged lymphocytes with atypical nuclei (so-called Downey cells), which present after a short period of time, but they usually follow the presence of heterophil antibodies, persisting after the disappearance of these antibodies.

HETEROPHIL ANTIBODIES—DESCRIPTION

Experimental work by Forssman (1911) revealed that emulsions of guinea-pig organs injected into rabbits provoked the formation of antibodies that lysed sheep erythrocytes in the presence of complement. Subsequently, the name "Forssman antigen" was used for any substance that would stimulate the formation of sheep hemolysin. The sheep antibody produced in this way is an example of a "heterophil" antibody, "heterophil" being the name given to several groups of antigens that occur in cells or fluids of apparently unrelated animals and microorganisms, yet that are so closely related that they cross-react with antibodies against any one member of the particular heterophil group. The Forssman antigen is found in the red cells of many species (horse, sheep, dog, cat, mouse, fowl) as well as in some bacteria such as pneumococci, certain strains of dysentery and paratyphoid bacilli, *Clostridium welchii,* and *Neisseria catarrhalis.* It is absent in humans, monkeys, rabbits, rats, ducks, and cows.

Although the Forssman antigen was the first example of a heterophil antigen, it is important to recognize that there are many heterophil systems, of which the Forssman is only one. Among some investigators, the terms *Forssman antigen* and *heterophil antigen* are used synonymously; yet the Forssman antigen is the antigen that was discovered in guinea-pig tissues, whereas the term *heterophil antigen* refers to a broad group of antigens in various plants and animals whose characteristics are similar to those of the Forssman antigen.

Apart from their intrinsic interest, heterophil systems are of some practical importance in that they can be put to (albeit limited) diagnostic use in some cases of typhus, primary atypical pneumonia, serum sickness, and infectious mononucleosis.

HETEROPHIL ANTIBODIES IN INFECTIOUS MONONUCLEOSIS

Paul and Bunnell (1932) observed that heterophil antibodies developed in patients suffering from infectious mononucleosis. The antibodies were found to react with a heat-stable antigen on sheep erythrocytes that is shared by ox (beef) erythrocytes but not by guinea-pig kidney (*i.e.,* they were non-Forssman in nature.)

The reasons for the development of heterophil antibodies in infectious mononucleosis are not clear, although it has been suggested that because the disease induces the formation in lymph nodes of lymphocytes and monocytes in increased numbers and abnormal forms and because lymphocytes may participate in the formation of globulin, this may be contributory. Agglutinins are usually observed within 2 weeks after the development of symptoms, lasting from 4 to 8 weeks and reaching maximal titers during the second and third weeks. The titer does not, in fact, correlate with the severity of the disease, and, because heterophil agglutinins appear in 50 to 80 per cent of cases of infectious mononucleosis, negative tests do not rule out the possibility of this infection.

SEROLOGIC TESTS FOR INFECTIOUS MONONUCLEOSIS

The Paul-Bunnell Test

Sheep erythrocytes carry an antigen associated with infectious mononucleosis, an antigen associated with serum sickness, and the Forssman antigen. The Paul-Bunnell test uses simple dilutions of patient's serum to which small amounts of sheep erythrocytes are added. Agglutination of the sheep cells is of limited value, however, because it reveals that one (or more) of the three types of antibodies mentioned is present in the test serum. The Paul-Bunnell test, therefore, is incapable of determining specificity and is only indicative of the presence or absence of heterophil antibodies. As a screening test, however, the test is useful, because it is simple and inexpensive, and, when negative results are obtained, it eliminates the need for further testing.

METHOD 1: THE PAUL–BUNNELL TEST FOR INFECTIOUS MONONUCLEOSIS (PRESUMPTIVE TEST [UNABSORBED])

Method

1. **Inactivate the patient's serum for 30 minutes at 56°C.**
2. **Prepare a 2 per cent suspension of washed sheep cells in normal saline (0.2 ml of packed cells and 9.8 ml of saline).**
3. **To a row of 10 test tubes (12 × 75 mm), add 0.4 ml of normal saline solution to the first tube and 0.25 ml of normal saline to each of the remaining 9 tubes.**
4. **Add 0.1 ml of patient's inactivated serum to tube 1, mix and transfer 0.25 ml to second tube 2, mix and transfer 0.25 ml to tube 3, repeating the transfer until the last tube is reached, and discard 0.25 ml.**
5. **Add 0.1 ml of 2 per cent sheep cell suspension to each tube. Shake the tubes thoroughly. In-**

cubate tubes for 1 hour at 37°C or at room temperature overnight.

6. Centrifuge for 1 minute at 1500 rpm.
7. Read macroscopically after gently shaking the tubes to resuspend the red cell sediment. Viewing with a low-power objective of the microscope is permissible.

Interpretation

A titer of 112 (*i.e.*, visible reaction at a 1:112 dilution; tube 5) or higher may be considered as a positive routine presumptive test in the presence of clinical and/or cytologic findings suggestive of infectious mononucleosis.

The Davidsohn Differential Test

Davidsohn (1937) designed a classic differential test to distinguish between heterophil sheep cell agglutinins in human serum due to Forssman antigen, serum sickness, and infectious mononucleosis. The principle of the test is based on the fact that some of the antigens that cause agglutination of sheep erythrocytes are carried on ox (beef) erythrocytes but not on the kidney cells of the guinea pig: therefore, exposure of the test serum to both guinea-pig kidney cells and ox (beef) erythrocytes causes absorption of either one or both of these antibodies. The absorbed agglutinins can be removed by centrifugation and aspiration of the resultant fluid, which is then tested with sheep erythrocytes. The actions of the two antigens in their absorption patterns are shown in Table 11–1.

METHOD 2: THE DAVIDSOHN DIFFERENTIAL TEST

Note: Beef cells and guinea-pig cells for this test are available from Baltimore Biologicals, Cockeysville, Maryland and from Difco Laboratories, Detroit, Michigan.

Materials

1. Test serum—inactivated at 56°C for 30 minutes
2. Diluent—0.85 per cent normal saline

3. Red cells—2 per cent suspension of sheep erythrocytes in saline. Cells should be between 24 hours and 1 week old.
4. Beef cells—20 per cent beef erythrocytes
5. Guinea-pig cells—20 per cent suspension of guinea-pig kidney cells
6. Test tubes—10 × 75 mm (round bottomed)
7. Positive and negative controls

Method

1. Place 1.0 ml of beef cells and 1.0 ml of guinea-pig cells into each of two test tubes.
2. Add 0.2 ml of test serum to each tube and shake.
3. Place at room temperature for 5 minutes, shaking periodically to bring the cells back into suspension.
4. Centrifuge at 1500 rpm for 10 minutes.
5. Carefully remove 0.25 ml of clear supernatant fluid from each tube, and place into separate tubes (marked 1 and 2, respectively).
6. Place tube 1 and tube 2 in row 1 and row 2, respectively, of a test tube rack.
7. Place seven additional tubes in each row.
8. Add 0.25 ml of diluent to each tube.
9. With a clean pipet, mix the contents of tube 1 and transfer 0.25 ml to tube 2 of row 1. Mix and transfer 0.25 ml from tube 2 to tube 3. Continue this process to tube 8, and discard 0.25 ml of the final dilution in tube 8. Repeat this step for row 2.
10. Add 0.1 ml of sheep erythrocytes to each tube.
11. Shake and leave at room temperature for 2 hours.
12. Read and record results.

Interpretation

The titer is recorded as the reciprocal of the highest dilution showing agglutination. Interpret the results of the tests as follows:

Infectious Mononucleosis

1. The titer of the Paul-Bunnell test is 1:56 or higher.
2. The titer in row 1 is reduced more than eightfold.
3. The titer in row 2 is reduced more than fourfold.

Serum Sickness

1. The titer of the Paul-Bunnell test is 1:56 or higher.
2. The titer in row 1 is reduced more than eightfold.
3. The titer in row 2 is reduced more than eightfold.

Table 11–1. ABSORPTION PATTERNS IN DAVIDSOHN DIFFERENTIAL TEST

Type of Heterophil Antibody	Absorbed by Guinea-Pig Kidney Cells	Absorbed by Beef Erythrocytes
Forssman	yes	no
Infectious mononucleosis	no	yes
Serum sickness	yes	yes

Forssman Antigen

1. **The titer of the Paul-Bunnell test is 1:56 or higher.**
2. **The titer in row 1 is not reduced.**
3. **The titer in row 2 is reduced more than eight-fold.**

Note: Positive and negative infectious mononucleosis serum controls should give the appropriate reactions when tested in parallel with the test. Results should not be considered valid unless controls give the expected results (see Table 11–1).

Rapid Differential Slide Tests (Spot Tests)

A number of rapid tests have been developed for which many commercial houses provide kits. These procedures can be divided into two main categories: those using papain-treated sheep erythrocytes, and those using horse erythrocytes.

The procedure using papain-treated sheep erythrocytes is based on Wallner's discovery that when papain is added to sheep erythrocytes, the receptors for the antibodies of infectious mononucleosis are specifically inactivated. The diagnosis of infectious mononucleosis is achieved in this test by testing the suspect serum with native as well as papain-treated sheep erythrocytes. Interpretation is as shown in Table 11–2.

Horse erythrocytes are used as an indicator in a rapid specific test for infectious mononucleosis. The test involves two stages: absorption of sera with guinea-pig kidney and with ox cells, followed by reaction with horse erythrocytes. The ox cells contain heterophil antigen to infectious mononucleosis but do not contain the Forssman antigen. Agglutination with the horse erythrocytes and the serum absorbed with guinea-pig kidney, therefore, indicates a positive reaction. The test is marketed under the name Monospot (Ortho Pharmaceuticals, Raritan, New Jersey). It is considered convenient because it is all performed on a glass slide,

and the agglutination occurs within minutes. It should be noted, however, that false-positive results with the Monospot test have been reported in patients with pancreatic carcinoma, rubella, and rheumatoid arthritis. The test can also be used to distinguish serum sickness from infectious mononucleosis.

Commercially produced kits for the rapid diagnosis of infectious mononucleosis include:

Bacto-Hetrol Slide Test (Difco)
Monostate (Colab)
Monotest (Wampole)
Heterocyte (Oxford)
Monosticon (Organon)
Monospot (Ortho)

Ox Cell Hemolysin Test

The ox cell hemolysin test detects the antibodies developed in the serum of patients with infectious mononucleosis. It is considered to be more sensitive than the sheep cell heterophil agglutination tests and is equal in specificity.

METHOD 3: THE OX CELL HEMOLYSIN TEST

Materials

1. **Preserved ox cells (Hyland Laboratories, Los Angeles, California). These are prepared by adding sterile ox blood to a modified Alsever's solution. Care should be taken not to contaminate the contents of the bottle. Store the cells at 5°C when not in use. When these precautions are observed, the cells should remain relatively free of hemolysin and should give satisfactory results for at least 10 weeks.**
2. **Infectious Mononucleosis Positive Control Serum (Hyland Laboratories, Los Angeles, California). This preparation is assayed for both sheep cell heterophil agglutinin and ox cell hemolysin titer and may be used as a control on technique in performing the test.**
3. **Saline. The saline solution used throughout the test is 0.85 per cent NaCl containing 0.1 gm $MgSO_4$.**
4. **56°C incubator**
5. **37°C incubator**
6. **Guinea-pig complement**
7. **Test tubes (10 × 75 mm)**
8. **Graduated pipets**
9. **Centrifuge**

Method

1. **Inactivate the patient's serum for 30 minutes at 56°C.**

Table 11–2. INTERPRETATION OF RAPID DIFFERENTIAL SLIDE TESTS USING NATIVE AND PAPAIN–TREATED SHEEP ERYTHROCYTES

Serum	Native Sheep Cells	Papain-Treated Sheep Cells
Normal serum (greater than 1:64) Infectious mononucleosis serum	Agglutination	No agglutination (occasional weak or late clumping)
Serum sickness or other heterophil antibodies	Agglutination	Agglutination (clump before N-cells)

Table 11–3. PROTOCOL FOR OX CELL HEMOLYSIN TITRATION

| | Tube No. | | | | | | | | | |
| | 1 | 2 | 3 | 4 | 5 | 6 | 7 | 8 | 9 | 10 |
										(Controls)
Serum	0.2 ml	*	*	*	*	*	*	*	0.1 ml	—
Saline	0.8 ml	0.5 ml	0.5 ml	0.5 ml	0.5 ml	0.5 ml	0.5 ml	0.5 ml	0.9 ml	0.5 ml
Resulting serum dilutions	1:5	1:10	1:20	1:40	1:80	1:160	1:320	1:640	1:10	—
Complement (1:15 dilution)	0.5 ml	0.5 ml	0.5 ml	0.5 ml	0.5 ml	0.5 ml	0.5 ml	0.5 ml	—	0.5 ml
2% ox cell suspension	0.5 ml	0.5 ml	0.5 ml	0.5 ml	0.5 ml	0.5 ml	0.5 ml	0.5 ml	0.5 ml	0.5 ml
Final serum dilution	1:15	1:30	1:60	1:120	1:240	1:480	1:960	1:1920	1:15	—
Titer	15	30	60	120	250	480	960	1920	—	—

*Serially transfer 0.5 ml of mixture from each preceding tube. Discard 0.5 ml from tube No. 8.

2. **Wash preserved ox cells three times, and prepare a 2 per cent suspension in saline.**
3. **Prepare a 1:15 dilution of complement.**
4. **Make dilutions of inactivated serum in a series of eight test tubes (10 × 75 mm) after placing 0.8 ml of saline in the first tube and 0.5 ml in the remaining tubes. Pipette 0.2 ml of serum into tube 1, mix, and transfer 0.5 ml to tube 2. Continue making serial dilutions through tube 8, and discard 0.5 ml from the final tube.**
5. **Add 0.5 ml of diluted complement and 0.5 ml of 2 per cent ox cell suspension to each tube. Shake the tubes well to ensure proper mixing.**
6. **Prepare two control tubes. In the first (tube 9), place 0.1 ml of inactivated serum, 0.9 ml of saline, and 0.5 ml of 2 per cent ox cell suspension. In the second (tube 10), place 0.5 ml of saline, 0.5 ml of diluted complement, and 0.5 ml of 2 per cent of ox cell suspension.**
7. **The protocol for ox cell hemolysin titration is given in Table 11–3.**
8. **Incubate the tubes at 37°C for 15 minutes, and centrifuge them at 2,000 rpm for 15 minutes.**
9. **Observe for hemolysis. The titer of the serum is the reciprocal of the highest dilution showing 50 per cent hemolysis. Reading of the end point is made by comparing tubes with a 50 per cent hemolysis standard prepared by adding 0.25 ml of the 2 per cent ox cell suspension to 1.25 ml of distilled water.**

Interpretation

A titer of 480 or above is considered significant in a presumptive diagnosis of infectious mononucleosis.

REVIEW QUESTIONS

MULTIPLE CHOICE

Choose the phrase, sentence, or symbol that completes the statement or answers the question. More than one answer may be correct in each case. Answers are given at the back of this book.

1. Infectious mononucleosis is a self-limiting disease caused by:
   (a) a virus
   (b) a bacterium
   (c) a fungus
   (d) EBV
   (Introduction)

2. The Epstein-Barr virus is:
   (a) a single-stranded RNA virus
   (b) a double-stranded RNA virus
   (c) a single-stranded DNA virus
   (d) a double-stranded DNA virus
   (The Epstein-Barr Virus)

3. The Epstein-Barr virus may be transmitted by:
   (a) blood transfusions
   (b) saliva
   (c) indirect contact
   (d) all of the above
   (The Epstein-Barr Virus)

4. Antibodies to the Epstein-Barr virus are found in:
   (a) 10 per cent of healthy adults
   (b) 50 per cent of healthy adults
   (c) 20 to 30 per cent of healthy adults
   (d) 80 to 90 per cent of healthy adults
   (The Epstein-Barr Virus)

5. Some of the characteristics of infectious mononucleosis include:
   (a) mild hepatitis
   (b) enlarged lymph nodes
   (c) the presence of Downey cells
   (d) the presence of heterophil antibodies
   (Characteristics)

6. The Forssman antigen is found in:
   (a) some bacteria
   (b) sheep
   (c) cows
   (d) *Clostridium welchii*
   (Heterophil Antibodies—Description)

7. Heterophil systems can be put to limited diagnostic use in some cases of:
   (a) infectious mononucleosis
   (b) typhus
   (c) primary atypical pneumonia
   (d) serum sickness
   (Heterophil Antibodies—Description)

8. Heterophil antibodies in infectious mononucleosis:
   (a) are usually observed within 2 weeks after the development of symptoms
   (b) are usually observed from 4 to 8 weeks after the development of symptoms
   (c) reach their maximal titers during the second and third weeks after the development of symptoms
   (d) are Forssman in nature
   (Heterophil Antibodies in Infectious Mononucleosis)

9. The Paul-Bunnell test for infectious mononucleosis:
   (a) uses small amounts of sheep erythrocytes
   (b) is capable of determining heterophil antibody specificity
   (c) is incapable of determining heterophil antibody specificity
   (d) is primarily useful as a screening test
   (The Paul-Bunnell Test)

10. The Davidsohn differential test for infectious mononucleosis:
    (a) can distinguish between heterophil sheep cell agglutinins in human serum due to Forssman antigen, serum sickness, and infectious mononucleosis
    (b) uses sheep erythrocytes and guinea-pig kidney cells
    (c) uses beef cells and guinea-pig kidney cells
    (d) is useful as a screening test for infectious mononucleosis only
    (The Davidsohn Differential Test)

ANSWER "TRUE" OR "FALSE"

11. Infectious mononucleosis may be confused with similar more serious diseases such as diphtheria, pharyngitis, Vincent's angina, lymphadenitis with scarlet fever, hepatitis, or pertussis.
    (Introduction)

12. The Epstein-Barr virus belongs to the family Herpetoviridae.
    (The Epstein-Barr Virus)

13. The Epstein-Barr virus is only associated with infectious mononucleosis and not with any other diseases.
    (The Epstein-Barr Virus)

14. In cases of infectious mononucleosis, enlarged lymphocytes with atypical nuclei (*i.e.,* "Downey cells") usually appear in the serum prior to the development of heterophil antibodies.
    (Characteristics)

15. "Forssman antigen" is a general term referring to all heterophil systems.
    (Heterophil Antibodies—Description)

16. Heterophil antibodies appear in 50 to 80 per cent of cases of infectious mononucleosis.
    (Heterophil Antibodies in Infectious Mononucleosis)

General References

Alba's Medical Technology, 9th ed. Anaheim, CA, Berkeley Scientific Publications, 1980.
Bennington, J. L. (Ed.): Saunders Dictionary and Encyclopedia of Laboratory Medicine and Technology. Philadelphia, W. B. Saunders Company, 1984.
Braude, A. I. (Ed.): Medical Microbiology and Infectious Diseases. Philadelphia, W. B. Saunders Company, 1981.
Widmann, F. K.: Clinical Interpretation of Laboratory Tests, 9th ed. Philadelphia, F. A. Davis Co., 1983.

TWELVE

AUTOIMMUNE DISEASES

OBJECTIVES

The student shall know, understand, and be prepared to explain:

1. The classification and characteristics of autoimmune diseases
2. The possible mechanisms in the initiation of autoimmune diseases
3. The criteria for autoimmune diseases
4. Genetic control of autoimmune diseases
5. The systemic autoimmune diseases, including:
   a. Systemic lupus erythematosus (characteristics, laboratory observations, etiology, serologic tests)
   b. Rheumatoid arthritis (characteristics of the disease, characteristics of rheumatoid factors, serologic tests)
   c. Ankylosing spondylitis
   d. Necrotizing angiitis (vasculitis)
   e. Polymyositis and dermatomyositis
   f. Progressive systemic sclerosis (scleroderma)
   g. Mixed connective tissue disease
   h. Sjögren's syndrome
6. The organ-specific autoimmune diseases, including:
   a. Autoimmune diseases of the blood (autoimmune hemolytic anemias, autoimmune thrombocytopenic purpura, neutropenia, lymphocytopenia, autoimmune aplastic anemia)
   b. Autoimmune diseases of the kidney (Types I, II, III, IV, and other forms)
   c. Autoimmune diseases of the endocrine organs (*i.e.,* thyroid, pancreas, adrenal, and parathyroid glands, including autoimmune thyroiditis (Hashimoto's thyroiditis), myxedema, thyrotoxicosis (Graves' disease)
   d. Autoimmune diseases of the nervous system (disseminated encephalomyelitis, idiopathic polyneuritis, Landry's paralysis, multiple sclerosis)
   e. Autoimmune diseases of the stomach and intestines (pernicious anemia, gastric atrophy, regional ileitis, ulcerative colitis, gluten-sensitive enteropathy)
   f. Autoimmune diseases of the liver (hepatitis, drug-induced liver diseases, primary biliary cirrhosis, portal cirrhosis)
   g. Autoimmune diseases of the muscle
   h. Autoimmune diseases of the eye
   i. Autoimmune diseases of the skin (pemphigus vulgaris, bullous pemphigoid, dermitis herpetiformis, systemic lupus erythematosus)
   j. Other autoimmune diseases (allergic architis, autoimmune diseases affecting the heart)

Introduction

In most individuals, there exists a tolerance and "self-recognition" of all body components; that is, normal individuals do not produce destructive responses to their own tissue antigens. In a minority of the population, however, disorders occur in which tissue injury is primarily caused by an apparent immunologic reaction of the host to his own tissues; these disorders are known as *autoimmune diseases*.

It should be noted that the terms *autoimmune disease* and *autoimmune response,* often used synonymously, do not refer to the same thing. In *autoimmune response*, an autoantibody directed against a "self" antigen can be demonstrated with respect to either erythrocytes or lymphocytes. The autoimmune response, although usually considered to be abnormal, often does not result in disease and frequently occurs in otherwise healthy individuals (*e.g.,* T-agglutinin, anti-I cold autoantibody, and antibodies to smooth muscle). Although it is thought that autoimmune diseases result from tissue injury by autoimmune responses, it is not known whether the autoimmune phenomena are a cause, a result, or an accompanying finding in autoimmune disease. It is common, for example, to see autoimmune phenomena in association with infectious diseases (*e.g.,* cold hemagglutinins in infection with *Mycoplasma pneumoniae*), yet there is no evidence that this response results in self-perpetuating protracted autoimmune disease.

POSSIBLE MECHANISMS IN THE INITIATION OF AUTOIMMUNE DISEASES

The precise mechanisms that initiate autoimmune diseases are not known, but several theories have been proposed:

Forbidden Clone Theory: The forbidden clone theory postulates a clone (*i.e.,* the progeny of a single cell) of changed or altered lymphocytes arising through cell mutation. Mutant cells carrying a foreign surface antigen would be destroyed by normal lymphocytes; mutant cells lacking foreign surface antigen would not be destroyed by normal lymphocytes. With the proliferation of these antigen-deficient mutants (so-called forbidden clones), these cells, because of genetic dissimilarity, would be capable of reacting with target tissues. The mutations responsible could occur at the level of the macrophage, T- or B-lymphocytes, or their progenitor cells.

Altered Antigen Theory: In addition to mutation (described previously), altered surface antigens (neoantigens) can be created by chemical, physical, or biologic means, possibly resulting in an autoimmune disease when a portion of the immune response is directed against the altered antigen. Altered antigens can be formed by autocoupling haptens, through physical forces (*e.g.,* visible and ultraviolet light, pressure, and cold), which cause the molecule to expose or create a new antigenic determinant, or through photosensitization.

Sequestered Antigen Theory: The sequestered antigen theory proposes that certain antigens are "hidden" (sequestered) in the circulation under conditions of normal health. The antigens often grouped as sequestered include lens proteins of the eye, milk casein antigens of the reproductive system (especially of the male), thyroglobulin, and so on. Exposure of the sequestered antigen to the lymphoreticular system in later life through trauma or infection results in autoimmune disease.

Immunologic Deficiency Theory: The concept of immunologic deficiency is based on a loss or deficiency of immunoregulation. The fact that T-helper and T-suppressor cells have pronounced effects on B-cells and certain T-cell subsets is now well recognized. This would suggest that a total or partial functional loss of these cells would result in diminished suppressor cell activities, reflected in heightened immunoglobulin levels or T-cell responses. Normal individuals, therefore, who develop autoimmune disease have an underlying immune deficiency that renders them susceptible to autoimmune states.

Loss of immunoregulation can be compared with loss of "tolerance." During embryonic life, antigens exposed to the lymphoreticular system (*i.e.,* prior to the time of immunologic maturation) are recognized as "self," whereas antigens not exposed to the lymphoreticular system during this time are regarded as "nonself." The body is "tolerant" of self antigens (*i.e.,* does not react immunologically to them) and "intolerant" of nonself antigens. The continued presence of self antigens ensures continued tolerance; however, mutation or the loss of immunoregulatory powers results in the condition in which self antigens behave as foreign antigens; this results in autoimmune disease.

The Cross-Reactive Antigen Theory: The cross-reactive antigen theory proposes that, because of the size of antigenic determinants, it is possible that complex foreign structures could possess structural parts that are similar or identical to self-structures, resulting in immunologic cross-reactivity. This cross-reactivity may, in certain circumstances, be sufficient to initiate autoimmune disease.

CRITERIA FOR AUTOIMMUNE DISEASES

Many different diseases are associated with autoimmune phenomena. These diseases can be *systemic* (involving more than one organ) or *organ-*

specific (in which the major effect involves a single organ).

With respect to these diseases, it is not always easy to determine whether the involved autoantibodies are merely associated with the disease or whether they play a central role in the cause. Certain criteria were devised by Koch (known as Koch's postulates) and by Witebsky to aid in this determination:

1. The autoimmune response must be regularly associated with the disease.
2. It must be possible to induce a replica of the disease in laboratory animals.
3. The immunopathologic changes observed in the natural and experimental diseases should parallel each other.
4. It should be possible to transfer the autoimmune illness from the diseased individual to a normal recipient through the transfer of serum or lymphoid cells.

In applying these criteria, it becomes clear that in certain of these diseases, the autoantibodies seem not to have any role in the origin or continuation of the disease and only serve as a convenient diagnostic support. In other diseases, any conclusion regarding the relationship of the immunologic phenomenon to the disease etiology is not possible with certainty, and, therefore, it can only be stated that autoantibodies are often associated with the disease.

GENETIC CONTROL OF AUTOIMMUNE DISEASES

Any hypothesis seeking to explain the development of the autoimmune state must recognize the genetic control of the immune system. It is well documented that certain immune disorders are characterized by predominance in the female and in families. The immune response gene is closely linked to the human leukocyte antigen (HLA) loci on chromosome number 6.

There are two approaches to determine whether an autoimmune disease is a genetic trait: family studies and population studies. A link between the disease and HLA is suggested when family members with a presumed autoimmune disease are found to share common HLA haplotypes. In cases in which family studies are not possible (due to death or where the family is small), population studies must be used. In this latter approach, antigen frequencies among large groups of patients with a specific illness are compared with those of a healthy group.

The autoimmune disease with the highest relative risk (the criteria for HLA-disease relationship) is ankylosing spondylitis. In this disease, the HLA-B27 antigen yields a relative risk of approximately 90 per cent. Other diseases showing varying levels of risk are given in Table 12–1.

SYSTEMIC AUTOIMMUNE DISEASES

Systemic Lupus Erythematosus

The autoimmune disease for which the most information is available is systemic lupus erythematosus (SLE), a disease of the connective tissue occurring primarily in women and having a strong hereditary tendency. The clinical differences between SLE and rheumatoid arthritis (discussed later in this chapter) are few, and the dividing line between the two would be difficult to draw.

Characteristics

Systemic lupus erythematosus is a generalized disorder that expresses itself as a vasculitis (*i.e.,* inflammation of a vessel), usually involving many organ systems. The disease affects females six to nine times more frequently than males and occurs primarily in young adults between the ages of 20

Table 12–1. RELATIONSHIP OF HLA AND AUTOIMMUNE DISEASES

Disease	Associated HLA Antigen	Patients Possessing Antigen (%)	Control Subjects Possessing Antigen (%)	Relative Risk
Ankylosing spondylitis	B27	79–100	4–13	90
Addison's disease	B8	20–69	18–24	1–7
Reiter's syndrome	B27	65–100	4–14	36
Graves' disease	B8	25–47	16–27	1.8–2.4
Yersinia arthritis	B27	58–78	9–14	18
Salmonella arthritis	B27	60–69	8–10	18
Sjögren's syndrome	Dw3	68–69	10–24	8–16
Adult rheumatoid arthritis	Dw4	38–65	18–31	4.4
Autoimmune thyroiditis	Bw35	63–73	9–14	16.8
Anterior uveitis	B27	37–58	7–10	9.4
MG	B8	38–65	13–18	4.4
Multiple sclerosis (MS)	B7	12–46	14–30	1.7

Modified from Barrett, J. T.: Textbook of Immunology, 4th ed. St. Louis, The C. V. Mosby Co., 1983.

and 40 years. The disease commonly manifests itself by skin lesions, usually in the form of a red rash across the nose and upper cheeks, the characteristic from which the disease gets it name (*lupus erythematosus,* the red wolf). More serious internal lesions involve the kidney, blood vessels, blood cells, and heart. In addition, there may be joint pain affecting several joints bilaterally. At least 50 per cent of patients have central nervous system involvement, arising from direct inflammation of the cerebral vessels or from the hypertension often found in these individuals. Widespread infarction of cerebral tissue may also be found, and SLE may present clinically as a seizure disorder or a psychiatric disturbance. The kidneys are involved in about 40 per cent of the cases, yet, in spite of this comparatively low percentage, the resultant decrease in kidney function is the primary cause of death in severe SLE.

There is no cure for SLE; however, steroids and immunosuppressive drugs are often helpful in controlling its course.

Laboratory Observations

Several immunologic phenomena are associated with SLE. The most striking feature of the disease, from a laboratory standpoint, is the appearance in the serum of numerous globulins with the properties of antibodies that are directed against various cell nuclei (anti-nuclear antibodies [ANA]). These

are usually IgG, but they may be IgM or IgA. Because of these anti-nuclear factors, patients with SLE may have false-positive serologic tests for syphilis (Wassermann reaction and Kahn flocculation test), hemolytic anemia with a positive antiglobulin test for antibody to red cell antigen, leukopenia, and thrombocytopenia.

The most relevant laboratory observation in SLE, however, is the lupus erythematosus (LE) cell phenomenon. This was first described in 1948 by Hargreaves, who detected unusual cells in the serum of SLE patients. The LE cell is a polymorphonuclear leukocyte found in the bone marrow and peripheral blood of patients with SLE, which is characterized by the presence of a homogeneous, cytoplasmic mass that often fills the cytoplasm of the phagocyte (Fig. 12–1). This mass (known as the LE body) is not always engulfed by the phagocyte and occasionally can be seen free in stained blood films (shown in Fig. 12–1). Often, free LE bodies that are not engulfed are surrounded by viable neutrophils, producing a rosette formation (Fig. 12–1). These viable phagocytes are apparently in competition with one another for phagocytosis of the deranged LE nucleus.

The development of these structures has been revealed by mixing the serum from an SLE patient with normal whole blood and then observing the changes using microcinematography. In these experiments, the nuclei of certain white blood cells lyse first, becoming homogeneous, and then swell

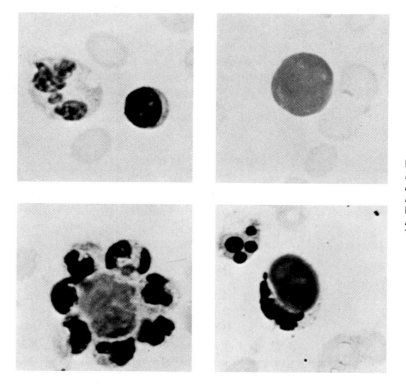

Figure 12–1. The LE cell phenomenon. *Upper left,* a normal neutrophil and lymphocyte; *upper right,* a free LE body; *lower left,* a rosette; and *lower right,* a single LE cell. (From Anderson, J. R., Buchannan, W. W., and Goudie, R. B.: Autoimmunity. Springfield, IL, Charles C Thomas, 1967.)

to as much as three or four times their normal size. The cells lose their dark staining quality, becoming paler and spherical. Those phagocytes that are unaffected approach the LE body (producing the rosette formation), strip away its cytoplasm, and engulf it. This final cell, the polymorphonuclear leukocyte with the lysed nucleus as an inclusion body, is an LE cell.

The LE *factor* (which is responsible for these changes) is a 7S IgG antibody, which reacts with deoxyribonucleoprotein (*i.e.,* anti-DNA) and complement, attaching to the nuclei from any source in agreement with the known nonspecificity of anti-DNA antibody. The LE factor is found in more than 95 per cent of SLE patients and in less than 4 per cent of normal individuals. It should be noted, however, that the LE factor is not specific as an indicator of SLE; it is also present (as are LE cells) in the serum of patients suffering from certain other autoimmune diseases (*e.g.,* rheumatoid arthritis, scleroderma, and polydermatomyositis).

Several different specifications of ANA have been found in patients suffering from SLE, mostly revealed through the use of fluorescent ANA techniques, which include antibodies to DNA, DNA-histone, RNA, and ENA (extractable nuclear antigen). ENA is known to be a mixture of several acidic antigens, few of which have been characterized chemically other than for the presence of dsDNA, dsRNA, ssDNA (or ssRNA), and protein. Certain ENAs (notably SM and MA antigens) appear to have a high degree of specificity for SLE.

Other antibodies found in SLE patients react with nRNP (nuclear ribonucleoprotein); PCNA (proliferating cell nuclear antigen); the Sjögren's syndrome antigens, SS-A and SS-B; the histone antigens, H1, H3, and H4; and others.

These autoantibodies do not cause tissue damage *directly;* tissue damage is triggered by the *depositing* of antigen-antibody *complexes* in the capillaries of affected organs. The removal of these complexes in the kidney accounts for the glomerulonephritis characteristic of the disease. The deposition of these complexes activates complement, leading to tissue destruction. As a result of this complement activation, about 75 per cent of SLE patients develop hypocomplementemia. The extensive antibody production results in hypergammaglobulinemia (an excess of gamma globulin), which is characteristic of many autoimmune diseases.

Etiology

In general, SLE arises spontaneously, caused by the formation of antibodies against the body's own tissues, probably due to a loss of Ts cells. This theory is supported by the success of immunosup-

pressive treatment. In some cases SLE may be induced by certain drugs (*e.g.,* hydralazine, penicillin, oral contraceptives and procainamide). Although this form of the disease may appear within a few weeks after the initiation of therapy, a prodromal period of several months is more common. The condition is usually reversible by discontinuance of the drug.

In individuals who are genetically predisposed to the disease (an association with HLA-B8 has been reported), viral infections are thought to be an important etiologic factor.

Serologic Tests

The laboratory tests for SLE involve two main procedures: the demonstration of the LE cell, and the detection of ANA. Although both procedures are discussed here, it should be noted that the LE test is no longer widely used because, although LE cell formation is a useful diagnostic aid when *positive,* many patients produce negative tests because of the difficulty in performing and interpreting these tests. For this reason, fluorescent antinuclear antibody (FANA) and other ANA tests have supplemented LE cell procedures.

FANA in the sera of SLE patients is identified by the indirect fluorescent antibody procedure. It should be noted, however, that the LE cell factor is only one of the *variety* of ANA that are directed against many nuclear antigens. These antibodies may be detected in 3 to 7 per cent of normal individuals (as well as about 40 per cent of elderly persons) and also as a result of inflammatory conditions, in 15 per cent of patients with rheumatoid arthritis, and (although usually at low titers), in some patients with chronic hepatitis, periarteritis nodosa, scleroderma, acute drug sensitivity, tuberculosis, lymphoma, and others. The detection of ANA, therefore, is not *diagnostic* of SLE; however, because these antibodies are so frequently found in patients with this disease, their absence can be used as a means of ruling out the disease.

There are several other methods that can be applied to the diagnosis of SLE, including methods for detecting antibodies to DNA and nucleoprotein, which include radioimmunoassay (RIA) and hemagglutination assays. Neither of these tests, however, is widely used in the clinical laboratory.

METHOD 1: INDIRECT FLUORESCENT ANTIBODY TEST FOR THE DETECTION OF ANTI–NUCLEAR ANTIBODIES IN HUMAN SERUM

An ANA Test Kit for qualitative and semiquantitative detection of ANA by the technique of indirect immunofluorescence is available from Meloy Laboratories Inc., Toronto, Canada. A similar test kit is available from Electro-Nucleonics Inc., Bethesda, Maryland. The following is a description of the use of the Meloy Test Kit.

Principle

Immunofluorescent techniques are used extensively to detect the presence of ANA activity in sera from patients with SLE and other connective tissue diseases. The indirect immunofluorescent assay is based on the use of fluorescein-conjugated antiglobulin. In the Meloy assay, a serum specimen or control is delivered into a well on a microscope slide containing a mouse liver substrate. If present, ANA will bind to nuclear antigens present in the nuclei of the liver sections. After a specific time, under controlled incubation conditions, the slide is carefully washed to remove nonspecific protein, and the antigen-antibody complexes are subsequently stained with fluorescein-conjugated antihuman globulins. A lattice or "sandwich" complex of nuclear antigen-human ANA and fluorescein-labeled antihuman globulins is thus formed. Several characteristic patterns of fluorescent staining emerge singly or in any combination. The most commonly encountered fluorescent staining patterns are homogeneous, peripheral, speckled, and nucleolar.

Reagents

1. **ANA Mouse Liver Substrate Slides:** These should be stored in the foil pouch at −20°C until ready for use. At the time of use, remove the required number of slides from the freezer (each slide contains 8 wells) and allow them to equilibrate to room temperature for 7 to 10 minutes. Carefully remove the slides by cutting the foil with scissors and lifting the foil away gently. The slides should not slide out of the foil pouch; this may cause the tissue to be dislodged.
2. **ANA Control Sera—Positive and Negative:** These should be stored at −20°C until first use, and thereafter at 2° to 5°C. They should not be refrozen. The prediluted control is ready for use when thawed.
3. **FITC Conjugate:** This should be stored at −20°C until first use, and thereafter at 2° to 5°C. Do not refreeze. The primary activity of FITC (fluorescein isothiocyanate–conjugated goat antihuman globulin), the conjugated antiserum, at its dilution is a reaction to human IgG. The reagent is prediluted and is ready for use when thawed.
4. **PBS Salts:** These should be stored either at

−20°C or at 2° to 5°C before reconstitution. Store at 2° to 5°C after reconstitution. One vial of PBS salts results in 1000 ml of reconstituted buffer (pH 7.0 ± 0.2). To reconstitute, place the PBS salts in a volumetric flask and bring to 1000 ml with distilled water. Mix thoroughly until salts are dissolved.
5. **Buffered Glycerol:** This should be stored at −20°C until first use and thereafter at 2° to 5°C. Do not refreeze. The kit contains 2 × 6.0 ml vials of buffered glycerol (pH 8.0). One per cent sodium azide is included as a preservative. The reagent is ready for use after thawing.

Precautions

1. **All human components have been tested by radioimmunoassay for hepatitis B surface antigen (HBsAg) and have been found to be negative. It should be noted, however, that this does not ensure the absence of HBsAg.**
2. **The sodium azide (0.1 per cent w/v) included in the reactive and nonreactive ingredients is toxic if ingested. It should also be noted that sodium azide may react with lead and copper plumbing to form highly explosive metal azides. If disposing of the agent through plumbing fixtures, flush with a large volume of water to prevent azide build-up.**
3. **Readings should be taken in the center of the substrate wells; avoid readings at the edge of the well.**
4. **Care should be taken that the wells are not subject to any abrasion.**
5. **Individual components in the kit are tested together to ensure compatibility; they should not be interchanged with components of kits that bear different lot numbers.**

Specimen Collection and Handling

The blood specimens for the test should be collected aseptically. Serum should be separated from the clot promptly to avoid hemolysis and should be stored between 2° and 5°C for analysis within 24 hours. If not tested within this time period, the sample should be stored frozen. Repeated freezing and thawing of the specimen should be avoided. Plasma may also be used and should be similarly stored.

Materials

The kit contains:
1. **10 ANA substrate slides**
2. **Positive ANA control serum**
3. **Negative ANA control serum**
4. **FITC antihuman globulin conjugate**
5. **Buffered glycerol**
6. **Phosphate buffered saline (PBS) salts**

Additional equipment required:

1. Fluorescent microscope with 250 × or greater capability
2. Magnetic stirring unit with bars
3. Coverslips—No. 1 glass coverslips
4. Staining dishes
5. Pasteur and serologic pipets
6. Squeeze bottle
7. Small test tubes with caps
8. 1000-ml volumetric flask
9. Distilled water

Method

1. **Slide preparation:** Remove the required number of slides from the freezer. Allow the slides to equilibrate to room temperature for at least 7 to 10 minutes. Remove from foil pouch by cutting with scissors.
2. **Sample application:**
   Screening Test: Dilute each patient's serum 1:20 with PBS. Save the undiluted sera for possible use in subsequent titration tests if positive screening test results are obtained.
   Titration Test: Sera found to be positive in the screening test should be titrated to end point. Prepare a fresh 1:20 dilution of each positive serum, then prepare serial twofold dilutions from this 1:20 dilution. Typically, sera strongly positive in the screening test should be assayed at serial dilutions ranging from 1:20 to 1:5120 in the titration test. Sera weakly positive in the screening test may be tested over the range of 1:20 to 1:640 dilutions.
3. Apply one drop (approximately 50 μL) of diluted patient sera to the wells, taking care not to overfill them. Include positive and negative control sera on each slide. Positive and negative control sera provided with the test kit are prediluted and should be applied without further dilution.
4. Incubate in a moist, covered chamber at room temperature for 30 minutes.
5. Hold the slide in a horizontal position, and tilt slightly toward you. Squirt the slide with PBS from a squeeze bottle back and forth between the wells to rinse sera off the bottom row of wells. Tilt the slide away from you, and repeat as above to wash off the top row of wells. Note: Do not aim directly at the wells. Wash in PBS for 5 minutes. Repeat the 5-minute wash with fresh PBS. (Note: Washing may be facilitated by placing the slides [up to four] upright against the sides of a staining dish containing 250 ml of PBS, adding a magnetic stirring bar and agitating on a magnetic stirrer. Thorough washing is essential to remove nonspecifically bound immunoglobulin, which may

subsequently bind fluorescein-conjugated antiglobulin to give a false-positive reaction).
6. Shake off the excess PBS, and apply prediluted conjugate to each well.
7. Incubate in a moist, covered chamber at room temperature for 30 minutes.
8. Squirt a light stream of PBS from a squeeze bottle above the wells as in step 5. Wash in PBS for 5 minutes. Repeat the 5-minute wash with fresh PBS.
9. Shake off excess PBS, and immediately apply one drop of buffered glycerol to each well.
10. Place a 24- × 50-mm coverslip over the glycerol saturated slide. Use only No. 1 glass coverslips for this purpose.
11. Examine for fluorescent nuclear reaction at a magnification of 250 × or greater. Slides should be read by fluorescent microscopy as soon as possible; however, they can be stored in the dark at 4°C for up to 48 hours prior to reading.
12. Sera positive in the screening test should be subsequently titrated to end point.

Interpretation

Note: Before reading, ensure that the positive and negative control results conform to the following specifications:

Negative Control: No green-gold fluorescence of greater than ± intensity.

Positive Control: Strong green-gold fluorescence of 3+ or greater intensity.

Negative Readings. In negative sera, the liver section nuclei contain no green-gold fluorescence.

Positive Readings. Results from the screening test should be recorded as positive or negative. The degree of fluorescence may be semiquantitated on a scale of 1+ to 4+. When titrating the serum, the end point should be considered as the highest dilution at which a definite fluorescent pattern may be distinguished. Positive samples show homogeneous, peripheral, speckled, or nucleolar fluorescence.

1. *Homogeneous (solid, diffuse):* The whole nucleus fluoresces evenly green-gold, although nonfluorescent vacuoles are sometimes seen.
2. *Peripheral (ring, membranous, shaggy, or thready):* This pattern is characterized by sharp green-gold fluorescence of the outer edge of the nucleus (nuclear membrane), with a gradually darkening inner border blending with a dark nuclear center.
3. *Speckled (mottled):* This pattern is characterized by numerous round speckles of green-gold nuclear fluorescence of various sizes against a dark background (giving the appearance of "pepper dots").

4. *Nucleolar:* This pattern is characterized by multiple round, smooth, green-gold fluorescing nucleoli of various sizes.

Note: Each laboratory should use its own judgment concerning the degree of fluorescence required for a positive test result. It is recommended that a panel of normal and abnormal sera be evaluated to determine a minimum fluorescent end point. If a minimum of 1+ reaction on a scale of 1+ to 4+ is considered positive, sera from apparently healthy individuals demonstrate negative results.

Limitations and Expected Values

The test system described should be interpreted keeping in mind the following:

1. ANA is a substance that has been shown to be present in several disease states and in some apparently normal individuals. The appearance of a positive ANA result, therefore, does not necessarily indicate a disease process. Further, data generated by this test should be reviewed in the framework of all available medical evidence.
2. Some positive reactions have been reported to be related to patients suffering from a connective tissue disease or in relatives of patients who may develop such a disease at a later stage. Various therapeutic agents have been shown to induce ANA in the serum of patients receiving these drugs.
3. Procainamide hydrochloride has been the most frequent and most accepted of the "systemic lupus erythematosus inducers" since 1965. After procainamide therapy, up to 50 per cent of patients develop ANA; however, most patients have remissions when the drug is discontinued. The following drugs have also been implicated as activators of SLE: aminosalicylic acid, diphenylhydantoin, griseofulvin, hydralazine, isoniazid, mephenytoin, methylthiouracil, penicillin, phenylbutazone, propylthiouracil, streptomycin, sulfate, sulfadimethoxine, sulfamethoxypyridazine, tetracycline, trimethadione, methyldopa, and ethosuximide.
4. In some patients, the ANA may not be detected if it is present as a complex with circulating antigen. Some evidence indicates its detection may occasionally be facilitated by treating the serum with the enzyme deoxyribonuclease (DNAse).
5. Sera shown to be positive at 1:20 should be titrated to end point. A homogeneous staining pattern may mask other fluorescent patterns. Upon titration of such sera, these other patterns may be observed.

Table 12–2. POSITIVE REACTIONS USING RECOMMENDED PROCEDURE FOR ANA IN SYSTEMIC LUPUS ERYTHEMATOSUS (SLE), PROGRESSIVE SYSTEMIC SCLEROSIS (PSS), AND RHEUMATOID ARTHRITIS (RA)

Titer	Normal Population	SLE	PSS	RA
Negative Tests				
1:10 (or lower)	96	1	4	15
Positive Tests				
1:20	0	0	2	0
1:49–1:80	0	2	4	4
1:160–1:320	0	4	3	1
1:640–1:1280	0	7	4	0
1:2560 (or higher)	0	6	0	0
Per cent positive	0	95	76	25

Expected values with this kit as prescribed with a 1:20 dilution of patient's serum are as follows:

1. The normal individual can be expected to give a negative reaction.
2. The patient population with SLE, progressive systemic sclerosis (PSS), and rheumatoid arthritis (RA) will give a positive test in approximately the same percentage as shown in the clinical survey in Table 12–2.

Note: Laboratory personnel are cautioned to consult and follow all manufacturer's recommended procedures for microscope and light source maintenance. It is further recommended that the laboratory maintain a log on lamp usage and change the bulb(s) after the elapsed usage time recommended by the manufacturer.

METHOD 2: THE LE TEST

Hyland's LE-test is a rapid slide test for the antinucleoprotein factors often found in SLE.

Materials

The materials for this test are available from Hyland Laboratories, Los Angeles, California, and include the following:

1. Latex-nucleoprotein reagent. This is prepared from polystyrene latex and deoxyribonucleoprotein obtained from calf thymus. This reagent has been standardized to give rapid and clear-cut reactions and can be used as a simple test for detection of the antinucleoprotein factors associated with SLE.
2. Positive control serum. This is obtained from patients with SLE.
3. Negative control. This is normal human serum.

Both reagent and control serums contain sodium azide 0.1 per cent as a preservative, but they should be stored at 2° to 10°C when not in use.

Method

1. **Resuspend the latex-nucleoprotein reagent thoroughly by gently shaking before use.**
2. **Using the capillary pipets provided, place one drop of the patient's serum in one of the ovals of the slide.**
3. **Add one drop of latex-nucleoprotein reagent. With a wooden applicator stick, mix and spread the reaction mixture completely over the area within the oval (approximately 20 × 40 mm).**
4. **From time to time, prepare positive and negative controls, each with one drop of appropriate LE-Test control serum and one drop of latex-nucleoprotein reagent. Use a separate capillary tube and slide for each mixture.**
5. **Tilt the slide slowly from side to side, and observe for macroscopic clumping. With a positive reaction, flocculation will be seen within 2 minutes.**

Rheumatoid Arthritis

Characteristics of the Disease

Rheumatoid arthritis (RA) is a chronic inflammatory disease, primarily affecting the joints and periarticular tissues. Although certain areas of the body show a particular susceptibility to inflammation, it appears likely that no body system or tissue is entirely exempt. Apart from the joints, the most commonly affected areas are other synovium-lined spaces such as tendon sheaths, the subcutaneous tissues at sites of pressure or friction, the heart and blood vessels, and the lungs. The highest incidence of the disease is in women between the ages of 20 and 40 years.

The pathologic changes during the disease process include a proliferation of a synovial membrane with the formation of granulation tissue that extends as a vascular "pannus" layer from the margin toward the center of the affected joint. The articular cartilage, too, gradually becomes replaced by fibrous granulation tissue; and focal collections of macrophages and lymphocytes are found in the synovial membrane, the joint capsule, and the periarticular tissues or in the form of subcutaneous nodules, which occur in approximately 20 per cent of patients and have a characteristic structure.

Other clinical manifestations of the disease include the following:

1. Hypochromatic anemia, often providing clear evidence of a hemolytic process without demonstrable erythrocyte abnormality.
2. Characteristic changes in the serum protein pattern.
3. Toxemia, demonstrated primarily by a considerably increased sedimentation rate of blood erythrocytes.
4. Generalized lymphadenopathy. Enlargement of the spleen and lymph nodes is occasionally seen, although in most cases of RA, the lymph node enlargement is restricted to nodes draining severely affected joints. A combination of anemia, arthritis, and splenomegaly is referred to as Felty's syndrome, although, in this disease, splenic enlargement is accompanied by other evidence of hypersplenism, and lymph node enlargement may be generalized. A similar state may occur in childhood in Still's disease, in which the spleen and lymph nodes are invariably enlarged. This disease, however, differs in so many of its clinical features from RA that it possibly represents a distinct entity.

Despite continued study of the disease throughout the world, the cause of RA remains unknown. An "autoimmune" etiology has received serious consideration for many years, yet convincing proof has not been forthcoming. It is generally accepted that the immunologic reactions (discussion follows) play an important, probably essential part in the pathogenesis of the disease, although the antigen(s) involved remain elusive.

Characteristics of Rheumatoid Factors

The clinical and histologic features of RA provide no more than suggestive evidence of immunologic involvement in the disease. A variety of immunologically oriented investigations, however, have provided more compelling evidence.

For more than 25 years, evidence has accumulated suggesting that several abnormal proteins circulate in the blood of patients with RA. These proteins, because of their obvious correlation with the disease, became collectively known as *rheumatoid factor* (RA factor). They are now generally accepted as a group of immunoglobulins that interact specifically with antigenic determinants on the IgG molecule (*i.e.*, *anti*-antibodies).

RA factor is characterized as a macroglobulin, or group of macroglobulins, with a sedimentation constant of 19S. The chemical, physical, and antigenic properties are very similar to those of the normal IgM class (although some patients with RA demonstrate RA factor of the same size as IgG [7S]; therefore, not *all* RA factor is in the form of macroglobulin). It is most probable that the antigenic determinants involved are actually present on the individual patient's own IgG molecules, and, therefore, the occurrence of such an antibody, an autoantibody, would lead to antigen-antibody reactions in the circulation. This indeed appears to be the case, and RA factors circulate in the blood as a complex, although some configurational alteration in the autoantigens from the native state may be necessary before the appropriate RA factors become detectable (Glynn, 1968, 1975). This complex has a sedimentation coefficient of approximately 22S and becomes dissociated with a change to acid pH, to 19S rheumatoid factor, and 7S normal immunoglobulin.

Rheumatoid factors can occur in nonrheumatoid individuals with chronic infective conditions (e.g., LE, infectious hepatitis, chronic hepatic disease, syphilis); likewise, animal homologues of these factors can be induced by repeated infection (Abruzzo and Christian, 1961). On the basis of these facts, the probable stimulus is the presence of IgG, configurationally changed by combination with antigen. The stimulus in cases of RA is presumably the same. It is interesting to note, however, that RA factors in chronic infective states virtually disappear when the infection is overcome by appropriate therapy, whereas in cases of RA, the RA factor persists indefinitely, providing evidence of a persistent infective agent or, alternatively, the persistence of another antigen whose combination with IgG constitutes an adequate stimulus.

The correlation between RA factor and the disease RA remains an intriguing, yet unsolved problem. Even if one accepts the autoantibody nature of RA factor, it does not obviously follow that any of the disease manifestations result from autoimmune processes. It is indeed possible that RA factors could be the *consequence* of infection with an *unrecognized agent* and are without any pathologic significance. Moreover, patients with various conditions, such as sarcoidosis, that are associated with hyperglobulinemia, may show high titers. Finally, RA may occur in patients with hypogammaglobulinemia; these patients lack detectable RA factor in their serum, as well as having very low levels of ordinary 7S gamma globulin.

Serological Tests

Tests for RA factors are designed to detect certain macroglobulins in the patient's serum that react with normal human IgG or normal animal IgG (i.e., RA factors). The majority of tests use particulate carriers (e.g., erythrocytes, latex and bentonite particles) that transform the reaction between RA factor and IgG into visible aggregation. In essence, all the tests are designed to detect antibody to immunoglobulin, but they are not identical, because sometimes human and sometimes animal immunoglobulin is used as the coating for the particles. In some circumstances, the different tests give different results; therefore, one can postulate

that a number of RA factors with different specificities are involved.

Included among the various serologic tests for the detection of RA factors are the latex fixation test (Singer and Plotz, 1965), the sheep cell agglutination test (Rose et al., 1948), the sensitized alligator erythrocyte test (Cohen et al., 1958), the bentonite flocculation test (Block and Bunim, 1959), and the concanavalin A and complement fixation test for the detection of IgG RA factor (Tanimoto et al., 1976).

Of these tests (with the exception of the last, which is specific for IgG RA factor), the latex fixation and the sheep cell agglutination tests are the most popular. A number of preparations for use in rapid slide tests are also available.

METHOD 1: THE LATEX–FIXATION TEST FOR RHEUMATOID FACTORS

Materials

1. **Test serum—The test serum need not be inactivated, although inactivated serum may be used.**
2. **Latex suspension—This is a standardized suspension of particles 0.81 μ in diameter, available from Difco Laboratories, Detroit, Michigan.**
3. **RA plasma fraction II—This is purified human IgG, available from Difco Laboratories, Detroit, Michigan.**
4. **RA buffer—This is an isotonic buffer with a pH of 8.2 when rehydrated, available from Difco Laboratories, Detroit, Michigan.**
5. **Test tubes—10 × 75 mm (round bottomed).**

Preparation of Antigen

1. **To determine the milliliters of buffer required, multiply the number of serum samples to be tested by three and add three (e.g., if 10 samples are to be tested, [10 × 3] + 3 = 33 ml of buffer).**
2. **Divide the number of milliliters of buffer required (e.g., 33) by 20 (1.65). This is the amount of RA plasma fraction II required.**
3. **Divide the number of milliliters of buffer required (e.g., 33) by 100 (0.33). This is the amount of latex suspension required.**
4. **In the example given above (i.e., with 10 samples), mix 33 ml of RA buffer with 1.65 ml of RA plasma fraction II and add 0.33 ml of latex suspension. This will be the "antigen" to use in the test.**

Method

1. **Set up three test tubes in a test tube rack for *each* test serum.**
2. **Add 1.9 ml of test serum in tube 1, mix and**

transfer 1.0 ml to tube 2, mix and transfer 1.0 ml to tube 3, and discard 1.0 ml from this tube.
3. Add 1.0 ml of the "antigen" (as previously prepared) to each tube.
4. Shake and incubate the tubes at 56°C for 2 hours.
5. Centrifuge at 2300 rpm for 4 minutes.
6. Read macroscopically for agglutination.

Interpretation

Any agglutination in tubes 2 and 3 is considered positive. The report will state "positive" or "negative"; no titer is reported.

Controls

1. Antigen control: 1.0 ml of RA buffer and 1.0 ml of antigen. This should give no agglutination.
2. Positive serum control: Using positive control serum (commercial), set up as with test serum. This should give agglutination in tubes 2 and 3.
3. Negative serum control: Using negative control serum (commercial), set up as with test serum. This should give no agglutination.

METHOD 2: THE SHEEP CELL AGGLUTINATION TEST FOR RHEUMATOID FACTORS

Materials

1. Test tubes—12 × 100 mm
2. Rabbit anti–sheep erythrocyte hemolysin (50 per cent glycerinated)
3. 2 per cent sheep erythrocytes
4. 0.85 per cent saline
5. Patient's serum—inactivated.

Estimation of the Minimal Hemagglutinating Dose (MHD)

1. Prepare the sheep erythrocytes by washing the cells three times with 0.85 per cent saline. After the third washing, centrifuge the cells for 10 minutes at 2500 rpm. Prepare a 2 per cent suspension.
2. Set up six test tubes. Place 0.5 ml of 0.85 per cent saline into tubes 2 through 6. Prepare a 1:100 dilution of anti-sheep erythrocyte hemolysin by adding 0.2 ml of 50 per cent glycerinated hemolysin to 9.8 ml of 0.85 per cent saline. Mix well and place 0.5 ml into tubes 1 and 2.
3. Mix the contents of tube 2 and transfer 0.5 ml to tube 3. Mix the contents of tube 3 and transfer 0.5 ml to tube 4. Continue mixing and transferring, and discard 0.5 ml from tube 6. The dilutions are 1:100 to 1:3200.
4. To each tube add 0.5 ml of 2 per cent sheep

erythrocytes and 1.0 ml of 0.85 per cent saline.
5. Mix the tubes and place in a 37°C water bath for 1 hour, followed by overnight incubation in the refrigerator at 2° to 4°C.
6. Observe for agglutination. The last tube in which agglutination is observed is the end point. The dilution of hemolysin in this tube corresponds to the agglutinating titer of the hemolytic serum (i.e., the MHD).

The Sensitization of Sheep Erythrocytes

1. Add one half MHD to an equal volume of 2 per cent sheep erythrocytes (e.g., if the MHD is 1:200, prepare a 1:400 dilution of anti-sheep erythrocyte hemolysin).
2. To a volume of 2 per cent sheep erythrocytes, add an equal volume of diluted hemolysin while constantly stirring. (The volume of sheep erythrocytes to be prepared will depend upon the number of tests to be performed.)
3. Incubate the suspension at room temperature for 45 to 60 minutes (for 10 minutes at 37°C followed by 30 minutes at room temperature). This now represents a 1 per cent suspension of sensitized erythrocytes.

Method

1. Collect a fasting blood specimen, allow to clot, and separate the serum.
2. Set up two sets of 10 test tubes (i.e., 20 tubes). Mark one set "sensitized" and the other set "unsensitized."
3. Place 0.9 ml of saline into the first tube of each set and 0.5 ml of saline into each of the remaining nine tubes of each set.
4. For each set, place 0.1 ml of the patient's serum into tube 1. Mix well and transfer 0.5 ml to tube 2. Continue mixing and transferring, and discard 0.5 ml from tube 9 of each set. The dilutions are 1:10 to 1:2560.
5. Place 0.5 ml of the 1 per cent suspension of sensitized sheep erythrocytes into each tube of the "sensitized" set. (The 1 per cent suspension is prepared by diluting the 2 per cent suspension 1:2 in saline).
6. Mix all tubes and incubate in a 37°C water bath for 1 hour, followed by overnight incubation in the refrigerator at 2° to 4°C.
7. Read for agglutination. The end point is the highest dilution of the serum giving at least a 1+ reaction. The results are expressed in terms of the geometric difference between serum titers with the "sensitized" and "unsensitized" erythrocytes. This "differential agglutination titer" (DAT) is calculated as follows:

$$DAT = \frac{\text{Serum titer with sensitized erythrocytes}}{\text{Serum titer with unsensitized erythrocytes}}$$

Interpretation

The DAT is reported in Rose units. A titer higher than 16 units is regarded as characteristic of sera from patients with RA.

Rapid Screening Tests for Rheumatoid Arthritis

Two test kits are in common use as rapid screening techniques for RA. These kits are provided by Wampole Laboratories, Cranbury, New Jersey, and are known as "Rheumatex" and "Rheumaton."

METHOD 3: THE 1–MINUTE LATEX AGGLUTINATION TEST FOR THE QUALITATIVE AND QUANTITATIVE DETERMINATION OF RHEUMATOID FACTOR IN SERUM (RHEUMATEX)

Specimen Collection and Preparation

Blood for this test should be collected aseptically by venepuncture into a clean tube without anticoagulant. The blood should be permitted to clot for at least 10 minutes at room temperature (20° to 25°C) before use. Rim the clot, and centrifuge at 1000 × g for 10 minutes or until the supernatant fluid is free of cells. No special preparation of the serum is required; however, specimens that are grossly hemolysed, that show gross lipemia or turbidity must not be used. (Note: Plasma must not be used for this test.)

If the specimen testing is delayed, the specimen should be stored refrigerated (2° to 8°C) for no longer than 24 hours. If the delay between the time that the specimen is collected and testing is longer than 24 hours, store the specimen frozen at −20°C. If the specimens are to be mailed, add sodium azide to a concentration of 0.1 per cent as a preservative. As with most biologic materials, repeated freezing and thawing should be avoided. If turbidity is apparent upon thawing, the specimen should be clarified by centrifugation prior to use.

Materials

The following materials are provided:
   Note: All materials must be stored in the refrigerator (2° to 8°C) when not in use. Do not freeze.

1. Rheumatex latex reagent (latex particles sensitized with human IgG)—contains buffer and preservative, 0.1 per cent sodium azide. Shake well before using.
2. Concentrated diluent 20 × (Glycine-saline buffer)—contains preservative; 0.1 per cent sodium azide. Dilute 1:20 with distilled water prior to use as required for assay.
3. Positive control (RA factor positive serum, human)—contains buffer, stabilizer, and preservative; 0.1 per cent sodium azide.
4. Negative control (RA factor negative serum, human)—contains buffer, stabilizer, and preservative; 0.1 per cent sodium azide.

The following materials are required but are not provided:

1. Stirrers
2. Conventional test tubes
3. Distilled water
4. Serologic pipets

Method

Note: The following precautions should be taken:

1. All reagents and specimens should be at room temperature prior to use.
2. Care should be taken to avoid contamination of reagents with each other or with the test specimens.
3. The latex reagent should be gently and well shaken prior to use. Expell the contents of the dropper, and refill.
4. The positive control and negative control should be run in parallel with the unknown specimen. Do not dilute the controls before testing.
5. Because traces of detergent or previous specimens may adversely affect the results, use only a thoroughly clean glass slide. Use only distilled water to clean the slide, and do not use detergent.
6. The results must be read at 1 minute; failure to do so may cause erroneous results.

Qualitative Procedure

1. Prepare a 1:20 working solution of the concentrated diluent with distilled water, as required.
2. Dilute specimen 1:20 with the prepared diluent. Place one drop (approximately 50 μL) of the diluted specimen on a section of the slide.
3. Place one drop of positive control on a section of the slide. On another section of the slide, place one drop of negative control.
4. Add one drop of well-shaken latex reagent to each section.
5. Mix each section separately. Use a new stirrer for each section.
6. Rock the slide back and forth gently and evenly for 1 minute at a rate of 8 to 10 times per minute.
7. Observe for agglutination *immediately* at 1 minute, using an indirect oblique light source.

Interpretation follows.

Quantitative Procedure

1. **Serum to be titrated should be serially diluted (1:20, 1:40, etc.) with prepared diluent. At least six more dilutions should be prepared.**
2. **Place one drop of each specimen dilution onto successive sections of the slide. Test each specimen dilution as described in the section entitled Qualitative Procedure, steps 4 through 7.**

Interpretation

Positive sera show readily visible agglutination. A weakly positive serum may show very fine granulation or partial clumping. Negative sera appear uniformly turbid.

In the quantitative procedure, the last dilution to show positive agglutination on the slide is taken as the RA factor titer. For example, if the 1:80 dilution of the specimen is positive while higher dilutions are negative, the titer is 1:80.*

Note: The qualitative test procedure described can also be performed using test tubes as follows:

Quantitative Tube Procedure
Materials
The following materials are required but are not provided:

1. **Test tubes—12 × 75 mm**
2. **37°C water bath**
3. **Centrifuge capable of 1000 × g**

Method

1. **Prepare a 1:20 working dilution of the concentrated diluent with distilled water as required.**
2. **Label 11 test tubes 1 through 11, and place them in a test tube rack.**
3. **Pipet 1.9 ml of prepared diluent into tube 1; 1.0 ml of prepared diluent into tubes 2 through 9, and 0.8 ml of prepared diluent into tubes 10 and 11.**
4. **Add 0.1 ml of specimen to tube 1. Mix and transfer 1.0 ml of this mixture to tube 2. Mix and transfer 1.0 ml of this mixture to tube 3. Continue serially diluting in this manner through tube 9. Discard 1.0 ml from tube 9. Pipet 0.2 ml of the positive control into tube 10**

Table 12–3. PREPARED DILUTIONS IN THE QUANTITATIVE TUBE PROCEDURE FOR THE DETECTION OF RHEUMATOID FACTOR IN SERUM

Tube No.	Dilution	Tube No.	Dilution
1	1:20	7	1:1280
2	1:40	8	1:2560
3	1:80	9	1:5120
4	1:160	10	Positive control
5	1:320	11	Negative control
6	1:640		

and 0.2 ml of the negative control into tube 11. The prepared dilutions are as shown in Table 12–3.
5. **Add one drop of well-shaken latex reagent to each tube.**
6. **Shake each tube, and incubate it for 15 minutes in a 37°C water bath.**
7. **Centrifuge the tubes at 1000 × g for 2 minutes.**
8. **Gently shake each tube until the sediment is dislodged from the bottom. Once the sediment is suspended, carefully tilt each tube back and forth until an even suspension is obtained. Do not use automatic mixing devices.**
9. **Examine all tubes for macroscopic agglutination against a dark background using an oblique light.**

Interpretation

The highest dilution at which agglutination can still be observed is considered the titer. If a secondary standard of the International Reference Preparation of Rheumatoid Arthritis Serum, such as Wampole's Rheumatoid Factor Reference Preparation is used, the results can be expressed in IU per ml, using the following equation:

When using RA factor latex tests, a titer of 80 or greater is generally considered a positive reaction, a titer of 20 or 40 is considered a weakly positive reaction, and, if there is no agglutination at 1:20, the specimen should be considered negative for RA factor, even if a subsequent dilution shows agglutination.*

Note: The tube dilution procedure is more sensitive than the slide procedure. Consequently, differences in the raw titers will be seen between the tube titration and slide procedures.

$$\text{IU RA factor/ml of specimen} = \frac{\text{IU/ml standard} \times \text{titer of specimen}}{\text{Titer of standard}}$$

---

*Reference: Rheumatex package insert. Wampole Laboratories, Cranbury, New Jersey.

*Reference: Rheumatex package insert. Wampole Laboratories, Cranbury, New Jersey.

METHOD 4: THE 2–MINUTE HEMAGGLUTINATION SLIDE TEST FOR THE QUALITATIVE AND QUANTITATIVE DETERMINATION OF RHEUMATOID FACTOR IN SERUM OR SYNOVIAL FLUID (RHEUMATON)

Specimen Collection and Preparation

Fresh serum should be used. If serum cannot be tested within 24 hours after collection, it should be stored frozen. If the sample to be tested is to be mailed, a preservative such as sodium azide (final concentration 0.1%) or thimerosal, 1:10,000, should be used. In the frozen state, serum may be kept for extended periods of time. Specimens must be clear and free from particulate material. Sera must be examined, and, if not clear, they should be centrifuged before use.

This test can also be performed using synovial fluid; comparable results have been reported with the sera of the same patients. Satisfactory results have been obtained using hyaluronidase to reduce the viscosity of the test material and without the use of enzyme pretreatment. In addition, the use of heparin in synovial fluid to prevent clots has been found not to interfere with the test.

Materials

The following materials are provided:

1. **Rheumaton reagent** (stabilized sheep erythrocytes sensitized with rabbit gamma globulin, 3 per cent)—contains buffer and 0.1 per cent sodium azide as preservative. Shake well before use.
2. **Positive control**—(RA factor positive serum, human)—contains saline and 0.1 per cent sodium azide as preservative.
3. **Negative control** (RA factor negative serum, human)—contains saline and 0.1 per cent sodium azide as preservative.
4. **Calibrated capillary tubes with rubber bulbs**
5. **Glass slides**

The following materials are required but are not provided:

1. Disposable stirrers
2. Distilled water or isotonic saline (0.85 per cent sodium chloride)

Qualitative Procedure

1. Fill the capillary to the mark with the patient's serum, and expel it into the center of a section of the slide.
2. Add one drop of Rheumaton reagent to the sample.
3. Mix with the disposable stirrer, spreading over the entire section. Use a clean disposable stirrer for each mixture.
4. Rock the slide gently with a rotary motion for 2 minutes, and observe immediately for agglutination.
5. If agglutination is evident, dilute the serum specimen one volume to 10 volumes using either distilled water or isotonic saline (0.85 per cent sodium chloride in distilled water) and repeat the test.

Quantitative Procedure

Dilute the serum sample with isotonic saline (0.85 per cent sodium chloride), starting with a 1:10 dilution and making progressive twofold serial dilutions up to 1:1280, as follows:

1. Place eight small test tubes (12 × 75 mm) in a test tube rack and label them 1 through 8.
2. To tube 1 add 1.8 ml of saline. To tubes 2 through 8 add 1.0 ml of saline.
3. Add 0.2 ml of serum to be tested to tube 1, mix and transfer 1.0 ml of this serum-saline mixture to tube 2. Mix the contents of tube 2, and transfer 1.0 ml of this mixture to tube 3. Continue mixing and transferring in this manner through tube 8. Discard 1.0 ml from tube 8.
4. Test each dilution (1:10 through 1:1280) as described under the Qualitative Procedure, previously given.

Interpretation

In the qualitative procedure, serum samples that contain serologically detectable RA factor will agglutinate with the Rheumaton reagent.

In the quantitative procedure, the last dilution to show positive agglutination on the slide is taken as the titer.

Note: Absence of agglutination with the diluted serum in the quantitative procedure (*i.e.*, 1:10) following a positive test with the undiluted serum indicates a very low RA factor titer such as may exist in a variety of other diseases, namely, LE, endocarditis, tuberculosis, syphilis, sarcoidosis cancer, viral infections, and diseases affecting the liver, lung, or kidney. RA factor has been detected in approximately 75 per cent of clinically diagnosed RA cases.

When testing undiluted serum, both RA factor as well as high-titer sheep agglutinins, as encountered in infectious mononucleosis and serum sickness, may also agglutinate in this test using Rheumaton reagent, by virtue of their reaction with cell antigens rather than with the rabbit gamma globulin coating the erythrocytes. In doubtful cases, tests for infectious mononucleosis should be carried out (see discussion earlier in this chapter).

Ankylosing Spondylitis

Ankylosing spondylitis (AS) is a systemic rheumatic disorder that affects 10 times more men than women and begins most often between the ages of 20 and 40 years. It is characterized by inflammation of the synovial and spinal apophyseal (synovial) joints, causing back pain. In some instances, however, the disease begins in peripheral joints and (although rarely) with acute iridocyclitis.

Evidence of an unusually high frequency of the inherited antigen HLA-B27 (96 per cent of patients, 50 per cent of first-degree relatives) in patients with AS has provided overwhelming confirmation of a genetic linkage in this disorder, as has been long been suspected, yet never proved.

The pathogenesis of AS is not fully understood, but it is suspected that variable inciting factors e.g., ulcerative colitis, regional enteritis, Reiter's syndrome, psoriasis), which have shown frequent, although hitherto unexplained associations with the disorder, might cause spondylitis in an individual possessing the HLA-B27 antigen. The disease may then result in a self-destructive attack of the immune response against "altered self."

Diagnosis of AS is based on the presence of the clinical and radiologic signs of the disease.

Necrotizing Angiitis (Vasculitis)

Necrotizing angiitis encompasses a group of disorders characterized by segmental inflammation of arteries, namely polyarteritis nodosa (PN), hypersensitivity angiitis, Henoch-Schönlein purpura, Wegener's granulomatosis, Takayasu's disease, and giant cell arteritis. Of these, PN and hypersensitivity angiitis are difficult to distinguish, although PN is seen more often in males and involves both medium and small arteries, whereas hypersensitivity angiitis involves only small arteries. Marked cutaneous involvement usually suggests hypersensitivity angiitis, which is often caused by drugs (notably penicillin and sulfonamides).

Henoch-Schönlein purpura affects the small arteries of the skin, joints, and gastrointestinal tract and is frequently accompanied by purpura, gastrointestinal bleeding, and focal glomerulonephritis. Deposits of IgA, C_3 and fibrin-fibrinogen in capillaries and connective tissue of the dermis have recently been reported and may prove useful in diagnosis. Of the other disorders mentioned, Wegener's granulomatosis is characterized by vasculitis in the upper respiratory tract, lung, and kidney; in Takayasu's disease, the vasculitis occurs in the aorta and its major branches; and in giant cell arteritis, it occurs in the temporal and other cranial arteries.

In PN, 30 to 40 per cent of patients reveal the presence of immune complexes of HBsAg (hepatitis B surface antigen) in affected tissues. Otherwise, the etiology of these conditions is unknown. At present, biopsy obtained from the affected area is the only means of confirming the diagnosis.

The laboratory diagnosis is aided by findings of elevated erythrocyte sedimentation rates (the most consistent finding in all types of vasculitis), anemia, moderate leukocytosis, and (possibly) reduced complement levels. When associated with other diseases (e.g., SLE), findings consistent with that disease are sought.

Polymyositis and Dermatomyositis

Polymyositis is a condition that is characterized by degeneration and inflammation of skeletal muscle, the disease being manifested by weakness of the muscles of the shoulders, hips, and neck, usually associated with muscle pain and tenderness. Common associated findings include dysphagia, Raynaud's phenomenon, and arthritis. The disease primarily affects females, its peak incidence occurring in the young and in those of late middle age. It is characterized histologically by myofiber necrosis, the phagocytosis of degenerating muscle cells and infiltration by chronic inflammatory cells. An associated connective tissue disease (e.g., SLE, RA) is found in some individuals. Laboratory findings include elevated serum muscle enzymes and abnormal electromyographic tracings. Diagnosis is aided by a finding of elevated creatine kinase levels and erythrocyte sedimentation rate (ESR), and by muscle biopsy.

Dermatomyositis is a form of polymyositis with involvement of the skin. In this condition, the symmetric weakening and atrophy of the muscles of the shoulders, hips, neck, and trunk is accompanied by a maculopapular or eczema-like skin rash. The etiology of the disease is unknown, although some cases are associated with malignant neoplasms or connective tissue disease. Dysphagia and symptoms typical of systemic sclerosis (discussion follows) may be produced by involvement of the esophagus.

Progressive Systemic Sclerosis (Scleroderma)

Progressive systemic sclerosis (PSS) (also called scleroderma) is a chronic disease of the connective tissue, characterized by diffuse fibrosis involving the skin and several internal organs (lungs, heart, kidney, and gastrointestinal tract), inflammatory and degenerative changes of the skin and viscera, and vascular abnormalities. The disease usually occurs in adults (20 to 60 years) and affects females two to three times more frequently than males. The disease may occur in a benign or rapidly progressive form, the latter form resulting in death within a few years, the major cause being irreversible renal disease.

Hematologic studies show anemia; urinalysis is usually normal (except in the presence of renal disease). Although the etiology is unknown, evidence for an antigen-mediated pathogenesis is suggested by increased levels of immunoglobulin (IgG) and ANA (40 to 70 per cent). Between 25 and 33 per cent of affected individuals have positive tests for syphilis; positive LE cell reactions also occur. Pulmonary function tests may show increased residual volume and decreased maximal breathing capacity. Esophageal hypomotility and diverticuli are often revealed by x-ray examination.

Mixed Connective Tissue Disease

Mixed connective tissue disease (MCTD) is a syndrome that has the combined clinical features of RA, SLE, PSS, and polymyositis. Typically, patients have positive ANA of the speckled pattern and high titers of antibody to extractable ribonucleoprotein (anti-RNP antibodies). In addition, RA factor, elevated ESR, and hypergammaglobulinemia are usually present, whereas anti-DNA and anti-Sm are usually absent.

Sjögren's Syndrome

Sjögren's syndrome (SS) most often occurs secondary to RA, scleroderma, polymyositis, or SLE. In its primary form, SS manifests itself in the form of dry eyes (keratoconjunctivitis sicca) and dry mouth (xerostomia).

Sjögren's syndrome is characteristically revealed through remarkable immunologic reactivity detected in the serum. LE cells, ANA, RA factor, and hypergammaglobulinemia are frequently present, and, in addition, antibodies against RNA, salivary duct, lacrimal gland, smooth muscle, mitochondria, and thyroid gland may be found. There is an increased frequency of renal tubular acidosis, and lymphoma may also develop, particularly in patients with the primary form of SS.

An association between the antigen HLA-Dw3 and primary SS has been found. Diagnosis is confirmed by salivary technetium pertechnetate scintiscanning, which is more sensitive than sialography and labial biopsy.

ORGAN-SPECIFIC AUTOIMMUNE DISEASES

Organ-specific autoimmune diseases are those diseases in which the major effect involves a single organ (Table 12–4). The diagnosis of these diseases is aided by serologic tests, which are used to detect the presence of antibodies to tissue-specific antigens.

Autoimmune Diseases of the Blood

The Autoimmune Hemolytic Anemias

All the formed elements of the blood may be involved in autoimmune reactions. The autoimmune hemolytic anemias (AHA) are a group of anemias characterized by a hemolytic process involving red cell specific antibodies in the serum.

Table 12–4. AUTOIMMUNE DISEASES THAT ARE ORGAN-SPECIFIC

Organ	Disease
Blood	Autoimmune hemolytic anemia Autoimmune thrombocytopenic purpura Neutropenia Lymphopenia Autoimmune aplastic anemia
Kidneys	Goodpasture's syndrome Acute streptococcal nephritis
Endocrine	Autoimmune thyroiditis (Hashimoto's disease) Primary myxedema Thyrotoxicosis (Graves' disease) Addison's disease Parathyroid disease Early onset diabetes
Nervous System	Disseminated encephalomyelitis Idiopathic polyneuritis Landry's paralysis Multiple sclerosis
Gastrointestinal	Pernicious anemia Gastric atrophy Regional ileitis (Crohn's disease) Ulcerative colitis Gluten-sensitive enteropathy Sjögren's syndrome
Liver	Chronic aggressive hepatitis Drug-induced liver diseases Primary biliary cirrhosis Portal cirrhosis
Muscle	Myasthenia gravis Demyelinating disease (MS)
Eye	Phacogenic uveitis Sympathetic ophthalmia Sjögren's syndrome
Dermis	Pemphigus vulgaris Bullous pemphigoid Cicatricial pemphigoid Dermatitis herpetiformis
Others	Allergic orchitis

The study of the AHA takes place primarily in the immunohematology laboratory. The brief description given here is included for the sake of completeness; readers are referred to the excellent texts by Mollison (1983) and by Petz and Garratty (1980) and also to Bryant (1982) for more detailed coverage. (See the list of General References at the end of this chapter.)

Autoimmune Hemolytic Anemia (Warm Type). This is the most common of the AHA, consisting of idiopathic and secondary types. The disease affects both sexes and people of all ages. The anemia is caused by antibodies primarily of the IgG class, which show limited complement-fixing ability and react (in the vast majority of cases) with Rh or extractable nuclear antigens. The idiopathic form accounts for more than half of all cases of AHA, and although the etiology remains obscure, on long-term follow-up some of these patients are found to have lymphoma. In the secondary type, anemia occurs in association with one of many diseases or after the use of drugs. In 30 to 40 per cent of cases, the patient's red cells are coated (sensitized) with IgG only; in 50 per cent of cases, the red cells are coated with IgG and complement; and in 10 to 20 per cent of cases, the red cells appear to be coated only with complement. In each case, IgG and complement are readily detected by the indirect antiglobulin (Coombs') test with broad-spectrum antihuman globulin.

Autoimmune Hemolytic Anemia (Cold Type). In the cold agglutinin group, antibodies are primarily IgM, reacting best at 0°C to 4°C, with lesser activity at higher temperatures, becoming dissociated at 37°C. These antibodies have the ability to fix complement and are usually directed against the I antigen, the i antigen, and (rarely) the Sp_1 antigen. These antibodies, particularly anti-I, are found in such diseases as primary atypical pneumonia *(Mycoplasma pneumoniae)*, infectious mononucleosis, and cold agglutinin disease. The clinical lesions include anemia, the severity of which is dependent upon the thermal activity of the antibody. Renal failure from hemolysis is rare. The disease is associated with cirrhosis, malignant diseases, infectious mononucleosis, mycoplasma infections, and sarcoidosis. On long-term follow-up, some patients are found to have overt lymphoma.

Paroxysmal Cold Hemoglobinuria. The cold autohemolysins (Donath-Landsteiner–type) found in this group of AHA were first described in patients with tertiary syphilis. The antibodies are cold agglutinins of the IgG class, which fix complement and are directed against the P antigen. Because complement fixation is avid, most cells are lysed before they reach phagocytic cells, and the result is rapid intravascular hemolysis when the body or

part of the body is cooled below the critical temperature (15° to 20°C). Hemolysis may occur, with hemoglobinuria, fever, chills, hypotension, and abdominal and back pain.

Etiology and Laboratory Diagnosis of AHA. The etiology of AHA is unknown. it has been postulated, however, that drugs and viruses may in some way alter the antigenic structure of the red cell membrane, rendering the erythrocyte susceptible to hemolysis. Genetically determined susceptibility to develop autoantibodies has also been postulated; this may be associated with certain immunologic abnormalities.

The major diagnostic criteria used in the laboratory to distinguish AHA from other forms of anemia are the presence of spherocytes in the peripheral blood smear and a positive direct antiglobulin (Coombs') test (for method, see Bryant, 1982). The type of AHA is determined by the temperature of the agglutination reactions.

Autoimmune Thrombocytopenic Purpura (AITP)

Patients with thrombocytopenia associated with normal, or possibly increased, numbers of megakaryocytes in the bone marrow were termed as having *idiopathic thrombocytopenic purpura (ITP)*. In view of evidence that the condition is due to the formation of autoantibodies, the term *autoimmune thrombocytopenic purpura* has now become more common, using the abbreviation AITP rather than ATP to avoid confusion with the abbreviation for adenosine triphosphate.

Harrington *et al.* (1951) were the first to demonstrate the presence of anti-platelet factor in the plasma of patients with AITP. These investigators found that plasma from an AITP patient, when transfused to an affected individual, resulted in a profound fall in the recipient's platelet count.

The serological tests for AITP include:

The Antiglobulin Consumption Test (Dixon *et al.*, 1975). This test gives a very high percentage of positive results; however, it is also positive in various disease states not necessarily associated with an increased rate of platelet destruction (*e.g.*, SLE). Certain modifications of the antiglobulin consumption test have been found to give varying, although encouraging results in cases of AITP. These include modifications suggested by Rosse *et al.*, 1980 and by Nel and Stevens, 1980, which used an enzyme-linked antibody.

Hymes *et al.* (1979) described an antiglobulin consumption test method in which platelets were frozen, thawed, and sonicated. The IgG was then extracted and applied to wells of microtiter plates, to which it stuck. Rabbit antihuman IgG was then added to the plates, followed by ^{125}I-labeled staphylococcal protein. The wells were then removed and counted. This method was found to be very sensitive and has the advantage of being able to use platelets stored at $-20°C$ before testing. A similar type of method found to be almost equal in sensitivity but using enzyme-linked antiglobulin serum was described by Hegde *et al.* (1981). In this technique, IgG was extracted from platelets and bound to antihuman IgG, previously coated onto polystyrene. The amount of platelet-associated IgG was then estimated by adding the enzyme reagent (antihuman IgG coupled with alkaline phosphatase) together with a suitable substrate.

The Platelet Immunofluorescence Test. The original platelet immunofluorescence test was plagued with the problem of nonspecific immunofluorescence. A modification of the technique was described by von dem Borne *et al.* (1978), which overcame this difficulty through the pretreatment of platelets with paraformaldehyde. In the latter method, paraformaldehyde-treated platelets are incubated with serum, then washed and incubated with antiglobulin serum labeled with fluorescein-isothiocyanate. After incubation, the cells are washed again, then examined under a fluorescence microscope. The test appears to be more sensitive than the antiglobulin consumption test, yet it also does not give positive results in all cases of AITP.

The Radioactive Antiglobulin Test. Soulier *et al.* (1975) and Mueller-Eckhardt *et al.* (1978) described the use of a ^{125}I-labeled antiglobulin test for the detection of platelet antibodies. The use of this test in cases of AITP revealed that only about 80 per cent of patients with the disease had a raised platelet-associated IgG (PAIgG) level, whereas an increased level of PAIgG was not confined to AITP but was also found in chronic liver disease, leukemia, myeloma, and other diseases (Mueller-Eckhardt *et al.*, 1980). Like the platelet immunofluorescence test, this test appears to be more sensitive than antiglobulin consumption, yet it does not give positive results in all cases of AITP.

Helmerhorst *et al.* (1980) performed a comparison test on a small number of patients using the three procedures just discussed and concluded that the platelet immunofluorescence test was the most sensitive of the three and that the higher percentage of positive results observed with the antiglobulin consumption test indicated the nonspecificity of that test in the detection of red cell–bound antibody. These investigators therefore recommend that a positive result with the immunofluorescence test (or the radioactive antiglobulin test) provides strong support for a diagnosis of AITP (although the diagnosis is not ruled out by a negative result), whereas a positive antiglobulin consumption test alone does not establish a diagnosis of AITP.

Neutropenia

This is a disease in which there is a decrease in the number of neutrophilic leukocytes in the blood below the lower reference limit of 2000 per mm^3 for caucasians and 1300 per mm^3 for blacks. The disease is therefore characterized by susceptibility to infection. The surface antigens of the neutrophil are probably causative, although it is possible that the disease is produced by several mechanisms, including decreased or ineffective neutrophil production in the bone marrow, increased loss of neutrophils from the peripheral blood, and "pseudo" neutropenia in which there is a shift from the circulating granulocyte pool to the marginal granulocyte pool.

The administration of drugs (particularly by cancer chemotherapy, but also as an idiosyncratic response to many other drugs) can cause neutropenia. It can also be caused by exposure to radiation. The disease is associated with acute leukemias, many infections, RA, congestive splenomegaly, and vitamin B_{12} deficiency. There are also several forms of congenital neutropenia, which, in young children, has a guarded prognosis. However, resistance to infection improves if children survive infancy, which is presumed to reflect compensatory development of antibody and cell-mediated responses, both of which are functionally intact in most of these patients.

The primary neutropenias can be diagnosed on the basis of age of onset, history of exposure to toxic substances or drugs, family history, and blood or bone marrow analysis. Immunologically mediated neutropenia is better established by determining the presence of serum leukoagglutinins or specific anti-neutrophil antibody.

Lymphocytopenia

This is a disease in which there is a decrease in the proportion of lymphocytes in the blood characterized by secondary immunodeficiency. The T-lymphocytes are preferentially depleted from the circulation to a greater extent than are the B-lymphocytes. In addition, there is a selective depletion of certain T-cell subpopulations, as determined by phenotypic markers as well as by functional capabilities. The probable antigens are lymphocyte-specific surface antigens; the antibody is much like heterologous anti-lymphocyte globulin.

Autoimmune Aplastic Anemia

This disease occurs in about one third of all patients with aplastic anemia (a type of anemia in which there is complete absence of reticulocytes in the blood and of all types of erythroblasts in the bone marrow). It is probable that the stem cell–specific antigens are involved. The immunity seems to be T-cell mediated.

Autoimmune Diseases of the Kidney

An inflammatory reaction within the kidney can result in any one of four types of immunologically mediated renal diseases:

Type I (Anaphylactic). Although no specific renal disease has been definitely ascribed to Type I hypersensitivity, it has been preliminarily implicated in mediating a form of renal disease associated with Henoch-Schönlein purpura, because IgE deposition in the glomeruli of patients with this disease has been noted. The acceptance of IgE as a pathogenic factor requires more extensive confirmation, however. It is likely that Type I hypersensitivity plays at least a contributing role in certain forms of reversible renal transplant rejection and in interstitial nephritis of methicillin-induced nephritis.

Type II (Cytotoxic). Injury to the kidney results from tissue antigen–antibody combination that activates complement and other systems of inflammation. Anti-GBM (glomerular basement membrane) disease is a good example in which antibody to GBM is produced and antibody and complement are deposited in linear fashion along the GBM. If the anti-GBM reacts with the other basement membranes (*e.g.,* the lung) as well, injury to the pulmonary capillary bed occurs. The syndrome of anti–GBM-mediated immune renal failure and pulmonary hemorrhage is known as *Goodpasture's syndrome.* The deposition of antibody and complement in linear fashion along the GBM can be shown by direct immunofluorescence (Fig. 12–2).

Tubulointerstitial renal disease occurs when the anti-basement membrane is directed against the tubular basement membrane (TBM). Anti-TBM antibodies are associated with such disorders as anti-GBM disease, SLE, and renal transplant rejection.

Hyperacute renal allograft rejection is a form of Type II–mediated renal disease that affects the entire kidney. It is associated with high levels of pre-existing HLA antibodies of the transplant. It is likely that the injury to the kidney results from a Type II attack by anti-HLA against HLA antigens of the renal transplant, which are widely distributed.

Type III (Immune Complex). Deposition of immune complexes formed in the glomeruli of kidneys is the basis of the majority of immunologically mediated renal diseases, even though the immunologic specificity is not directed toward the antigens of the kidney itself. The antigen-antibody complexes deposit in the glomerular capillary wall (immune-complex glomerular renal disease) or in the tubulointerstitium (immune-complex tubulointerstitial renal disease).

A classic example of immune complex disease of the kidney is SLE, in which the antigen-antibody–complement complexes form in the blood, deposit in the glomeruli in granular distribution, and activate complement, thus inducing inflammation and activating the clotting system.

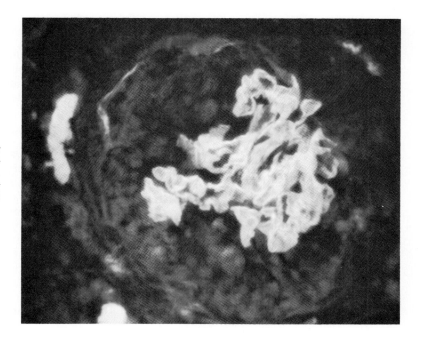

Figure 12–2. A photomicrograph of the kidney of a patient with Goodpasture's syndrome demonstrated by direct fluorescence microscopy. (From Bellanti, J. A.: Immunology III. Philadelphia, W. B. Saunders Company, 1985, p. 432.)

Acute post-streptococcal glomerulonephritis is another form of immune-complex disease. In this, the antigen resides in the wall of the streptococcus (usually group A beta-hemolytic streptococci, particularly types 12 and 49). Infection induces the production of antibody that combines with the streptococcal antigens, and these complexes deposit in the glomerular capillary wall. An acute glomerular inflammatory response ensues, with activation of complement, release of lysozymes from polymorphonuclear cells, and subsequent tissue injury.

Both exogenous antigens (*i.e.*, bacterial, viral, parasitic, foreign serum, and drugs) and endogenous antigens (*i.e.*, nuclear antigens and tumor antigens) may induce immune-complex glomerulonephritis (Table 12–5).

Type IV (Cell-Mediated). Cell-mediated immune renal injury is best exemplified by renal allograft rejection, in which sensitized lymphoid cells attack the graft, with immune renal injury resulting. The reaction occurs throughout the kidney, and soluble substances are released by lymphoid cells. These soluble substances (called *lymphokines*) may cause an inflammatory response, thus inducing tissue injury.

It is also possible that chronic glomerulonephritis may fall into the category of Type IV hypersensitivity. It has been hypothesized that the release of renal tissue antigens after acute glomerulonephritis may result in cell-mediated hypersensitivity to those antigens. This hypothesis is supported by studies showing that, on exposure to renal tissue antigens by lymphoid cells from patients with chronic glomerulonephritis, migration inhibitory factor (MIF) is released.

Table 12–5. EXOGENOUS AND ENDOGENOUS ANTIGENS ASSOCIATED WITH TYPE III IMMUNE RENAL INJURY

Antigen	Examples
Exogenous	
Bacterial	Post-streptococcal GN Staphylococcal
Viral	Chickenpox Hepatitis B
Parasitic	Malaria Toxoplasmosis
Foreign serum	Serum sickness
Drugs	Heroin nephropathy (?)
Endogenous	
Nuclear antigens	Systemic lupus erythematosus
Tumor antigens	Carcinoembryonic antigen

Slightly modified from Bellanti, J. A.: Immunology III. Philadelphia, W. B. Saunders Company, 1985, p. 434.

Other Forms of Immune Renal Disease

A number of renal diseases have been described that do have apparent immunologic bases, yet do not fit into any of the categories just described. Two of them are IgG-IgA nephropathy (Berger's disease) and membranoproliferative or mesangiocapillary glomerulonephritis.

In IgG-IgA nephropathy (Berger's disease), renal biopsy shows IgG and IgA deposits in mesangial areas of the glomerulus, with subsequent mesangial cell hyperplasia. The cause of deposition in this disease is not known. It has been suggested, from studies in rabbits, that the mesangium may be capable of clearing small amounts of immune complexes during early antigen-antibody production when the level of complexes is small, but that after saturation of other mononuclear phagocytic systems (*e.g.*, the liver and spleen), complexes may begin to accumulate in the capillary wall and extraglomerular sites.

Membranoproliferative glomerulonephritis appears to result from the deposition of activated complement components within the kidney, the complement possibly activated through the alternative pathway (see Chapter 3). The direct activation of C3 is likely to be related to a heat-stable gamma globulin in the serum known as *nephritic factor,* which is capable of cleaving C3 to C3b directly. In this form of renal disease, C3 is deposited densely within the capillary wall of the glomerulus. The disease does not in all instances proceed to kidney failure, but patients who do develop renal failure and receive transplants are at risk of the disease recurring in the transplant.

Autoimmune Diseases of the Endocrine Organs

Autoimmune disease has been associated with all the endocrine organs, although the most extensively studied and most frequently occurring are diseases involving the thyroid gland.

Autoimmune Diseases of the Thyroid

The diseases of the thyroid gland in which autoimmune factors are involved are *lymphocytic thyroiditis (Hashimoto's thyroiditis)* and *thyrotoxicosis (Graves' disease).*

Autoimmune Thyroiditis (Hashimoto's Thyroiditis). This is the most common form of thyroiditis, occurring at any age, although it usually occurs in patients between the ages of 35 and 55 years. It is 5 to 10 times more frequent in females than in males.

Initially, the symptom is enlargement of the thyroid gland, which is usually painless and may develop gradually over a number of years. If the enlargement is great, dysphagia, choking, and dyspnea may result. The enlargement is generally diffuse, although it may be nodular; in some cases, the lesion may occur as a solitary nodule.

The disease is characterized histologically by an intense infiltration of the thyroid stroma and follicles by lymphocytes and plasma cells, and by degeneration and regeneration of the thyroid parenchyma. Immunologically, circulating antibodies as well as lymphoproliferative responses to various constituents of thyroid are commonly seen. In addition to these circulating antibodies (which may represent autoimmune phenomena), antibodies have been described in this disease (and in Graves' disease, discussion follows), that appear to regulate cellular activity and may in fact contribute to the hyperthyroidism. These include:

1. Long-acting thyroid stimulator (LATS). This has an *in vivo* ability to enhance the release of thyroid hormone. It is an IgG immunoglobulin that is detected by means of bioassay. The antibody is formed against a thyroid protein and mimics most actions of thyrotropin. Not all patients with Hashimoto's thyroiditis have detectable levels of LATS; none is detected in normal individuals.
2. LATS protector activity (LPA). This has the ability to prevent the neutralization of LATS by an inactivator normally present in human thyroid extract.
3. Thyroid-stimulating immunoglobulins (TSI). These appear to represent autoantibodies directed against thyrotropin receptors, which are capable of binding to the receptor and stimulate the production of cyclic AMP and the excessive production of thyroid hormone. TSI has been detected in 15 per cent of patients with Hashimoto's thyroiditis.

Whether or not these activities represent three distinct antibodies (or whether they may be different manifestations of the same antibody specificity differing only in the methods required for their detection) remains unclear.

There are many immunologic tests that are useful in the detection of thyroid antibodies. Antithyroglobulin antibodies can be detected by precipitation, latex agglutination, the tanned red cell (TRC) test, and radioimmunoassay. Microsomal antibodies can be detected using complement fixation, cytotoxicity tests, immunofluorescence of unfixed thyroid epithelial cells, radioimmunoassay, and hemagglutination tests. The second antigen of acinar colloid, a protein that is distinct from thyroglobin, is also detected by immunofluorescence. This antibody is not specific for Hashimoto's thyroiditis and is seen in patients with thyrotoxicosis and cancer of the thyroid. Immunofluorescence on living suspensions of human thyroid cells has revealed thyroid-specific cell surface antibodies; the significance of these antibodies is unknown.

Tests of thyroid function, including T_3 and T_4 levels, T_3-resin uptake, and ^{131}I uptake are usually in the range of low to normal in this disorder; in such cases, the most sensitive test for hypothyroidism is the measurement of thyroid-stimulating hormone (TSH) levels.

A useful test for the detection of anti-thyroid antibody (ATA) in the sera of patients with chronic thyroiditis (including Hashimoto's thyroiditis and Graves' disease) is the CSI ATA Immunopath Fluoro-Kit (Clinical Sciences Inc., Whippany, NJ 07981), which uses an indirect fluorescent antibody method and is designed as a screening test for all three ATA. This test should be run on every patient with a goiter, because 10 to 20 per cent of the adult patients with chronic thyroid disease may have negative results when tested with the hemagglutination technique, because the latter test is only reactive with the thyroglobulin antigen, whereas the CSI ATA Immunopath test is capable of detecting all three organ-specific antibodies simultaneously.

Myxedema. This is a condition associated with hypothyroidism and characterized by the collection of hydrated mucopolysaccharides in the dermis and in other tissues of the body. The diagnosis of this disease is based on the clinical signs and measurement of the serum levels of thiiodothyronine (T_3) and thyroxine (T_4). Frequently, there is also hypercholesterolemia and increased serum levels of TSH.

Thyrotoxicosis (Graves' Disease). An association between Hashimoto's thyroiditis and Graves' disease is becoming more and more frequently recognized, because the two conditions frequently exist together in the same patient and may represent different manifestations of a common spectrum. Graves' disease is now considered to be a multisystem disorder consisting of three components:

1. Hyperthyroidism due to diffuse goiter
2. Infiltrative ophthalmopathy (exophthalmos)
3. Infiltrative dermopathy (localized pretibial myxedema)

These components may present in combination with each other or, in some cases, individually. Infiltrative ophthalmopathy and infiltrative dermopathy occur most frequently in adult patients in whom a higher incidence of antibodies is found.

The three ATA previously described (see Hashimoto's thyroiditis) are also present in Graves' disease. LATS is detected in about 50 per cent of patients with Graves' disease, and TSI is detected in about 90 per cent of these patients.

The CSI ATA Immunopath Fluoro-Kit, just described (see Autoimmune Thyroiditis [Hashimoto's Thyroiditis]) is also used for the detection of ATA in Graves' disease.

Autoimmune Diseases of the Pancreas

Antibodies to insulin have been found in the sera of diabetic patients. If IgE, these antibodies may contribute to insulin allergy, or, if IgG, IgA, or IgM, they may contribute to insulin resistance. Radioimmunoassay of insulin concentrations is a useful test, facilitated through the production of insulin antibodies in animals.

Thyroid and gastric autoantibodies have also been found in the sera of diabetic patients without clinical thyroid disease or pernicious anemia. These antibodies are primarily found in juvenile-onset diabetes and are usually insulin-dependent and often insulin-resistant. They are more frequently detected in females.

Autoimmune Disease of the Adrenals

Autoantibodies to adrenal tissues, detectable by immunofluorescence or complement fixation, have been reported in patients with Addison's disease. The significance of these findings is not known.

Autoimmune Disease of the Parathyroids

Antibodies to thyroid, adrenal, and gastric tissues have been detected in a disorder known as *idiopathic hypoparathyroidism,* which occurs more frequently in children than in adults and is more common in females than in males. Hypoparathyroidism may be accompanied by certain associated disorders, including idiopathic Addison's disease, pernicious anemia, alopecia totalis, and moniliasis. When clusters of two or more of these associated diseases are present, it appears that an autosomal recessive mode of transmission of an underlying defect may be involved. Hypoparathyroidism is also associated with developmental failure of the thymus-dependent immune system in DiGeorge's syndrome.

Autoimmune Diseases of the Nervous System

The best-studied autoimmune disease of the central nervous system is acute disseminated encephalomyelitis. Other autoimmune conditions of the nervous system include acute idiopathic polyneuritis (Guillain-Barré syndrome), Landry's paralysis, and multiple sclerosis (MS).

Disseminated Encephalomyelitis. This is a disease characterized by fever, photophobia, blindness, muscle weakness, decreased consciousness, seizures, paresis, loss of appetite, and sphincter disturbance. Increased protein and lymphocytosis is seen in the cerebrospinal fluid. The condition may develop susequent to infection by either bacterial or viral agents, but viral infections (*e.g.,* measles, mumps, and rubella) are much more common as predisposing causes. Following infection, there is a latent period of 5 to 30 days before the onset of disease. Various immunizations (notably smallpox or rabies) may precipitate the disease.

Circulating antibody to encephalitogenic factors has been demonstrated by a number of techniques, but now there is rather clear evidence that the *major* pathologic change in experimental allergic encephalomyelitis (EAE) is mediated by sensitized lymphocytes.

Idiopathic Polyneuritis. Also known as Guillain-Barré syndrome, idiopathic polyneuritis is another form of neurologic disease that has immunologic features. The disease, which is of unknown etiology, is characterized by peripheral nerve involvement. The disease may follow a variety of infectious diseases, or it may occur subsequent to immunization (*e.g.,* swine influenza immunization).

Landry's Paralysis. This is another form of polyneuritis that produces a weakness and sensory loss in the limbs as a result of inflammation in the peripheral nerves.

Multiple Sclerosis. This is a slowly progressive disease of the central nervous system of unknown cause, usually beginning in early adult life, which is characterized by disseminated, patchy demyelination of the brain and spinal cord. The disease results in a number of neurologic symptoms and signs, and it may relapse and remit over long periods of time. A number of infectious disease pathogens have been implicated in MS, but the precise cause remains unclear. The finding of an elevated spinal fluid gamma globulin in 80 per cent of patients is a distinguishing feature of the disease. No specific treatment of MS is available, and death is usually due to some intercurrent disease.

Autoimmune Diseases of the Stomach and Intestines

Diseases of the stomach and intestines that are triggered by an immunologic response include pernicious anemia, gastric atrophy, regional ileitis, ulcerative colitis, and gluten-sensitive enteropathy (celiac disease).

Pernicious Anemia. This is a disorder characterized by inflammation of the gastric mucosa with inability to secrete hydrochloric acid, intrinsic factor, and pepsin, followed by the development of macrocytic anemia. The disease is characteristically associated with the presence of parietal cell antibody or intrinsic factor antibody or both in patients with atrophic gastritis. Antibody has recently been found in the gastric juice, and lymphoid cells have been found in infiltrate gastric mucosa. An antibody that, when mixed with intrinsic factor, interferes with the absorption of vitamin B_{12} has been found in the sera of patients with pernicious anemia (PA). Whether these antibodies are the cause or the result of the disease is not known. The clear link, however, between the presence of these antibodies and the clinical disease and the fact that pernicious anemia will respond to steroid therapy lend evidence for the autoimmune nature of the disease.

Serologic tests in cases of PA include complement fixation or immunofluorescence (for the detection of antibodies directed against the microsomal fraction of gastric mucosal cells) and blocking and binding antibody tests (to detect the antibodies that bind with preformed intrinsic factor B_{12} complex, binding antibody, or those that block the combination of intrinsic factor with antibody, blocking antibody). The tests for these antibodies are important in differentiating PA from other causes of megaloblastic anemia.

Gastric Atrophy. Atrophic gastritis affects about 20 to 30 per cent of the adult population, apparently progressing from a lesion of superficial gastritis. The incidence of the disorder increases with age, as do the gastric autoantibodies. Parietal cell antibodies and intrinsic factor antibody occurring in this case would cause PA. Their presence is particularly associated with other diseases of autoimmunity (*e.g.,* Graves' disease, myxedema, insulin-dependent diabetes, Addison's disease), and they occur with increased frequency in the families of patients with PA, thyroid diseases, and other autoimmune disorders.

Regional Ileitis (Crohn's Disease). Although suspected, an autoimmune basis has not been substantiated in this disease, which is characterized by granulomatous inflammatory changes of the ileum that sometimes also involve other parts of the gastrointestinal tract. Antibodies to heterologous colon have been demonstrated in regional ileitis.

Ulcerative Colitis. The pathogenesis of ulcerative colitis is unknown, but it is thought to be autoimmune on the basis of circulating antibody to colonic tissue, possibly triggered by enteric infection. The fact that females are more affected than males suggests a genetic predisposition in this disorder. The disease primarily affects the large bowel and is characterized by bloody diarrhea, abdominal pain, weight loss, and anemia.

An IgM hemagglutinin, a precipitating antibody, and an immunofluorescent antibody are the three kinds of antibodies that have been demonstrated against colonic tissue, although their significance in the pathogenesis of ulcerative colitis is not clear. The lymphocytes from affected patients cause cytotoxicity to cells in culture (although antibody-containing serum does not); this suggests that cell-mediated immune mechanisms may be more important than humoral antibody in the pathogenesis of this disease.

Gluten-Sensitive Enteropathy (Celiac Disease). This disorder is characterized by malabsorption of fats and carbohydrates. The ingestion of the gliadin fraction of gluten (a protein found in grains) appears to cause diarrhea in these patients, although it is not known how this effect is mediated. A hypersensitivity reaction may also occur to the gliadin fraction itself. High-titer antibodies to gliadin (IgA and IgM) have been detected in affected patients. In addition, the finding that IgA deficiency occurs more frequently in celiac patients than in the general population is probably related to common factors underlying the two conditions. An association between gluten-sensitive enteropathy (GSE) and HLA-Dw3 and B8 has been reported.

Autoimmune Diseases of the Liver

Liver diseases with immunologic features include viral hepatitis (acute and chronic), drug-induced liver disease, biliary cirrhosis, and portal cirrhosis. Of these, the most important are infectious hepatitis (type A) and serum hepatitis (type B; see Chapter 7).

Hepatitis. (See Chapter 7.)

Drug-Induced Liver Diseases. The use of a number of different drugs can induce liver disease in hypersensitive individuals. Two forms of drug-induced liver disease are seen: (1) a toxic form and (2) a true hypersensitivity reaction. Antibodies have been detected in the toxic form, although not in the hypersensitivity form. The disease can only be treated through the discontinuation of the offending drug.

Primary Biliary Cirrhosis. The term *cirrhosis* refers to liver disease characterized pathologically by loss of the normal microscopic lobular architecture with fibrosis and nodular regeneration. The term is sometimes used to refer to chronic interstitial inflammation of any organ. Primary biliary cirrhosis is a rare form of biliary cirrhosis of unknown etiology, occurring without obstruction or infection of the major bile ducts, sometimes occurring after the administration of certain drugs (*e.g.,* chlorpromazine, arsenicals). The disease primarily affects middle-aged women and is characterized by chronic cholestasis with pruritus, jaundice, and hypercholesterolemia, with xanthomas and malabsorption.

Portal Cirrhosis. Also known as *Laennec's cirrhosis*, this is the form of liver disease that is closely associated with chronic excessive alcohol ingestion.

Autoimmune Diseases of the Muscle

Polymyositis (dermatomyositis) has been discussed with the systemic autoimmune conditions; the other muscular disorder considered to be autoimmune in nature is *myasthenia gravis*, which is associated with thymic abnormalities and affects the voluntary muscles, causing muscle weakness and fatigability. The disease can occur in a transitory neonatal form and has been described in infants born of myasthenic mothers. It commonly affects young females, with a peak incidence in those between 10 and 20 years; the peak incidence in males is between the ages of 60 and 70 years. Juvenile and adult cases are chronic, although signs and symptoms are variable. Thymic abnormalities consisting of hyperplasia and plasma cell infiltration occur in 80 per cent of patients. Evidence indicates that there is a thymic polypeptide factor that acts to inhibit neuromuscular transmission at the myoneural junction. Antibodies to neuromuscular receptors have also been described.

Serum antibodies directed against muscle may be detected by a variety of tests, including direct and indirect immunofluorescence, complement fixation, precipitation, and tanned-cell hemagglutination.

MS can also be classified as an autoimmune disease affecting the muscles (see earlier discussion in this chapter).

Autoimmune Diseases of the Eye

Autoimmune phenomena have been implicated in three diseases of the eye: (1) phacogenic uveitis, which affects the lens; (2) sympathetic ophthalmia, which affects the uvea; and (3) autoimmune reaction involving the lacrimal gland (Sjögren's syndrome).

The eye is isolated anatomically and contains a variety of antigens that normally are not in contact with the circulation (so-called sequestered antigens). The release of lens protein into the circulation as a result of trauma or surgery may result in both inflammatory and immunologic events leading to the destruction of the lens. Inflammatory cells are found within the lesions, and anti-lens antibody is found within the circulation and aqueous humor of the affected individual.

Sympathetic ophthalmia typically follows penetrating injuries of the globe. The injured eye subsequently may develop an endophthalmitis characterized by diffuse lymphocytic infiltration of the uvea. The unaffected eye (sympathetic eye) may spontaneously develop a similar lesion several days or weeks later. Anti-uveal antibody has been demonstrated in some patients.

Autoimmune Diseases of the Skin

The typical immunologic fluorescent staining patterns seen in those diseases of the skin that have an autoimmunologic basis are shown in Table 12–6.

Pemphigus Vulgaris. In this disease, the loss of intracellular bridges in the epidermis is associated with autoantibodies directed against antigens located in the intercellular zones between adjacent epidermal cells.

Bullous Pemphigoid. This is another skin disease in which blisters arise subepidermally, but the autoantibodies react with constituents in the zona pellucida of the basement membrane in the epidermis rather than the intercellular cement.

Dermatitis Herpetiformis. This disease is characterized by grouped vesicles surmounted on an erythematous base involving predominantly the

Table 12–6. IMMUNOFLUORESCENT STAINING PATTERN IN AUTOIMMUNE DISEASES OF THE SKIN ILLUSTRATING DEMONSTRATION OF IMMUNOGLOBULINS (Ig) AND COMPLEMENT (C)

	Direct					Indirect		
	Intercellular		Basement Membrane					Basement Membrane
Disease	IgG	C	IgG	IgA	IgM	C	Intercellular	
Dermatitis herpetiformis	−	−	+	+ + + +	0	+	0	0
SLE (involved and uninvolved skin)	−	−	+ + + +	+	+	+	0	0
Discoid lupus (uninvolved skin only)	−	−	+ + + +	+	+	+	0	0
Bullous pemphigoid	−	−	+ + + +	+	+	+	0	+
Pemphigus vulgaris	+ + + +	+	−	−	−	−	+	0

From Bellanti, J. A.: Immunology III. Philadelphia, W. B. Saunders Company, 1985, p. 439.

extensor surfaces of the back and arms. The HLA-B8 antigen has been found in approximately 75 to 80 per cent of patients with the disease. The examination of the perilesional skin of patients with the disease has shown a granular deposition of IgA (in 95 per cent of patients) as well as C3, C5, properdin, and properdin factor B. IgG and early components of complement are infrequently noted. These findings suggest that the major activation of complement in the disease may be via the alternative pathway.

Systemic Lupus Erythematosus. The skin manifestations of SLE are seen in both the systemic and the chronic discoid forms of the disease. In chronic discoid lupus, the skin lesions consist of a sharply circumscribed scaling erythematous dermatitis in which follicular plugging, telangiectasia, and atrophy are commonly seen. In both SLE and discoid lupus, immunoglobulins and complement are found in granular deposition at the dermal-epidermal junction. In chronic discoid lupus, this deposition is confined to the involved areas of skin, whereas in SLE, the deposition is seen both in involved and uninvolved areas.

Other Autoimmune Diseases

Other diseases that have autoimmune mechanisms as their basis include:

Allergic Orchitis. This disorder may occur because of autosensitization to spermatozoa following vasectomy or vas repair or after traumatic injury to the testicle. Hypospermia or aspermia, caused by the presence of sperm-immobilizing antibodies excreted into the seminal fluid, may result in infertility.

Autoimmune Diseases Affecting the Heart. Injury to the myocardium appears to result in subsequent autoimmune disease of the heart. When this follows surgery, it is known as *postcardiotomy syndrome,* and, when it follows coronary occlusion, it is known as *postmyocardial infarction (Dressler's syndrome).* In both conditions, there is an association with autoantibodies against heart muscle.

CONCLUSION

The autoimmune diseases are in effect a collection of disorders that have in common the activation of autoimmune phenomena. The relationship of these autoimmune phenomena to the disease is not well understood. It is possible that these diseases are under *genetic* control, as evidenced by the abnormal sex ratios that several of them show and that they represent disorders of suppression or regulation of the lymphoid system.

REVIEW QUESTIONS

MULTIPLE CHOICE

Choose the phrase, sentence, or symbol that completes the statement or answers the question. More than one answer may be correct in each case. Answers are given at the back of this book.

1. The theories that have been proposed to explain the mechanisms that initiate autoimmune diseases include:
   (a) the forbidden clone theory
   (b) the altered antigen theory
   (c) the altered antibody theory
   (d) the immunologic deficiency theory
   (Possible Mechanisms in the Initiation of Autoimmune Diseases)

2. Which of the following represent Koch's postulates:
   (a) All autoimmune diseases are either systemic or organ-specific
   (b) The autoimmune response must be regularly associated with the disease
   (c) It must be possible to induce a replica of the disease in laboratory animals
   (d) The autoantibodies in autoimmune disease must play a central role in the cause
   (Criteria for Autoimmune Diseases)

3. The immune response gene is closely linked to the:
   (a) Rh locus on chromosome 1
   (b) ABO locus on chromosome 9
   (c) HLA locus on chromosome 6
   (d) none of the above
   (Genetic Control of Autoimmune Diseases)

4. Systemic lupus erythematosus:
   (a) is a disease of the connective tissue
   (b) occurs primarily in women
   (c) has a strong hereditary tendency
   (d) occurs primarily in adults between the ages of 20 and 40 years
   (Systemic Lupus Erythematosus)

5. The LE cell:
   (a) is a polymorphonuclear leukocyte
   (b) is found in the bone marrow and peripheral blood of patients with systemic lupus erythematosus
   (c) is always engulfed by the phagocyte and fills its cytoplasm
   (d) when free in stained blood, is often surrounded by viable neutrophils, producing a rosette formation
   (Systemic Lupus Erythematosus: Laboratory Observations)

6. The LE factor:
   (a) is a 7S IgG antibody
   (b) reacts with DNA
   (c) is found in 4 per cent of SLE patients
   (d) is found in 60 per cent of normal individuals
   (Systemic Lupus Erythematosus: Laboratory Observations)

7. RA factor:
   (a) represents proteins found in the blood of patients with rheumatoid arthritis
   (b) shows no particular correlation with rheumatoid arthritis
   (c) is generally thought to be a group of immunoglobulins that react with antigenic determinants on the IgG molecule
   (d) has a sedimentation coefficient of 19S
   (Rheumatoid Arthritis: Characteristics of Rheumatoid Factors)

8. The tests for rheumatoid arthritis:
   (a) are designed to detect rheumatoid factors
   (b) usually use particulate carriers that transform the reaction between RA factor and IgG into visible aggregation
   (c) are designed to detect antibody to immunoglobulin
   (d) always give identical results
   (Serologic Tests for Rheumatoid Factors)

9. Which of the following would be classified as systemic autoimmune disease?
   (a) autoimmune aplastic anemia
   (b) ankylosing spondylitis
   (c) vasculitis
   (d) mixed connective tissue disease
   (Other Systemic Autoimmune Diseases)

10. Autoimmune hemolytic anemia of the warm type:
    (a) is the most common form of AHA
    (b) affects both sexes and all ages
    (c) is more prevalent in males than in females
    (d) is caused by antibodies primarily of the IgM class
    (Autoimmune Diseases of the Blood)

11. The serologic tests for autoimmune thrombocytopenic purpura include:
    (a) the antiglobulin (Coombs') test
    (b) the antiglobulin consumption test
    (c) the platelet immunofluorescence test
    (d) the radioactive antiglobulin test
    (Autoimmune Thrombocytopenic Purpura)

12. Neutropenia:
    (a) is an autoimmune disease of the blood
    (b) is characterized by susceptibility to infection
    (c) is probably caused by surface antigens on the neutrophil
    (d) may be caused by decreased neutrophil production in the bone marrow
    (Neutropenia)

13. Among the four types of immunologically mediated renal diseases are:
    (a) anaphylactic
    (b) cytotoxic
    (c) genetic
    (d) systemic
    (Autoimmune Diseases of the Kidney)

14. Long-acting thyroid stimulator (LATS):
    (a) is an IgG immunoglobulin
    (b) can be detected by means of bioassay
    (c) is found in 30 per cent of normal individuals
    (d) is found in detectable levels in all patients with Hashimoto's thyroiditis
    (Autoimmune Diseases of the Thyroid)

15. LATS is detected in:
    (a) about 50 per cent of patients with Graves' disease
    (b) all patients with Hashimoto's thyroiditis
    (c) about 20 per cent of patients with Graves' disease
    (d) all patients with Graves' disease
    (Thyrotoxicosis [Graves' Disease])

16. Which of the following diseases affects the nervous system?
    (a) pernicious anemia
    (b) Landry's paralysis
    (c) multiple sclerosis
    (d) gastric atrophy
    (Autoimmune Diseases of the Nervous System)

17. Autoimmune diseases of the skin include:
    (a) pemphigus vulgaris
    (b) bullous pemphigoid
    (c) dermatitis herpetiformis
    (d) systemic lupus erythematosus
    (Autoimmune Diseases of the Skin)

ANSWER "TRUE" OR "FALSE"

18. In systemic autoimmune diseases, the major effect involves a single organ.
    (Criteria for Autoimmune Diseases)

19. There is a relationship between the presence of the HLA-B27 antigen in an individual and the occurrence of the disease ankylosing spondylitis.
    (Genetic Control of Autoimmune Diseases)

20. Systemic lupus erythematosus and rheumatoid arthritis are two distinct diseases showing completely different clinical signs and symptoms.
    (Systemic Lupus Erythematosus)

21. About 75 per cent of patients with systemic lupus erythematosus develop hypocomplementemia.
    (Systemic Lupus Erythematosus: Laboratory Observations)

22. Rheumatoid factors can occur in non-rheumatoid individuals with chronic infective conditions.
    (Rheumatoid Arthritis: Characteristics of Rheumatoid Factors)

23. Necrotizing angiitis is a systemic autoimmune disease that affects the arteries.
    (Necrotizing Angiitis [Vasculitis])

24. Portal chirrhosis is closely associated with chronic excessive alcohol ingestion.
    (Autoimmune Diseases of the Liver)

25. Autoimmune diseases affecting the heart are not associated with autoantibodies against heart muscle.
    (Other Autoimmune Diseases)

General References

Alba's Medical Technology, 9th ed. Anaheim, CA, Berkeley Scientific Publications, 1980.

Bellanti, J. A.: Immunology III. Philadelphia, W. B. Saunders Company, 1985.

Bennington, J. L. (Ed.): Saunders Dictionary and Encyclopedia of Laboratory Medicine and Technology. Philadelphia, W. B. Saunders Company, 1984.

Bryant, N. J.: An Introduction to Immunohematology. Philadelphia, W. B. Saunders Company, 1982.

Petz, L. D., and Garratty, G.: Acquired Immune Hemolytic Anemias. New York, Churchill Livingstone, 1980.

THIRTEEN

THE SEROLOGY OF ESCHERICHIA, SHIGELLA, AND SALMONELLA

OBJECTIVES

The student shall know, understand, and be prepared to explain:

1. The general aspects of the family *Enterobacteriaceae*
2. Escherichia, specifically:
   a. Antigenic properties
   b. Pathogenicity
   c. General aspects of *Escherichia* serotyping
   d. The slide agglutination test
   e. The tube agglutination test
3. Shigella, specifically:
   a. Characteristics
   b. Pathogenicity
   c. Antigenic properties
   d. General aspects of *Shigella* typing
   e. The slide agglutination test
   f. The tube agglutination test
   g. A general understanding of the identification of shigella
   h. Problems encountered in *Shigella* typing
4. Salmonella, specifically:
   a. Characteristics
   b. Antigen variation
   c. The technique of phase suppression
   d. Pathogenicity
   e. General aspects of *Salmonella* typing
   f. General procedure for the serologic identification of salmonella
   g. The Spicer-Edwards Tube test
   h. The tube agglutination test
   i. The technique of absorption
   j. The Widal test (rapid slide and tube test)

The family Enterobacteriaceae is composed of a number of gram-negative bacilli. The serologist, however, is primarily interested in those enteropathogenic escherichiae (*i.e.,* those microorganisms that cause infections of the intestines), salmonellae, and shigellae. This chapter, therefore, is confined to these areas of discussion; the interested student is referred to the list of general references at the end of this chapter for more detailed information.

THE FAMILY ENTEROBACTERIACEAE—GENERAL ASPECTS

The family Enterobacteriaceae is composed of interrelated gram-negative, non–spore-forming facultatively anaerobic bacilli that inhabit the large intestines of vertebrates and that exhibit a capacity to break down one or more carbohydrates rapidly, producing either acid (lactic, formic, or acetic) or acid and gas (carbon dioxide, hydrogen, or hydrogen sulfide). They are either motile (with peritrichous flagella) or nonmotile. All members of this family ferment glucose, reduce nitrates to nitrites, are oxidase-negative, and (with the exception of Erwinia species) do not liquify sodium pectinate.

The antigens of this family may be represented as a mosaic, falling into the following major categories:

1. K Antigens. The K (German *Kapsel* = capsule) or envelope antigens are those that surround the cell. They are (with certain exceptions) heat labile. In some genera, K antigens are given an alternate designation (*e.g.,* the Vi antigens of *Salmonella typhi* and *S. paratyphi* C) or are subdivided by physical characteristics and labeling (*e.g.,* in the genus *Escherichia*, the L, A, and B antigens).
2. O Antigens. The O (German *ohne Hauch* = nonspreading) or somatic antigens are heat stable. Those that cause agglutination are located at the surface of the cell. Note that K antigens mask the somatic antigens of the cell and can cause live cells to be rendered inagglutinable in O antisera.
3. H Antigens. The H (German *Hauch* = spreading) antigens are heat labile and are located in the flagella.
4. F Antigens. The F (or fimbrial) antigens are fine peritrichous hairlike appendages. They are numerous and extremely small (0.1 μ in width and 0.3 μ to 1.0 μ in length). F antigens have been demonstrated in escherichiae, shigellae, and salmonellae, as well as in certain other species of the family Enterobacteriaceae. In addition, some Pseudomonas strains also show

fimbriae. The reaction caused by fimbriae is not unlike H agglutination. Fimbrial antigens are not species-specific, and intrageneric reactions occur (*e.g.,* between escherichiae and shigellae). "O" agglutination of a fimbriated bacterial antigen suspension may be masked in an antiserum produced from a similar nonfimbriated species.

ESCHERICHIA

Antigenic Properties

Only one *Escherichia* species is known, *E. coli*. Several serologic types of this species exist, which are divided into groups according to their O antigens. Each group contains a varying number of species, which are differentiated by specific K and H antigens.

E. coli is known as the "colon bacillus," because it is the predominant facultative species in the large bowel. Tests for its presence are widely used in public health laboratories, because its presence in a water supply is usually indicative of fecal contamination.

Approximately 162 different O antigens of *E. coli* have been identified by specific agglutination reactions. These are designated by number (*e.g.,* O26, O120, and so on). In addition, more than 50 H antigens and more than 100 different capsular K antigens have been described. A typical *Escherichia* species formula, therefore, is written as follows:

$$O26:K60(B6).$$

(Note: The K antigens of Escherichiae are divided into three varieties, namely, L, A, and B, on the basis of their physical behavior. The L-type antigen is described as an "envelope" antigen and the A-type antigen as a "capsule" antigen; B-type antigen occurs as an envelope or capsule (Kauffmann, 1965). Some species may possess an O antigen that consists of two separate and slightly different fractions, in which case the small letters a, b, and c are used to distinguish them (*e.g.,* O127a, O127b:K65(B10) (Ewing *et al.,* 1956). The presence of K antigens on the cell surface, as mentioned, often masks the deeper O antigens. This property is destroyed by heating to temperatures varying from 60° to 120°C.

Escherichiae are widely spread throughout nature, and it is possible that strains with O, K, or H antigens exist that are similar to the known enteropathogenic varieties. Full serologic analysis is therefore necessary to determine whether an *E. coli* is the etiologic agent of a diarrhea: O antigen grouping is insufficient (Ewing and Davis, 1961).

Pathogenicity

Diseases of the urinary tract are commonly caused by *E. coli*. Most often, in these diseases, the bacilli move from the urethra through the bladder and up the ureters to the kidneys. When the bacterial count in the urine is greater than 100,000 per milliliter, bacterial disease of the urinary tract is usually present. This occurs most commonly in infants (in the diaper period), in pregnant women, and in patients with obstructive lesions of the urinary tract or neurologic diseases affecting micturation. Catheterization and other forms of urethral instrumentation are often precipitating factors.

Certain strains of *E. coli* cause acute diarrhea in humans, especially in infants. These "enteropathogenic *E. coli*" are divided into three types, based on the mechanisms of pathogenicity:

1. Enterotoxigenic *E. coli* (ETEC). These are toxin-producing strains. They are associated with diarrhea in infants and adults (Rowe *et al.*, 1977; Sack, 1975). The ETEC strains that have been described belong to one of eight O groups (*i.e.*, 6, 8, 16, 25, 27, 78, 148, and 159) (Ørskov *et al.*, 1976).
2. Enteroinvasive *E. coli*. These strains are associated with invasion of intestinal epithelium. They also produce diarrheal disease in adults and infants, and they, too, are associated with only nine serogroups of *E. coli* (*i.e.*, 28, 112, 115, 124, 136, 143, 144, 147, and 152)(Sakazaki, *et al.*, 1967).
3. Enteropathogenic *E. coli* (EPEC). These strains may produce enterotoxins. The involved O groups (26, 55, 86, 111, 114, 119, 125, 126, 127, 128, and 142) are primarily associated with infantile diarrhea, although they may cause enteric disease in adults (Guerrant and Dickens, 1974; Sack, 1976).

The frequency with which dysentery-like and toxigenic strains of *E. coli* cause human diarrhea is not clear, but it is probable that such organisms play a large role in the acute diarrhea of infants, in "traveler's diarrhea," and in "food poisoning" episodes.

E. coli is frequently found in peritonitis, appendicitis, and infections of the gallbladder and biliary tract, along with other enteric bacteria. It occurs on the skin of the perineum and genitalia and often infects wounds that become contaminated with urine or feces. *E. coli* is now the most frequently encountered species in gram-negative sepsis resulting in bacteremia and severe shock.

General Aspects of *Escherichia* Serotyping

In the past it was customary to determine whether or not *E. coli* isolated from fecal material from infants belonged to an enteropathogenic serotype. Although epidemiologically associated with newborn nursery outbreaks of diarrhea, strains belonging to these serotypes have not been found to elaborate enterotoxin or to invade. Routine serotyping of strains isolated from fecal material of infants is therefore considered unnecessary.

In the event that it is necessary to distinguish the enteropathogenic *E. coli*, this can be accomplished in the clinical laboratory using specific antisera to each of the strains of enteropathogenic *E. coli*. In routine testing, pools of type-specific antisera are more practical, because the individual testing of each suspect enteropathogenic *E. coli* with type-specific sera would be both wasteful and impractical. To facilitate testing procedures, therefore, any number of type-specific antisera may be pooled together.

One such system is outlined in Table 13–1. Five polyvalent antisera (*i.e.*, containing antibodies of more than one type) are tested against the culture material, thus limiting the number of total tests required to arrive at a final result. If an enteropathogenic *E. coli* isolate agglutinates, for example, with Poly E and not with any other polyvalent antiserum, only the four type-specific antisera listed under Poly E (Table 13–1) need to be used for the final identification. If, conversely, the *E. coli* isolate is nonpathogenic, negative results will be obtained with all five polyvalent antisera.

METHOD 1: THE SLIDE AGGLUTINATION TEST FOR THE IDENTIFICATION OF ENTEROPATHOGENIC *E. COLI*

(Note: The technique given is old enough to be considered established. Modifications of the test

Table 13–1. SCHEME FOR THE TESTING OF THE ENTEROPATHOGENIC *E. COLI* SEROTYPES

Poly A	Poly D
O26:K60 (B6)	O2:K56 (B1)
O55:K59 (B5)	O8:K25 (B2)
O111:K58 (B4)	O9:K57 (B3)
O127a:K63 (B8)	O18a O18b:K76 (B20)

Poly B	Poly E
O86a:K61 (B7)	O112a O112b:K68 (B13)
O119:K69 (B14)	O113:K75 (B19)
O124:K72 (B17)	O:127a O127b:K65 (B10)
O125:K70 (B15)	O136:K78 (B22)
O126:K71 (B16)	
O128:K67 (B12)	

Poly C	
O18a O18c:K77 (B21)	
O20a O20c:K61 (B7)	
O20a O20b:K84 (B)	
O28:K73 (B18)	
O44:K74	
O112aO112c:K66 (B11)	

exist, but the serologist is cautioned to test adequately the effects of these modifications before using them routinely.)

Method

1. Mark off two areas on a clean glass slide with a grease pencil. Label the one area T (test) and the other C (control).
2. Place a 3-ml loopful of saline on the test area and two loopfuls on the control area.
3. Remove enough culture material from a triple sugar iron agar (TSI) slop or infusion agar to prepare a heavy suspension on both areas of the slide. (The suspension should appear milky on the slide.)
4. Add one loopful of appropriate serum to the test suspension, and quickly mix with the loop.
5. Hold the slide against a dark background and rock gently.
6. Specific agglutination should occur within 1 minute: the control suspension should remain homogeneous.

Discussion

1. Organisms in the rough stage of dissociation are unsuitable for any agglutination test. Roughness can be determined by autoagglutination of the strain in 1/500 trypaflavine or acriflavine.
2. Agglutination that occurs *after* 1 minute should be ignored, especially if it does not grow any stronger within 3 minutes. Doubtful results should be checked by tube agglutination tests, which are less likely to show cross-reactions. Results obtained with antigen suspensions prepared from bile salt media should be treated with reserve.
3. Reagent volumes should be kept to a minimum to avoid cross-reaction.
4. Work close to a jar of disinfectant so that the slide can be safely and conveniently discarded, or use alcohol-treated "O" suspensions and formalin-treated "H" suspensions.

METHOD 2: THE TUBE AGGLUTINATION TEST FOR THE IDENTIFICATION OF ENTEROPATHOGENIC *E. COLI*

Preparation of Heated "O" Antigen Suspension

1. Inoculate an infusion broth, and incubate at 37°C for 4 to 6 hours. Adjust opacity to Brown's Opacity Tube number 1 (750 million organisms per milliliter). Heat the broth in a boiling water bath for 1 hour, and then cool and use, *OR*
2. Harvest the growth from an infusion agar and suspend in saline and adjust opacity as above. heat for 1 hour, cool, and then use.

Preparation of K O Antigen Suspension

As above, but instead of heating, add three drops of 40 per cent formalin.

Method

1. Serially dilute the "OB" antiserum at a 1:5 dilution, continuing to at least 1:640. (Include a saline control.) Use 0.5-ml amounts.
2. After adding 0.5 ml of the heated "O" antigen, shake gently and incubate for 16 to 18 hours at 50°C. (OB tests are incubated at 37°C for 2 hours and refrigerated overnight.)
3. Read and record results.

Discussion

In spite of the fact that the value of serotyping of enteropathogenic *E. coli* has been questioned, the fact that other pathogenic mechanisms are also involved and the disagreement among experts suggests that serotyping should not be totally abandoned, especially in situations in which very young children are involved.

SHIGELLA

Characteristics

In humans, shigellae cause a disease known as *bacillary dysentery* (Greek = sick gut), a common illness that spreads rapidly under conditions of poor sanitation and overcrowding. The first species of this group was isolated by the Japanese bacteriologist Shiga in 1898.

The genus *Shigella* should, as determined by DNA-relatedness analysis, be included with the genus *Escherichia*. Because of the possible confusion that this would generate, however, *Shigella* has been retained as a separate genus.

As a group, shigellae are gram-negative rods that are nonmotile and, with a few exceptions (biotypes of *Shigella flexneri* 6), they are anaerogenic. Although many shigellae produce catalase (Carpenter and Lachowicz, 1959), this is an inconsistent property within the genus. *Shigella dysenteriae* 1, the type species of the genus, is usually negative. Some shigellae are late lactose fermenters. On TSI, the reaction is A1K/A gas − H_2S − .

Colonies of shigellae, on enteric media, are usually smaller than those of salmonellae, but occasionally, mucoid variants may be found in subgroup C.

Aside from bacillary dysentery, *Shigella* may occasionally cause bacteremia, pneumonia, or other infection.

The genus is divided into the following four species (or subgroups):

Shigella dysenteriae—serologic subgroup A
Shigella flexneri—serologic subgroup B
Shigella boydii—serologic subgroup C
Shigella sonnei—serologic subgroup D

Each of these four species possesses specific polysaccharide O antigens, and certain smooth (S) strains possess heat-labile K antigens. They are, however, nonmotile, and therefore possess no H antigens. They are differentiated from other *Enterobacteriaceae* by biochemical reactions and from each other by biochemical and antigenic characteristics. Each species is further divided into serologic subtypes, on the basis of biochemical and somatic (O) antigen characteristics (Table 13–2).

Pathogenicity

All known species of the genus *Shigella* are pathogenic for humans. Shigella dysentery is characterized by the sudden onset of abdominal cramps, diarrhea, and fever, following an incubation period of 2 to 3 days. The organisms are ingested in contaminated food or drink. In infants and young children, the loss of water and salts may cause dehydration and electrolyte imbalance. Blood and mucus are commonly seen in the feces.

Shigellae commonly produce mucosal ulcerative lesions in the gastrointestinal tract, mostly confined to the terminal ileum and colon. These lesions are covered by a pseudomembrane made up of polymorphonuclear leukocytes, cell debris, and bacteria enmeshed in fibrin; they are believed to arise when the organisms cross the epithelial barrier and enter the lamina propria. Metabolic products accumulate locally, and endotoxin is released; the result is death of the epithelial cells. During recovery, granulation tissue fills the ulcerations, which eventually heal. Scar formation is sometimes seen in cases of unusually extensive ulcers.

Shigella dysenteriae type 1 (Shiga bacillus) is known to produce (in addition to the endotoxin common to all shigellae) a heat-labile exotoxin known as *Shiga neurotoxin,* which, when injected parenterally into rabbits, mice, or guinea pigs, causes paralysis, diarrhea, and death and, in addition, elaborates a potent enterotoxin that causes fluid accumulation in ligated segments of rabbit ileum. This neurotoxin therefore appears to be responsible for the pathogenicity of Shiga's bacillus. The factors responsible for pathogenicity in the other shigellae are not clearly defined.

During convalescence, specific agglutinins appear in the blood, and antibodies can often be demonstrated in the feces (so-called coproantibodies); circulating antibodies appear to have no effect on the course of the disease, but coproantibodies may play a role in the recovery.

Shigella dysentery varies in severity according to species. The general order is, from least to most severe, *S. sonnei, S. boydii, S. flexneri,* and *S. dysenteriae.*

Antigenic Properties

Nomenclature. The *Shigella* serotypes are numbered with arabic numerals, beginning at one and continuing consecutively (see Table 13–2). Each serotype is referred to by the subgroup heading followed by the serotype number (*e.g., S. flexneri* 5 or *S. dysenteriae* 1). Smooth (S) and rough (R) forms of *S. sonnei* are referred to as *S. sonnei* I and II, respectively.

Antigens. Almost all shigellae possess a K antigen of the B variety (Edwards and Ewing, 1972) that is subgroup-specific. The usefulness of the K antigens in shigellae differentiation has not been fully studied. The *Shigella* and *Escherichia* species are similar in many biochemical properties; therefore, it is not surprising to find antigenic similarities as well. Biochemical differentiation of these two genera is, however, a simple matter, and laboratories usually experience no difficulty in this regard.

Table 13–2. CLASSIFICATION OF THE SHIGELLAE

Species	Subgroup Designation	Serotype Designation	Antigen Formulae
Shigella dysenteriae	A	1	
		2	
		3	
		4	
		5	
		6	
		7	
		8	
		9	
		10	
Shigella flexneri	B	1A	I:4
		1B	I:4,6
		2A	II:4
		2B	II:7,8,9
		3A	III:6,7
		3B	III:4,6,7
		3C	III:(4),6
		4A	IV:4
		4B	IV:6
		5	V:7
		6	IV:(4)
Shigella boydii	C	1	
		2	
		3	
		4	
		5	
		6	
		7	
		8	
		9	
		10	
		11	
		12	
		13	
		14	
		15	
Shigella sonnei	D	I Sh. sonnei (S)	
		II Sh. sonnei (R)	

Shigellae do not possess flagella, and antigenic identity is based entirely on somatic components.

General Aspects of *Shigella* Typing

With the use of polyvalent antisera against each of the four species, it is a simple matter to distinguish a *Shigella* isolate. Because all four *Shigella* species are biochemically, physiologically, and morphologically similar, they are best distinguished by their serologic characteristics.

The best method of obtaining specimens for culture is by means of a rectal swab. Specimens obtained from ulcerative intestinal lesions, under direct vision through a sigmoidoscope, are most likely to contain organisms. Cultures are best made of MacConkey, xylose-lysine-deoxycholate or eosin methylene blue agar. (Note: Deoxycholate citrate and *Salmonella-Shigella* (SS) agars are often inhibitory.) Final identification of the organism is based on biochemical and specific agglutination tests.

A suspension of a *Shigella* isolate is prepared by mixing a loopful of culture in a drop of saline on a microscope slide. A drop of one of the four antisera (A, B, C, or D) is added to the suspension, and the mixture is gently rotated by hand. The test is repeated until one of the suspensions gives clearly visible clumping of the bacteria in suspension. All the polyvalent antisera should be tested, even if a positive result is obtained early in the series. The frequency of certain serotypes in certain geographical locations will determine which antiserum should be used first. In the United States, it is advisable to start with *S. flexneri* or *S. sonnei* forms I and II, because these are more prevalent. Agglutination in any one of these polyvalent antisera will indicate a *Shigella* species and its respective group. By using monospecific antisera systematically and in turn, a serotype identification can be made.

Biochemical tests should be completed in full, and the results must coincide with the serologic findings before a final result is reported.

METHOD 3: THE SLIDE AGGLUTINATION TEST

(This method is exactly the same as that described for *E. coli*.)

METHOD 4: THE TUBE AGGLUTINATION TEST

Preparation of Antigen Suspension

1. **Add three drops of 40 per cent formalin to an overnight infusion broth culture, and adjust opacity to Brown's Opacity Tube number 1 (750 million organisms per milliliter), OR**

2. **Suspend the growth from an infusion agar in 0.5 per cent formol-saline, and adjust opacity as previously described.**

Method

1. **Double dilute the antiserum serially in 0.5-ml amounts, commencing at a 1:10 dilution and continuing until the titer of the serum is reached.**
2. **Add 0.5 ml of antigen to each tube and a saline control.**
3. **Incubate in a water bath at 50°C for 4 hours.**
4. **Read and record results.**

Notes of the Identification of the Shigellae

S. dysenteriae. Intersubgroup relationships exist between *S. dysenteriae* 2 and 10 and *S. boydii* 1 and between *S. dysenteriae* 8 and *S. boydii* 15 (Ewing and Johnson, 1961). *S. dysenteriae* 1 also displays minor antigenic similarities to alkalescens-dispar (A-D) group 01. Full investigation of the biochemical characteristics of a strain that agglutinates in unabsorbed *Shigella* antisera is therefore essential to effect identification. (The A-D group of organisms includes nonmotile anaerogenic enterobacteria that ferment lactose late [*B. dispar*] or not at all [*B. alkalescens*] but otherwise resemble *E. coli* in their biochemical reactions.)

S. flexneri. The *S. flexneri* subgroup members contain common as well as specific antigens. The antigenic formula, therefore, of *S. flexneri* 1B, for example, is written as 1:4,6 (See Table 13–2). The formulae appearing in Table 13–2 are abbreviated as suggested by Ewing (1949). For example, *S. flexneri* 5 contains antigens 1 and 5 as well as 7, but, to avoid confusion, it is only necessary to identify *S. flexneri* by its 7 component.

Because of interserotype and intersubserotype reactions with *S. flexneri*, monospecific antisera preparation requires extensive absorption. Cross-reactions occur with some commercial antisera. In some instances, cross-reactions in *S. flexneri* antisera with strains of *S. boydii* and A-D can be eliminated by dilution of the antisera. More often, however, further absorption with A-D is necessary.

S. boydii. There is a reciprocal relationship between *S. boydii* 6 and *S. sonnei* II, and cross-reactions can be expected unless the *S. boydii* 6 is prepared from a freshly isolated strain. In spite of these relationships, however, there is no evidence of significant intrageneric or extrageneric sharing of antigens.

S. sonnei. Freshly isolated *S. sonnei* strains appear in two forms, sometimes even within the same culture. They are called *smooth* (S-form 1) and *rough* (R-form II) and, in most cases, are easily distinguishable. The colonies of the smooth form are similar to those of other enteric organisms; colonies of the rough form are two to six times larger and fairly flat, and they have an irregular edge with raised section and lobate concentrate striations about the raised portion of the colony (like a bomb burst). Antisera prepared from each form are form-specific.

As mentioned previously, close similarities exist between *S. sonnei* II and *S. boydii* 6, and care must be taken in this regard in identification procedures.

Problems Encountered in Shigella Typing

If no agglutination of any of the subgroup polyvalent antisera is seen, attempts should be made to agglutinate the strain with a polyvalent A-D antiserum. If agglutination occurs and biochemical tests agree, the strain can be reported as an A-D. If no agglutination of the subgroup polyvalent antisera or A-D polyvalent antiserum is seen, the strain is neither one of the currently known serotypes nor an A-D. Note, however, that the strain may be an encapsulated shigella or A-D. As mentioned, encapsulated strains prevent somatic agglutination in sera containing only somatic antibodies. Any strain biochemically resembling a shigella, therefore, that fails to agglutinate in O antisera, should be heated for 1 hour at 100°C to destroy this inhibiting effect.

Finally, if agglutination in more than one subgroup or monospecific antiserum is seen, only strong agglutination should be accepted as valid. Weak reactions must be ignored because of antigenic relationships previously discussed. Biochemical tests can also be of great help in doubtful situations.

SALMONELLA

Characteristics

The genus *Salmonella* is composed of motile organisms that do not ferment lactose or sucrose; they do not produce urease or gelatinase, nor do they use malonate. In general, they ferment dulcite and do not grow in KCN medium. They grow easily on blood agar and on MacConkey and Hecktoen agars. On the last two of these, they are colorless (on MacConkey) or blue green (on Hecktoen), possibly with black centers, and, after overnight incubation at 35°C, they are about 5 mm in diameter, circular, convex, and soft and smooth if the colony is in a smooth phase.

By systematic testing with antisera absorbed with one strain after another to detect and analyze antigenic differences, Kauffmann and White provided an extraordinarily detailed scheme for classification of the salmonellae, now known as the Kauffmann-White scheme (Edwards and Ewing, 1972). Originally, salmonellae were named according to the disease they caused or the animal from which they were first isolated. Now the species epithet is taken from the name of the city, suburb, area, province, or state in which the serotype is first isolated.

Recent United States usage recognizes only three species of salmonella, *S. choleraesuis*, *S. typhi*, and *S. enteritidis*. The first two *S. choleraesuis* and *S. typhi* do not contain bioserotypes or serotypes, but *S. enteritidis* contains more than 100 bioserotypes and serotypes (note: A serotype indicates a group of organisms having a common antigenicity, whereas a bioserotype indicates a group with common biochemical reactions.) The differentiation of the *Salmonella* species is shown in Table 13–3.

The salmonellae have both somatic (O) and flagellar (H) antigens, both of which are used to identify the serotypes. In some instances, capsular (Vi) antigens are also useful *(e.g., S. typhi)* The O antigens are designated numerically, and the H antigens are designated both alphabetically and numerically. A salmonella formula would be written, for example, as *S. heidelberg* 1,4,5,12:r:1,2. The 1,4,5,12 portion of the formula (before the first colon) designates the O antigens, and r:1,2 are the H antigen designations. Salmonella serotypes with similar O antigens are grouped together, and each separate group is designated with consecutive alphabet letters (a, b, c, and so on). Groups C and E are further subdivided into groups C_1 and C_2 and E_1, E_2, E_3, and E_4. Because the number of salmonella groups exceeds the number of alphabet letters, it is customary to use Z_1, Z_2, Z_3 and so on to accommodate the overflow. The two H portions of the formula (as in *S. heidelberg*, r:1,2) are associated with H antigen phase variation. Variation also occurs in O, Vi, and fimbrial antigens. These phenomena are described in the following section.

Table 13–3. DIFFERENTIATION OF *SALMONELLA* SPECIES

Test	S. enteritidis	S. choleraesuis	S. typhi
H_2S	+	+/−	+W
Citrate	+	(+)	−
Ornithine	+	+	−
Dulcite	+	d	d
Gas from glucose	+	+	−

From Raphael, S. S.: Lynch's Medical Laboratory Technology, 4th ed. Philadelphia, W. B. Saunders Company, 1983, p. 378.

Antigen Variation

There are six types of antigenic variation in salmonellae. These are associated with (1) change in the H antigen (phase variation); (2) loss of the H antigen (H-O variation); (3) change from smooth to rough forms (S-R variation); (4) a quantitative change in the O antigens (form variation); (5) a loss or change of the Vi antigen (V-W variation); and (6) fimbrial-nonfimbrial variation. Each of these variations will be discussed.

Phase Variation. A "phase" can be described as a distinct antigenic entity. The majority of salmonellae are diphasic (*i.e.*, consisting of two antigenic entities), although they can be monophasic (consisting of a single antigenic entity) or multiphasic (consisting of a number of antigenic entities). For example, *S. enteritidis,* 9,12:gm, is monophasic, because each organism in an *S. enteritidis* culture has the antigenic properties 9,12:gm. On the other hand, *S. heidelberg,* 1,4,5,12:r:1,2 is diphasic, because it is a mixed population consisting of 1,4,5,12:r and 1,4,5,12:1,2 individuals. Each of these individuals (or antigenic entities) is described as a phase. A culture of diphasic salmonellae will contain proportions of each phase. The rapidity and strength of the reactions will therefore vary according to the proportions of the two antigenic entities present in the particular colony; this is referred to as *phase variation.* In serotyping of salmonellae, both antigenic entities should be identified. In some cases, it is necessary to suppress the predominant phase before identifying the alternate phase, using the technique of phase suppression. The two phases of biphasic salmonellae are commonly referred to as *phase 1* and *phase 2.*

METHOD 5: THE TECHNIQUE OF PHASE SUPPRESSION

Method

1. **Heat to melt 5 ml of sterile infusion agar (0.2 to 0.5 per cent), and then cool to 48° to 50°C.**
2. **Mix in two drops of phase one or two serum (depending upon the phase to be inhibited), and then carefully drop a dry sterile tube (open at both ends with the bottom end jagged) to the tubed agar. (Note: This open-ended tube must be long enough to protrude at least 1/2 inch above the agar surface.) Care should be taken not to splash agar up the sides of the inserted tube.**
3. **Seed the agar surface within the inserted tube with a shallow prick using a pick-off needle. (The growth should be harvested from an infusion agar slope half covered with infusion broth. A moist slope is more conducive to**
flagella formation than a dry slope. Broth cultures provide too few organisms for this procedure.)
4. **Incubate the tube for 24 hours at 37°C. (During the incubation, the antibody in the serum in the agar will immobilize those organisms that have homologous antigens, and the alternate phase can be isolated from the agar surface outside the glass tubing.)**
5. **Remove a small amount of the infusion agar with a sterile pipet, and transfer it aseptically to an infusion broth and another infusion agar slope half covered with broth.**
6. **Incubate both tubes for a further 24 hours at 37°C.**

After incubation, the agar or broth tube cultures can be used to determine the identity of the alternate phase. The culture may require a further passage through the Craigie tube if agglutination of the alternate phase is unsatisfactory. The agar-slope culture obtained from the Craigie tube will then serve as the source of the inoculum for a further passage.

H–O Variation. The loss of H antigens occurs rarely in flagellated salmonellae as a result of loss of flagella. In most cases, however, the loss of H antigen is due to use of a medium for cultivation that reduces their motility and therefore their capacity to react in specific antisera. Media that are likely to *enhance* motility (*e.g.*, infusion broth or moist infusion agar) should therefore always be used for the identification of H antigens.

S–R Variation. When repeatedly subcultured salmonella cultures undergo changes in growth characteristics and the O antigen characteristics and tend to cross-react with previously unrelated organisms and to autoagglutinate in saline, this is known as S-R variation, because colonies of unchanged organisms appear smooth, whereas colonies of changed organisms appear rough. The change from S to R forms is a gradual process, and smooth colonies may contain rough forms. When suspended in 1/500 typaflavine or acriflavine, rough forms tend to agglutinate, and this rapid test may prove useful in handling suspect cases.

Form Variation. This refers to a quantitative change in O antigens and is usually associated with the 1, 6, 12, 22, 23, 24, and 25 antigens. Variation may occur within a strain and from strain to strain, so that specific antisera for these factors could yield reactions of varying strength with cultures known to contain these factors. Moreover, antigens 6 and 12 contain subfractions named 6 and 6_2 and 12, 12_2, and 12_3, respectively. The 6 and 12_2 antigens are subject to form variation, whereas 6_2, 12, and 12_3 are not.

V–W Variation. Colonies of *S. typhi* that agglutinate in Vi antiserum are known as *V colonies;*

those that do not are known as *W colonies* (Kauffmann, 1965). The fact that V colonies do not agglutinate in O antiserum, whereas W colonies do, indicates that Vi antigen has a masking effect on O antigens. This inhibition (or masking) can be destroyed by boiling or by standing the culture in phenolyzed saline for a few hours.

Fimbrial–Nonfimbrial Variation. Fimbriae possessed by many salmonellae are unlikely to affect serotyping, because the methods used to prepare antigen suspensions for animal immunization do not allow for fimbrial formation.

Pathogenicity

Salmonella infection is almost always due to the ingestion of contaminated food or water, the organisms entering the tissues from the intestines via the lymphatics. The incubation period varies with the individual and the number of organisms ingested. Salmonellosis is particularly common in children younger than 10 years of age, suggesting that an acquired immunity prevents a large number of infections. Infection with *Salmonella* is common; in 1979, more than 33,000 cases were reported, a figure that is believed to represent only about 1 per cent of all infections.

Three principal syndromes result from salmonella infection in humans:

1. Enteric fever (characteristic of *S. typhi,* but also seen with some serotypes of *S. enteritidis*)
2. Gastroenteritis (characteristic of *S. enteritidis* serotypes)
3. Extraintestinal focal infections in one or more organs accompanied by septicemia (usually reflecting bacteremia with *S. enteritidis* serotypes).

Enteric Fever. Among the enteric fevers, the classic example is typhoid fever. The typhoid organisms, *S. typhi,* produce the disease only in humans and chimpanzees. After an incubation period of 7 to 14 days, clinical signs begin to appear. Malaise, anorexia, and headache usually appear first and are followed by the onset of fever, which rises in a steplike manner and is accompanied by relative bradycardia. During the first week, prostration may be marked, and the patient may have diarrhea, although constipation is more common, with abdominal tenderness and distention. At this time, the patient may have a cough and bronchitis, rose spots frequently appear on the trunk, and splenomegaly and leukopenia are common. In severe cases, the sensorium is dulled, and the patient may become delirious and show the so-called typhoid state for which the disease was named. After the third week, the fever usually subsides by gradual lysis. During the later stages of the disease, there may be severe intestinal hemorrhages or perforation of the bowel, causing peritonitis.

The kinetics of the bacteremia, shedding of organisms in the feces and urine and formation of antibodies, are as follows:

1. Blood cultures are often positive in the first and second weeks and are less frequently so in the third week.
2. Stool cultures may be positive from the beginning and often remain positive until convalescence has been completed.
3. Urine cultures are often positive during the second and third weeks and may remain so for a considerable period after convalescence.
4. Antibodies are usually formed during the second week, reaching a peak in the fifth or sixth week.

Note: Cultures of the bone marrow may show typhoid bacilli when blood cultures are negative. Organisms may also be found in the rose spots.

Ingested *S. typhi* multiplies in the gastrointestinal tract; some organisms enter the intestinal lymphatics, from which they are disseminated throughout the body by the blood stream and are excreted in the urine. The bile provides a good culture medium for *S. typhi,* and luxuriant growth occurs in the biliary tract and provides a continuous flow of organisms into the small bowel, where they tend to localize in Peyer's patches. Their ability to persist in the biliary tract may result in a chronic "carrier" state, in which they continue to be excreted in the feces.

On postmortem examination, lesions (ulcerations) are seen in the small intestine, as is lymphoid hyperplasia involving the lymph nodes, Peyer's patches, and the spleen. Focal necrosis of the liver, inflammation of the gallbladder, and patchy inflammatory lesions in the lungs, bone marrow, and periosteum are also often seen.

Relapses occur in 10 per cent of cases, and the disease is fatal in 10 per cent of cases.

Enteric fevers caused by other salmonellae (so-called parathyhoid fevers) are usually milder and have a shorter incubation period. In such cases, bacteremia occurs early, fever lasts for 1 to 3 weeks, and rose spots are rare. Enteric fever may be caused by almost any salmonella; in the United States, the most common agents are *S. paratyphi* B *(S. schottmülleri)* and *S. typhimurium.*

Gastroenteritis. Gastroenteritis caused by Salmonella occurs 4 to 48 hours after the consumption of contaminated food. The disease is confined to the gastrointestinal tract and is characterized by diarrhea, ranging from mild to a fulminant form with sudden onset ("food poisoning"). Fever usually lasts from 1 to 4 days. Symptoms include headache, chills, abdominal pain, nausea, and vomiting. Blood cultures are rarely positive; stool cultures are usually positive. In the United States, the most common cause of salmonella gastroenteritis is *S. typhimurium*.

Septicemia. Salmonella septicemias are characterized by high, remittent fever, bacteremia (usually without apparent involvement of the gastrointestinal tract), and focal suppurative ulceration, which may develop in the biliary tract, kidneys, heart, spleen, meninges, joints, and lungs. Prolonged septicemia of this type is commonly caused by *S. choleraesuis*.

General Aspects of *Salmonella* Typing

The majority of *Salmonella* isolates in the United States fall within groups B to E_4 (Table 13–4). The growing multiplicity of serotypes of salmonella, however, and the numerous antisera required for complete characterization of all of them make it impractical for many laboratories to attempt complete serologic typing of all salmonellae. A compromise is therefore made, and smaller laboratories possess a minimal number of antisera that allow them to identify the more important salmonellae that are endemic in human populations.

For practical purposes, polyvalent antisera containing antibodies to the group antigens of the most commonly isolated serotypes of *Salmonella* are available from a number of commercial houses. When agglutination occurs with an isolate in the presence of such polyvalent serum, further identification may be made with factor-specific antisera that contain antibodies to single H, O, or Vi diagnostic antigens.

Polyvalent salmonella O and H antisera will agglutinate any organism that is a salmonella. The polyvalent O antiserum contains antibodies to all O groups; the polyvalent H antiserum contains

Table 13–4. THE ANTIGENIC FORMULAE AND GROUPING OF THE MORE COMMON SALMONELLAE

		H	
	O	*Phase 1*	*Phase 2*
Group B			
S. typhimurium	1,4,5,12	i	1,2
S. heidelberg	1,4,5,12	r	1,2
S. saint-paul	1,4,5,12	eh	1,2
S. paratyphi B	1,4,5,12	b	1,2
S. java	1,4,5,12	b	(1,2)
S. derby	1,4,5,12	fg	—
S. bredeney	1,4,5,12	lv	1,7
S. san-diego	4,5,12	eh	enz 15
Group C_1			
S. infantis	6,7	r	1,5
S. thompson	6,7	k	1,5
S. montevideo	6,7	gms	—
S. oranienburg	6,7	mt	—
S. tennessee	6,7	Zng	—
S. bareilly	6,7	y	1,5
S. choleraesuis	6,7	c	1,5
Group C_2			
S. newport	6,8	eh	1,2
S. blockley	6,8	k	1,5
S. muenchen	6,8	d	1,2
S. kentucky	(8),20	i	Z_6
Group D			
S. typhi	9,12,Vi	d	—
S. enteritidis	1,9,12	gm	—
S. panama	1,9,12	lv	1,5
Group E_1			
S. anatum	3,10	eh	1,6
Group E_2			
S. newington	3,15	eh	1,6
Group E_4			
S. senftenberg	1,3,19	Z_{27}, Z_{43}, Z_{45}, Z_{46}	
Group G			
S. worthington	1,13,23	Z	12

antibodies to almost all the H antigens. Although polyvalent O antiserum is more widely used (since some cases fail to develop H antigens), polyvalent H antiserum can serve to determine the cross-activity of the H antigens of the strain under study, thus indicating whether H antigen analysis can proceed or whether motility needs to be enhanced by cultivation in a suitable medium.

Before serologic investigations are attempted, nonlactose fermenters on planted agar should be subcultured on a differential medium such as TSI and tested for phenylalanine deamination and urease production. Serologic test results should be regarded as tentative until these biochemical tests are complete.

All O agglutination tests should be carried out on slides. Preliminary H agglutination tests may be carried out on slides, but the result should be confirmed by tube test. The slide agglutination test is performed with an O polyvalent salmonella antiserum. If this test is positive, the strain should be tested against individual O group antisera. If negative, the strain should be further tested against Vi, polyvalent Arizona, and polyvalent Bethesda-Ballerup antisera. (Note: If agglutination occurs with Vi antiserum, a heated suspension [20 minutes to 1 hour at 100°C] should be tested against the polyvalent O antiserum or O Group C or D antiserum. Agglutination in D antiserum would then indicate *S. typhi*, provided that biochemical analysis is supportive.) Negative agglutination in Vi or Arizona serum rules out currently known salmonellae and Arizonae. If the organism biochemically resembles a salmonella or Arizona, it should be submitted to a reference center for further study to confirm the findings and to consider the possibility of a new serotype.

Because group B salmonellae are prevalent in the United States, the salmonella under study should first be tested with group B antiserum, and then each of the other salmonella group antisera should be used in turn. Testing should be performed with each group antiserum, even when strong agglutination is observed early in the series, to ensure correct grouping and, further, to ensure that cross-agglutination is not occurring. (Note: Cross-agglutination is usually weak, but interpretation is sometimes difficult unless a strong specific reaction is available for comparison.)

Once the group determination is complete, the strain should be tested in polyvalent H antisera to determine whether the H antigens are sufficiently well developed. A negative reaction to the polyvalent H antiserum would indicate a salmonella devoid of flagella, in which case a motility test or a flagellum strain might lend support to the serologic findings.

In the Widal or agglutination test (procedure that follows), a rising titer of specific agglutinins is accepted as definite evidence of infection with a particular salmonella strain. If only a single specimen is available, an O agglutination titer of more than 50 (dilution 1:50) during the first 10 days of illness is considered strong presumptive evidence if the patient has not been vaccinated within 2 years.

General Procedure for the Serologic Identification of Salmonella

1. Perform the slide agglutination test. (Note: This test procedure is exactly the same as that described earlier for *Escherichia* [see Method 1]. If this test is positive, it is probable that the organism is a salmonella, although some species of *Enterobacteriaceae* may include salmonella antigens.
2. If biochemical results suggestive of *S. typhi* have been obtained with the organism, the O antigen may be masked by its capsular Vi antigen and a false-negative result may be obtained with O antisera. In such cases, a slide agglutination test using anti-Vi serum should be used. (Note: The slide agglutination test is exactly as described for *Escherichia*, earlier in this chapter). Positive agglutination in this test confirms the presence of Vi antigen. The combination of a positive test with Vi antiserum and typical biochemical pattern is diagnostic of *S. typhi* or *S. enteritidis* bioser Paratyphi C. The demonstration of the Vi antigen alone, however, is *not* conclusive, because other "coliform" organisms may possess this antigen. The Vi antigen may be destroyed, if desired, by boiling a saline suspension of the organism for 1 hour, followed by washing by centrifugation, which leaves the O antigens unmasked.
3. If polyvalent agglutination is observed, proceed using group antisera. It should be noted that certain antisera are supplied, which are directed against the entire O component of a particular organism, whereas others are absorbed out so as to be specific. Specific antisera are, of course, preferable, because they eliminate troublesome cross-reaction.
4. After the identity of the group to which the organism belongs has been established, it is necessary to identify the flagellar antigens. This can be accomplished using the Spicer-Edwards tube test, which uses seven commercially prepared antisera against the bacterial suspension. The precipitation pattern obtained allows for the identification of 17 types and groups of H antigens (phase 1 and phase 2). The availability of this method eliminates the need to retain a large collection of individual H antisera in the laboratory.

METHOD 6: THE SPICER-EDWARDS TUBE TEST

Reagents

Spicer-Edwards antisera (available from commercial houses)
Formalized saline (prepared as follows):

Commercial formalin	**6ml**
Sodium chloride	**8.5 gm**
Distilled water	**to 1 L**

Method

1. **Label seven test tubes 1, 2, 3, 4, 1-7, L, and en.**
2. **Place 5 ml of formalized saline in each tube.**
3. **To tube 1, add 2 drops of Spicer-Edwards serum 1; to tube 2, add 2 drops of Spicer-Edwards serum 2, and so on with the other tubes. This produces an approximate 1:75 dilution with the formalized saline.**
4. **From an overnight culture of the organism on a nutrient agar slant, make a heavy suspension of the organism by adding 3 ml of formalized saline and mixing by gentle rotation. Transfer into a sterile tube.**
5. **Label seven Kahn tubes the same way as the original seven tubes. Add 5 drops of formalized suspension of the organism to each tube. Then add an equal quantity of each diluted antiserum to each tube.**
6. **Incubate the tubes at 56°C for 3 hours.**
7. **After incubation, allow the tubes to stand at room temperature overnight, covered with a clean cloth.**
8. **Read the tubes the following morning, noting those with typical fluffy H agglutination.**

Interpretation

Agglutination may occur in both phase 1 and phase 2 antisera, thus yielding a complete flagella-antigen formula as shown in Table 13–5. If the organism can be found only in one phase and if identification requires knowledge of the other phase, perform the technique of phase suppression (see Method 5).

It should now be possible to state the antigenic formula of the organism and possibly its identity. In most cases, the possibilities have been narrowed down to a few organisms, and more specific antisera are necessary to establish identity. To this end, further anti-O antisera testing may be performed.

Other Test Methods

METHOD 7: THE TUBE AGGLUTINATION TEST (used for checking doubtful results in the slide agglutination test)

Preparation of H Antigen Suspension

1. **Inoculate an infusion broth with a pick-off needle, and incubate for 24 hours. Dilute the culture with equal portions of 0.6 per cent formol-saline, OR**
2. **Inoculate an infusion broth and incubate for 4 hours. Add three drops of formalin, and then dilute with sterile broth to an opacity equal to**

Table 13–5. INTERPRETATION OF SPICER-EDWARDS TUBE TEST (See text)

H Antigen	Spicer-Edwards Antisera				
	1	*2*	*3*	*4*	
a	+	+	+	−	
b	+	+	−	+	
c	+	+	−	−	
d	+	−	+	+	
e,h	+	−	+	−	
G complex	+	−	−	+	
i	+	−	−	−	Phase 1 antigens
k	−	+	+	+	
r	−	+	−	+	
y	−	+	−	−	
z	−	−	+	+	
z_4 complex	−	−	+	−	
z_{10}	−	−	−	+	
z_{29}	−	+	+	−	
e,n,x, e,n, z_{15}	e,n complex antiserum				Phase 2 antigen
l,v.l,w.l,z_{13}.l,z_{28}	L complex antiserum				
1,2 1,5, 1,6, 1,7	1 complex antiserum				

Note: the G complex includes flagellar antigens f,g, f,g,t, g,m, g,m,s, g,m,t, g,p, g,p,u, g,q, g,s,t, m,s, and t. The z_4 complex includes z_4,z_{23}, z_4, z_{24}, and z_4,z_{32}.

From Raphael, S. S.: Lynch's Medical Laboratory Technology, 4th ed. Philadelphia, W. B. Saunders Company, 1983, p. 379.

Brown's Opacity Tube number 1 (750 million organisms per milliliter).

Preparation of O Antigen Suspension

1. Suspend the growth from an infusion agar slant in absolute ethyl alcohol and heat to 60°C for 1 hour; then centrifuge it for 10 minutes to pack the cells so that the alcohol can be poured off. Resuspend in saline, and adjust opacity to Brown's Opacity tube number 1 (750 million organisms per milliliter), *OR*
2. Transfer the growth from an infusion agar slant to 0.5 ml of saline in a test tube and stopper. Place in a boiling water bath for 10 minutes, and then dilute to the required opacity (Brown's Opacity Tube number 1, 750 million organisms per milliliter).

Method

1. Dilute appropriate serum 1/25 with normal saline.
2. Place 0.5 ml of this into a clean, dry tube, and add 0.5 ml of the antigen suspension.
3. Incubate H and O agglutination tests at 50°C for 2 and 4 hours, respectively.

Discussion

A single dilution is all that is necessary except when distinguishing closely related antigens, in which case a series of dilutions should be set up to cover the titer of the serum.

A saline control tube with antigen suspension should be set up to check for autoagglutination of the strain and to act as a negative control.

The tubes should be submerged so that approximately one third of the fluid in the tubes is above the level of water in the water bath.

METHOD 8: THE TECHNIQUE OF ABSORPTION

Method

1. Seed moist, thick infusion agar plates in 100-mm Petri dishes with 0.5 ml of a 24-hour broth culture of the absorbing strain.
2. Incubate the Petri dishes for 24 hours with their medium surfaces facing up.
3. After incubation, flood the plates with 0.25 per cent phenol-saline and scrape off the growth into a centrifuge tube.
4. Centrifuge at high speed (2000 to 3000 rpm) for 15 minutes to pack the cells so that the supernatant fluid can be poured off.
5. Resuspend the cells in 1.0 ml of phenol-saline.

6. Add serum to be absorbed, and mix well.
7. Incubate for 2 hours at 50°C.
8. After incubation, centrifuge and remove the absorbed serum.
9. Titrate the absorbed serum against a suspension of the absorbing strain and one or more serotypes containing the selected factors. A check against the absorbing strain is made to ascertain whether the absorption has been satisfactorily achieved. A check against the selected serotypes is made to ascertain the titer of the selected factor(s). If the absorbed antiserum is to be used in slide tests, these checks must be carried out on slides.

METHOD 9: THE WIDAL TEST (RAPID SLIDE)

Method

1. Pipet 0.8, 0.04, 0.01, and 0.005 ml of test and control sera onto separate areas on a ruled glass plate that is blackened on the opposite side.
2. Add one drop of the appropriate antigen suspension (undiluted) to each serum. (Take care to resuspend the antigen properly before it is dispensed.) Final serum dilutions of 1:20, 1:40, 1:80, and 1:320 are thus achieved.
3. Mix each suspension with an applicator stick, starting with the highest dilution and working toward the lowest.
4. Tilt the glass plate back and forth for a minute, and then read under a bench lamp.
5. If agglutination is seen, confirm with the tube test (description follows).

METHOD 10: THE WIDAL TEST ("O" TUBE TEST PROCEDURE)

Method

1. Set up eight tubes in a test tube rack.
2. To the first tube, add 1.9 ml of 0.25 per cent phenol-saline. Add 1.0 ml of phenol-saline to the remaining seven tubes.
3. Add 0.1 ml of the patient's serum to tube 1, mix and transfer 1 ml to tube 2. Repeat for each tube, finally discarding 1 ml from tube 7. The final dilutions are 1:20 through 1:1280. Tube 8 will act as a control. (Note: A positive control should be set up with the patient's tests. Salmonella polyvalent antiserum should be used for this purpose.)
4. Add 0.05 ml of the appropriate antigen suspension to all tubes. Mix by shaking the racks.
5. Incubate tests at 37°C for 2 hours.
6. Refrigerate overnight, and then let stand at room temperature for 2 hours.
7. Read and record results.

METHOD 11: THE WIDAL TEST ("H" TUBE TEST PROCEDURE)

Method

1. Set up eight tubes in a test tube rack.
2. To the first tube, add 0.9 ml of 0.25 per cent phenol-saline. Add 0.5 ml of phenol-saline to the remaining seven tubes.
3. Add 0.1 ml of the patient's serum to tube 1. Mix and transfer 0.5 ml to tube 2. Repeat for each tube, finally discarding 0.5 ml from tube 7. The final dilutions are 1:20 through 1:1280. Tube 8 will act as a control. (Note: A positive control should be included with the patient's tests. Polyvalent specific and nonspecific H antiserum should be used for this purpose.)
4. Add 0.5 ml of the appropriate antigen suspension to all tubes. Mix by shaking the racks.
5. Incubate at 50°C for 2 hours.
6. Read and record results.

REVIEW QUESTIONS

MULTIPLE CHOICE

Choose the phrase, sentence, or symbol that completes the statement or answers the question. More than one answer may be correct in each case. Answers are given at the back of this book.

1. Which of the following is not true of the bacilli in the family *Enterobacteriaceae?*
   (a) They are gram-negative bacilli
   (b) They are gram-positive bacilli
   (c) They are non–spore-forming bacilli
   (d) They are incapable for breaking down carbohydrates
   (The Family Enterobacteriaceae—General Aspects)

2. The O antigens of the family *Enterobacteriaceae:*
   (a) are capsular antigens
   (b) are located at the surface of the cell if they cause agglutination
   (c) are heat labile
   (d) are heat stable
   (The Family Enterobacteriaceae—General Aspects)

3. *E. coli:*
   (a) is the predominant facultative species of *Escherichia* in the large bowel
   (b) is known as the "colon bacillus"
   (c) may be the etiologic agent of a diarrhea
   (d) is one of many species of *Escherichia*
   (Escherichia–Antigenic Properties)

4. The enteropathogenic *E. coli:*
   (a) are divided into three types, based on the mechanisms of pathogenicity
   (b) cause diarrhea in humans, especially in infants
   (c) are of no clinical significance
   (d) are now the most frequently encountered species in gram-negative sepsis
   (Pathogenicity of E. coli)

5. Serologic tests for enteropathogenic *E. coli:*
   (a) are essential in all cases
   (b) are only essential when infants are involved
   (c) are considered unnecessary
   (d) are performed using 24 type-specific antisera for each suspect case
   (General Aspects of Escherichia Serotyping)

6. The genus *Shigella* is divided into four species. Which of the following is known as serologic subgroup D?
   (a) *Shigella dysenteriae*
   (b) *Shigella sonnei*
   (c) *Shigella flexneri*
   (d) none of the above
   (Shigella)

7. Shigella:
   (a) causes bacillary dysentery in humans
   (b) does not possess flagella
   (c) does not possess somatic components
   (d) possesses flagella
   (Shigella)

8. The majority of salmonellae are:
   (a) diphasic
   (b) monophasic
   (c) multiphasic
   (d) none of the above
   (Salmonella—Antigen Variation)

9. H-O variation in salmonellae refers to:
   (a) loss of H antigen
   (b) loss of O antigen
   (c) a loss or change in the Vi antigen
   (d) a change in the H antigen
   (Salmonella—Antigen Variation)

10. In cases of typhoid fever:
    (a) blood cultures are usually positive before the disease is symptomatic
    (b) blood cultures are usually positive during the sixth to eighth week
    (c) urine cultures are often positive during the second and third weeks and may remain so for a considerable period after convalescence
    (d) stool cultures are usually nonreactive
    (Salmonella—Pathogenicity)

ANSWER "TRUE" OR "FALSE"

11. All members of the family *Enterobacteriaceae* ferment glucose.
    (The Family Enterobacteriaceae—General Aspects)

12. Only one *Escherichia* species is known.
    (Escherichia)

13. Shigella organisms are gram-negative, motile rods.
    (Shigella)

14. The majority of species of the genus *Shigella* are nonpathogenic for humans.
    (Shigella—Pathogenicity)

15. The salmonellae have both somatic and flagellar antigens.
    (Salmonella)

16. Prolonged septicemia due to salmonella is commonly caused by *S. typhimurium.*
    (Salmonella—Septicemia)

General References

Alba's Medical Technology, 9th ed. Anaheim, CA, Berkeley Scientific Publications, 1980.

Bennington, J. L. (Ed.): Saunders Dictionary and Encyclopedia of Laboratory Medicine and Technology. Philadelphia, W. B. Saunders Company, 1984.

Braude, A. I.: Medical Microbiology and Infectious Diseases. Philadelphia, W. B. Saunders Company, 1981.

Raphael, S. S.: Lynch's Medical Laboratory Technology, 4th ed. Philadelphia, W. B. Saunders Company, 1983.

FOURTEEN

FUNGAL ANTIBODY TESTS, FEBRILE ANTIBODY TESTS, AND VIRAL ANTIBODY TEST

OBJECTIVES

The student shall know, understand, and be prepared to explain:

1. The fungal antibody tests for histoplasmosis, aspergillosis, coccidioidomycosis, North American blastomycosis, candidiasis, and sporotrichosis
2. The febrile antibody tests
3. The viral antibody tests, specifically:
   a. Complement fixation
   b. Latex fixation
   c. Precipitation
   d. Neutralization
   e. Immunofluorescence
   f. Hemagglutination

FUNGAL ANTIBODY TESTS

Several species of fungi are associated with respiratory diseases in humans that are acquired by inhaling spores from exogenous reservoirs, including dust, bird droppings, and soil. A selected number are briefly described here, including mainly those for which serologic tests can be performed.

Histoplasmosis

This disease is a granulomatous infection caused by *Histoplasma capsulatum*. It is often difficult to diagnose, because it presents as a broad spectrum, ranging from an asymptomatic or mild infection, to an acute fulminating disease, to a chronic pulmonary disease of long duration. A definite diagnosis requires the isolation in culture and microscopic identification of the fungus, as well as serologic evidence.

Kauffmann (1966) described the use of immunodiffusion for the detection of histoplasmin antibodies. The test is useful for screening purposes. Carlisle and Saslaw (1958) described a latex agglutination test for histoplasmosis that is of diagnostic value. A complement fixation test for histoplasmosis was described by Hazen *et al.* (1970). It is generally considered that a diagnosis made with a combination of history, physical examination, and delayed hypersensitivity skin testing is confirmed by a rise in complement-fixing antibodies to *Histoplasma* antigens.

Aspergillosis

This refers to any disease of humans and animals that is caused by species of the genus *Aspergillus*.

Of the many species recognized, only seven or eight are pathogenic for humans, and, of these, *Aspergillus fumigatus* is the most important (Fig. 14–1), being responsible for about 90 per cent of infections. The disease caused by *Aspergillus fumigatus* is an acute or chronic inflammatory granulomatous infection of the sinuses, bronchi, lungs, and (occasionally) other parts of the body. It has been recognized as an occupational disease among those who handle and feed squabs and among the handlers of furs and hair.

In culture, *Aspergillus* grows rapidly at 37°C on common mycologic laboratory media; however, it is sensitive to cyclohexamine. Species identification of *Aspergillus* is made microscopically.

Serologically, skin reactions and immunodiffusion are useful tools for identification, especially if the culture is negative. Precipitin formation by immunodiffusion is useful in patients with pulmonary eosinophilia, severe allergic aspergillosis, and aspergillomas. When aspergillomas are surgically removed, the precipitin bands disappear. For invasive aspergillosis, the patient is usually immune deficient; therefore, antibody detection is complicated. The sensitivity of immunodiffusion can be increased by using a battery of antigens from several species of *Aspergillus*, as well as serum concentration. The ELISA procedure is currently being used to detect both IgE and IgG antibodies in patient's sera (see further discussion earlier in this text).

Coccidioidomycosis

This disease is also known as desert fever, San Joaquin fever, and valley fever. It occurs in acute, chronic pulmonary, and disseminated forms. It is generally contracted from the inhalation of soil or dust containing the arthrospores of the causative agent, *Coccidioides immitis*.

In culture, *C. immitis* grows on Sabouraud's glucose agar from arthrospores or spherules. After 3 or 4 days of incubation, a cottony white, moist colony with aerial mycelia develops and gradually turns brown with age.

Several serologic tests are available; the tube precipitin test, complement-fixation test, latex agglutination test, and immunodiffusion. Of these, the tube precipitin test is positive in more than 90 per cent of the primary symptomatic cases. The complement fixation test becomes positive later than the tube precipitin test and is more effective in determining disseminated disease. Immunodiffusion tests give results that usually correlate with those observed with the complement fixation test. The latex agglutination test is highly sensitive and rapid but is not as specific as the tube precipitin test.

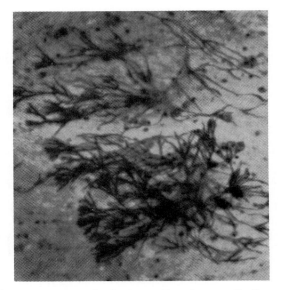

Figure 14–1. *Aspergillus fumigatus.* (From Freeman, B.: Burrows Textbook of Microbiology. Philadelphia, W. B. Saunders Company, 1985.)

North American Blastomycosis

This chronic systemic fungal disease is usually secondary to pulmonary involvement. The causative agent is *Blastomyces dermatitidis*. It is marked by suppurating tumors in the skin or by lesions in the lungs, bones, subcutaneous tissues, liver, spleen, and kidneys.

On incubation at room temperature in Sabouraud's glucose medium or in blood agar without cyclohexamine at 37°C, a white, filamentous colony forms, with white mycelia. Growth of *B. dermatitidis* is slow and may range from a few days to a month. Serologic diagnosis is problematic due to high cross-reactivity with antigenic components of the organisms causing histoplasmosis and coccidioidomycosis. Two tests, immunodiffusion and complement fixation, have been used in serodiagnosis. Immunodiffusion, in this regard, is claimed to yield better results than complement fixation (Busey and Hinton, 1967); however, the complement fixation test may provide prognostic value. There is a good fluorescent antibody test specific for the yeast phase of *B. dermatitidis*.

Candidiasis

The genus *Candida* contains many species, including *C. albicans*, *C. tropicalis*, *C. krusei*, *C. parakrusei*, *C. stellatoidea*, and *C. guilliermondi*. It is a genus of yeastlike fungi characterized by production of mycelia but not ascospores. The term *candidiasis* refers to any fungal infection involving the genus *Candida*. Of the many species, only *C.*

albicans is considered to be pathogenic for humans, but other species are encountered in pathologic conditions. The fungus is found in the lesions of thrush.

Candida grows on most laboratory media at room temperature. *C. albicans* produces a germ tube after incubation in serum at 37°C for 2 hours. On cornmeal agar, *C. albicans* produces chlamydospores.

Chew and Theus (1967) described a precipitation test for the detection of antibodies to *Candida,* but the test appears to be of little practical value because of the high incidence of Candida antibodies in apparently healthy individuals.

Precipitating antibodies prepared from protoplasts are more specific an indicator of Candida antibody than are antigens prepared from whole cells (Venezia and Robertson, 1974). Agglutination tests using suspensions of *C. albicans* are of little value because of the incidence of antibodies in normal individuals. Moreover, an inhibitor of agglutination has been found in some individuals with candidiasis (Louria *et al.,* 1972); therefore, even negative agglutination tests are of dubious value.

In spite of these difficulties, however, the serologic diagnosis of candidiasis is evolving as a tool for laboratory diagnosis, mainly because high titers of antibodies to intracellular antigens of *Candida* are indicative of systemic disease.

Sporotrichosis

This chronic progressive, subcutaneous lymphatic (rarely respiratory) mycosis is caused by the fungus *Sporotrichum schenckii.* The disease takes three forms: lymphatic, disseminated, and respiratory—the lymphatic form being the most common. It is characterized by a "sporotrichotic chancre" at the site of inoculation followed by the development and formation of subcutaneous nodules along the lymphatics draining the primary lesions. The infection is associated with injuries caused by thorns or splinters. Handlers of peat moss are susceptible to the disease, especially when working in rose gardens. The fungus also grows saprophytically on mine timbers as well as on other pieces of wood.

In culture, *S. schenckii* grows readily in Sabouraud's glucose agar at room temperature or in blood agar at 37°C. At 37°C, the organism exists as a cigar-shaped yeast, whereas at room temperature, it is mold. *Sporothrix* is resistant to cyclohexamine.

Serologically, a fluorescent antibody staining technique is available for the identification of *S. schenckii.* Two of the most sensitive identification tests are the yeast cell and the latex particle agglutination tests (Welsh and Dolan, 1973), which utilize lyophilized whole yeast cells in a buffer suspension and several dilutions of patient serum with agglutination checked after 1 hour. There is also a skin test available that uses a derivative of *S. schenckii* called *sporotrichin,* which produces a tuberculin-type reaction.

FEBRILE ANTIBODY TESTS FOR DISEASES OTHER THAN SALMONELLOSIS*

Several diseases are detected by the so-called Weil-Felix test (Table 14–1). These diseases as well as several others are collectively known as the *febrile diseases.*

One of the earliest tests of diagnostic value, known as the Widal test, was developed by Widal and Sicard in 1896. This test is still widely used for the detection of antibodies in typhoid fever, brucellosis, and tularemia (Corbel and Cullen, 1970; Damp *et al.,* 1973). (Note: The Widal Test is described in Chapter 13.)

---

*See also Chapter 13.

Table 14–1. WEIL-FELIX REACTIONS IN RICKETTSIAL DISEASE

Organism	Disease	*Proteus* Strain Used and Degree of Reaction		
		OX-2	OX-19	OX-K
R. prowazekii	Epidemic typhus, Brill's disease	+	+ + + +	0
R. mooseri (R. typhi)	Murine typhus	+	+ + + +	0
R. rickettsii	Rocky Mountain spotted fever	+	+ + + +	0
R. akari	Rickettsialpox	0	0	0
R. tsutsugamushi	Tsutsugamushi disease (scrub typhus)	0	0	+ + + +
R. quintana	Trench fever	0	0	0
R. burnetii (Coxiella burnetii)	Q fever	0	0	0

The Weil-Felix test, developed by Weil and Felix (1916), is based on the fact that certain strains of *Proteus vulgaris* most probably share antigens with several of the Rickettsia species that produce febrile diseases, such as typhus. Three strains of *Proteus vulgaris* have been found to be useful in diagnosing rickettsial diseases; these have been labeled OX-2, OX-19, and OX-K. By testing suspension of all three strains, it is possible to detect antibodies against a number of rickettsial diseases (Table 14–1).

As will be noted in Table 14–1, the Weil-Felix test does not distinguish between antibodies to *Rickettsia prowazekii, R. mooseri,* and *R. rickettsii.* Clinical symptoms must therefore be studied in conjunction with serologic results.

Q fever agglutinins may be detected by a capillary agglutination test described by Luoto (1953). This test uses embryo-cultured *Coxiella burnetii,* which is suspended in saline, inactivated with formalin, and finally stained with hematoxylin and standardized. Similar test antigens have been developed for psittacosis or ornithosis, but they are not widely available. Laboratory diagnosis of Q fever, however, is preferably made using the complement fixation test.

VIRAL ANTIBODY TESTS

Many diseases of humans now recognized as caused by viruses, such as smallpox and yellow fever, have been known for centuries. Several additional major illnesses of humans (and other animals) are viral in nature, including influenza, measles, mumps, and poliomyelitis.

Serologic tests used for the detection of viral antibodies include complement fixation, latex fixation, precipitation, neutralization, immunofluorescence, and hemagglutination. These tests vary greatly in their diagnostic usefulness.

Complement Fixation

The interaction of viral protein and antibody often fixes complement, and because sensitive methods for the titration of complement are available, this provides a convenient and accurate method of measuring the amount of either viral antigen or antibody to such antigens. Complement fixation is useful, too, in the detection of viral antibodies, because it is less complex, less time consuming, and less costly than other techniques.

Latex Fixation Tests

Aubert *et al.* (1962) reported studies of viral antibody titrations using latex suspensions. These tests have not gained wide acceptance, however, except in the detection of HBsAg, in which latex fixation is often used as a screening test for blood donors.

Precipitation

Because of the difficulty in preparing purified antigens, few satisfactory precipitation tests have been developed. Chew and Theus (1967) described a double-diffusion test for adenoviral antibody, and Mata (1963) described an agar cell culture precipitation test, which is an adaptation of the Elek diffusion test using Eagle's medium. Although these methods have merit, they have never been widely used.

Neutralization

A number of distinctly different neutralization techniques have been developed in the field of virology. Lennette and Schmidt (1969) have described these procedures in some detail. Another method, essentially the same as the *in vivo* tests, uses embryonated eggs instead of animals for the inoculation of virus and of antibody mixtures. This *in ovo* method is now mainly of historic value. Some viruses produce distinct "pocks" on some of the membranes of embryonated eggs; this fact has been used in the development of so-called pock reduction tests. In this technique, the allantoic membrane is dropped to allow the outer surface to be inoculated. Inocula of certain virus suspensions may be titrated to produce a determinable number of pocks during a specific time period and then mixed with test sera just prior to inoculation. When the test serum contains antibodies to the pock-producing virus, a reduction in the number of pocks produced is an indicator of the quantity of antibody present.

The tissue-culture neutralization test is useful in virology and has been adapted to a microtitration method (Rosenbaum *et al.*, 1963). Sterile microplates are available for this test from Baltimore Biological Laboratories, Baltimore, MD, and Cooke Engineering, Alexandria, VA. The test, while economically practical, is highly sophisticated and requires extensive experience to perform. (Note: This tissue culture neutralization test has been adapted for use in the determination of diphtheria antibodies; Quevillon and Chagnon, 1973).

Dulbecco (1952) used plaque reduction tests with some success in viral antibody determination. In this technique, monolayers of cell cultures are inoculated with virus suspensions and immediately overlaid with an agar-gel medium, which prevents the virus particles released from infected cells from moving via the medium to cells other than the immediately adacent ones. Patches of infected cells (plaques) therefore develop underneath the agar surface. Each live virus particle will, in theory, produce one plaque, and the plaques may be counted to determine the number of viable viruses. To determine the number of antibodies in a test serum, viral suspensions are mixed with dilutions of test serum prior to inoculation onto the cell culture; this results in a reduced number of plaques. The reduction is proportional to the number of antibodies in the test serum. Kenyon and McManus (1974) have shown that the number of plaques produced by *Rickettsia,* unaffected by some antisera, can be reduced in the presence of antiglobulins to the antisera.

A metabolic inhibition test was proposed by Salk *et al.* (1954). It has some distinct advantages over the conventional tissue-culture neutralization test, but it also has serious shortcomings that greatly limit its practical usefulness. The test is based on the fact that certain viruses inhibit the metabolic processes of living cells that are suspended in a culture medium, resulting in a readily observable pH change of the cell culture medium. When viruses are mixed with antisera, no pH change occurs. The test is easy to read and appears to be more sensitive than other tissue culture neutralization tests; only a few viruses bring about the pH change, however, and, in some instances, pH changes may occur in the absence of virus.

Immunofluorescence

Immunofluorescence has been widely used in the detection of rubella-specific IgM (Iwakata *et al.,*

1972), cytomegalic inclusion virus in smears from urinary sediments (Hanshaw, 1969), herpes simplex in clinical specimens (Nahmias *et al.,* 1971) and IgM specific for Epstein-Barr virus (Banatvala *et al.,* 1972). These tests are highly useful and have become important tools in viral diagnostic testing. Practical limitations include the difficulty in maintenance and standardization of virus-infected cells, the stability of these cells, and the problem of nonspecific reactions.

Hemagglutination

Hirst's report (1942) of the phenomenon of viral hemagglutination quickly led to the development of the hemagglutination-inhibition (HI) test for the detection and titration of viral antibodies in patient's sera and for the identification of specific viruses. This test has, in recent years, become the most practical for determining the immune status of an individual against rubella and in the serologic diagnosis of rubella viral infections. The HI test can be used in any situation involving viruses that agglutinate (*e.g.,* influenza, mumps, vaccinia, smallpox, Newcastle disease, rubella). In principle, the test involves the attachment of antibody molecules to the viral particles, subsequently hindering the absorption of viral particles to erythrocytes. Failure of hemagglutination to occur constitutes a positive test. HI can also be useful in the identification of virus isolates by mixing known antiserum dilutions with fixed quantities of unknown hemagglutinating viral suspensions.

REVIEW QUESTIONS

MULTIPLE CHOICE

Choose the phrase, sentence, or symbol that completes the statement or answers the question. More than one answer may be correct in each case. Answers are given at the back of this book.

1. The detection of histoplasmin antibodies can be achieved using:
   (a) the immunodiffusion test
   (b) hemagglutination tests
   (c) neutralization tests
   (d) none of the above
   (*Histoplasmosis*)

2. The serologic tests that are considered useful in the serologic diagnosis of aspergillosis include:
   (a) skin tests
   (b) immunodiffusion
   (c) precipitation
   (d) ELISA
   (*Aspergillosis*)

3. The causative agent of coccidioidomycosis is known as:
   (a) *Coccidioides immitis*
   (b) *Coccidioides amitis*
   (c) *Coccidioides dermatitidis*
   (d) *Coccidioides* guilliermondi
   (*Coccidioidomycosis*)

4. Which of the following members of the genus *Candida* is considered to be pathogenic for humans?
   (a) *C. tropicalis*
   (b) *C. parakrusei*
   (c) *C. albicans*
   (d) *C. guilliermondi*
   (*Candidiasis*)

5. Which of the following fungal diseases is caused by *S. schenckii?*
   (a) coccidioidomycosis
   (b) sporotrichosis
   (c) blastomycosis
   (d) none of the above
   (*General*)

6. The Widal test is used for the detection of:
   (a) Q fever agglutinins
   (b) strains of *Proteus vulgaris*
   (c) antibodies in typhus fever
   (d) antibodies in typhoid fever
   (Febrile Antibody Tests)

7. In which of the following fungal diseases is the fungus encountered in the lesions of thrush?
   (a) North American blastomycosis
   (b) candidiasis
   (c) aspergillosis
   (d) histoplasmosis
   (Fungal Antibody Tests)

8. Which of the following is not a strain of *Proteus vulgaris* useful in diagnosing rickettsial disease?
   (a) OX-2
   (b) OX-19
   (c) OX-K
   (d) OX-4
   (Febrile Antibody Tests)

9. The pack reduction test is:
   (a) a neutralization technique
   (b) a complement fixation technique
   (c) an immunofluorescence technique
   (d) a precipitation technique
   (Viral Antibody Tests)

ANSWER "TRUE" OR "FALSE"

10. Histoplasmosis is caused by *Histoplasma capsulatum*.
    (Fungal Antibody Tests)
11. Aspergillus is sensitive to cyclohexamine.
    (Fungal Antibody Tests)
12. Complement fixation cannot be used as a test for coccidioidomycosis.
    (Fungal Antibody Tests)
13. Growth of *B. dermatitidis* on blood agar or in Sabouraud's glucose medium may take as long as 1 month.
    (Fungal Antibody Tests)
14. The genus *Candida* contains only one species, *C. albicans*.
    (Fungal Antibody Tests)
15. Immunofluorescence has been widely used in the detection of rubella-specific IgM.
    (Viral Antibody Tests)

General References

Alba's Medical Technology, 9th ed. Anaheim, CA, Berkeley Scientific Publications, 1980.
Bennington, J. L. (Ed.): Saunders Dictionary and Encyclopedia of Laboratory Medicine and Technology. Philadelphia, W. B. Saunders Company, 1984.
Braude, A. I.: Medical Microbiology and Infectious Diseases. Philadelphia, W. B. Saunders Company, 1981.
Raphael, S. S.: Lynch's Medical Laboratory Technology, 4th ed. Philadelphia, W. B. Saunders Company, 1983.

FIFTEEN

THE DETECTION OF COMPLEMENT LEVELS

OBJECTIVES

The student shall know, understand, and be prepared to explain:

1. The clinical significance of complement deficiency, including:
   a. C1q deficiency
   b. C1r deficiency
   c. C1s and C1s INH deficiency
   d. C4 deficiency
   e. C2 deficiency
   f. C3 deficiency
   g. C5 deficiency
   h. C6 and C7 deficiency
2. The measurement of complement components (general aspects), including:
   a. Hemolytic assays
   b. Functional assays
   c. Immunoassays

The nine major components of complement (C1 to C9) and various inhibitors can be measured in human serum. Clinically useful assays of complement consist primarily of CH_{50} or total hemolytic assay and specific functional and immunochemical assays for various components.

CLINICAL SIGNIFICANCE OF COMPLEMENT DEFICIENCY

The complement system is significant both in the diagnosis of disease and in the understanding of pathophysiology of several human disease states. Reduced amounts of serum complement activity have been reported in a variety of disease states (*e.g.*, systemic lupus erythematosus [SLE], with glomerulonephritis; acute glomerulonephritis; acute serum sickness; advanced cirrhosis of the liver). Other diseases (*e.g.*, obstructive jaundice, thyroiditis, acute rheumatic fever, rheumatoid arthritis) are associated with elevated serum complement concentrations.

Inadequate amounts of the various components of the complement system (including the inhibitors and inactivators that regulate the activation cascade) may arise from genetic conditions in which the component is not synthesized at all or is produced at subnormal levels. It is also possible that the molecule may be synthesized normally, yet may be defective in some structural way, rendering it functionally inert. A deficiency of one of the complement proteins may also be produced by hypercatabolism (*i.e.*, an increased rate of breakdown or degradation), and this may be difficult to distinguish from activation of the molecule, particularly if only a late-acting component is involved.

The elevation of complement levels has been reported in a number of conditions, yet the significance of this observation is not clear. The most likely explanation is simply overproduction.

In the case of genetic disorders, the absence of the complement component follows simple mendelian inheritance patterns and is inherited as an autosomal recessive trait. Therefore, patients who are heterozygous tend to have half normal levels and patients who are homozygous have little or no detectable complement component activity.

Deficiencies involving almost every component of the classical activation sequence are known. The majority of these patients present with one or another manifestation of autoimmune disease. The role of complement deficiency in the development of these diseases is not yet clear, although it has been hypothesized that autoimmunity may be a manifestation of chronic viral illness, and, if complement aids in viral neutralization, an interruption of those pathways of activation may promote chronic viral infection.

C1q Deficiency

Human deficiency of C1q was originally reported in 1961, and many other examples have been added since that time. Most of these cases have been associated with a sex-linked agammaglobulinemia or a combined immunodeficiency disease. C1q deficiency is frequently associated with a loss of B- and T-lymphocytes (and therefore with depressed levels of IgG in the circulation); therefore, it is difficult to recognize any single defect associated with it. C1q deficiency has also been described in one patient with an SLE–like syndrome and increased susceptibility to bacterial infection (Wara et al., 1975).

C1r Deficiency

Normal C1q levels have been noted in those few individuals in whom markedly depressed levels of C1r have been detected. All these patients had extensive medical histories, revealing multiple episodes of upper respiratory tract disease, chronic kidney disease, or a lupus erythematosus (LE)–like syndrome.

C1s and C̄1s INH Deficiency

Patients with C1s deficiency may have a loss of almost 50 per cent of their C1s. Very little is known about the association of C1s deficiency and human health, although several of the individuals studied had an LE–like syndrome and an increased susceptibility to bacterial infection (Day et al., 1973).

C1s INH deficiency, however, is clearly associated with hereditary angioneurotic edema (HANE). This disease is transmitted as an autosomal dominant deficiency in which the subjects average 31 μg per ml of C̄1s INH, compared with 180 μg per ml for normal individuals.

C4 Deficiency

Only two examples of C4 deficiency in humans have been reported. One of the victims had a pronounced skin rash of uncertain cause. C4 deficiency, however, has been recognized as an autosomal recessive characteristic in guinea pigs. In guinea pigs, the homozygous condition reveals absolutely no C4, whereas in the heterozygous state, up to 30 per cent of the normal values were observed. The alternative complement pathway is intact in these animals and may be their major source of protection against bacterial and viral infections.

C2 Deficiency

This is the most common of the human complement deficiencies; more than 40 cases, revealing both heterozygous and homozygous origins, have been described. The heterozygous individuals have 30 to 70 per cent of the normal C2 levels, whereas the homozygous-deficient individuals range below 4 per cent of normal values, based on hemolytic assays. The frequency of hypersensitive disease such as LE and dermatomyositis and repeated infectious disease exceeds that which would be expected on the basis of random distribution in C2-deficient individuals. Patients with C2 deficiency have chronic renal disease and antibody directed against DNA. C2 deficiency has been associated with the HLA haplotype A10, B18.

C3 Deficiency

Approximately a half dozen C3-deficient individuals are recorded in the medical literature, yet only one individual is known to have total C3 deficiency (2.5 μg per ml of serum compared with a normal level of 1250 μg per ml). Five other children in this same family plus the mother had about half-normal C3 levels. The patient had experienced a considerable number of infections, which emphasizes the critical role of C3 not only in linking the classic and alternative pathways but also in immune adherence, opsonization, and chemotaxis, all of which are important defense functions.

Two forms of C3 deficiency exist: type I and type II. In type I, C3 is probably deficient as a result of a deficiency of C3 inactivator. Type II C3 deficiency is the type reported in the individual just described (Alper et al., 1973). This patient's decreased level of C3 was found to be associated with increased destruction and decreased synthesis.

C5 Deficiency

Familial C5 dysfunction has been described in patients presenting with failure to thrive, diarrhea, seborrheic dermatitis, and susceptibility to infection with bacterial organisms (Miller and Nilsson, 1970). Only three examples of C5 dysfunction are known, and, in these, the C5 level as determined immunochemically was normal, but hemolytic titrations of complement could detect no C5. A depression of phagocytic activity, which could be restored to normal with human C5, was noted in these individuals. The higher incidence of infectious disease in these patients is related to this loss of phagocytic activity.

C6 and C7 Deficiency

Human C6 deficiency has been described in four individuals who lacked hemolytically or immunochemically active C6. The parents and siblings of these individuals had half-normal serum levels of C6. C6 deficiency appears to be associated with increased susceptibility to *Neisseria* infections.

Several patients have been described who are deficient in C7, and another group lacking C8 has also been identified.

MEASUREMENT OF COMPLEMENT COMPONENTS

Hemolytic Assays

Hemolytic assay provides a crude screening test for complement activity in human serum. The test uses sheep erythrocytes, rabbit antibody to sheep erythrocytes, and fresh guinea pig serum as a source of complement. Hemolysis of the sheep erythrocytes is measured spectrophotometrically as the absorbance of released hemoglobin and can be directly related to the number of red blood cells lysed. For clinical purposes, measurement of total hemolytic activity of serum is taken at 50 per cent of the hemolysis level. The CH_{50} is an arbitrary unit that is defined as the quantity of complement necessary for 50 per cent lysis of red cells under rigidly standardized conditions of red blood cell sensitization with antibody. These results are expressed as the reciprocal of the serum dilution giving 50 per cent hemolysis.

The test has limited usefulness, because a drastic reduction of complement is necessary to produce a reduction in hemolytic assay. The reduction of specific complement components may give normal hemolytic assay results or slightly depressed results, even when reduction of individual components is marked.

THE MEASUREMENT OF INDIVIDUAL COMPLEMENT COMPONENTS

In order to establish that a deficiency of some complement molecule exists, it is necessary to have a reliable method for quantitating the individual components or the whole complement system. At the present time, accurate methods are available for measuring all the nine classical pathway components, most of the alternative pathway components, and several enzymes and inhibitors that regulate the complement system. Many of these methods, however, are still considered to be research techniques and are not available routinely. This discussion will be confined to techniques that do not require a laboratory skilled in complement research for their performance. Two types of techniques are in use: those that measure the complement proteins as antigens in serum, and those that measure the functional activity of the components.

Functional Assays

Functional complement assays can be considered to be both sensitive and precise tools for measuring the activity of a complement component. Some of these methods can be used to quantitate activity at the molecular level, whereas others express complement components in arbitrary titration units. The level of activity is measured by using pure preparations of each component added sequentially to antibody-coated erythrocytes until the step is reached in the activation sequence just prior to addition of the component to be measured. The test sample is then added, and the degree of hemolysis is related to the presence of later-acting components. This test is described in detail by Rapp and Borsos (1970). The disadvantages of functional assays include the fact that they are complex and time consuming and require relatively highly purified reagents, which are costly when compared with those required for immunochemical tests.

Immunoassays

Immunochemical analyses (*i.e.*, antigenic) are generally simpler to perform than those for evaluating functional activity.

These antigenic assays are highly specific and require fewer specialized reagents and considerably less time. The reagents that are required are commercially available, either serum or plasma can be used, and the commonly available methods of freezer storage (*i.e.*, $-20°C$) are sufficient. It should be noted, however, that antigenic assays have the disadvantage of not being able to provide information on the activity of a component because they may detect degradation products as well as functionally active components. Also, in general, antigenic assays are not as sensitive as functional assays and may not detect the presence of a complement component in certain body fluids whose presence *can* be shown by its functional activity. The sensitivity of assays depends to some extent upon the strength of the antisera used, and, with usual assays, as little as 1 to 10 μg per ml of a protein antigen can be measured. It should also be noted that, whereas antisera to many of the complement proteins are available commercially (*e.g.,* C1q, C4, C3, C5, properdin factor B, C1 inhibitor), the others are not generally available except as research reagents.

REVIEW QUESTIONS

MULTIPLE CHOICE

Choose the phrase, sentence, or symbol that completes the statement or answers the question. More than one answer may be correct in each case. Answers are given at the back of this book.

1. Reduced amounts of serum complement activity have been reported in cases of:
   (a) systemic lupus erythematosus with glomerulonephritis
   (b) acute glomerulonephritis
   (c) acute serum sickness
   (d) advanced cirrhosis of the liver
   (Clinical Significance of Complement Deficiency)

2. Elevated serum complement concentrations are associated with:
   (a) systemic lupus erythematosus
   (b) obstructive jaundice
   (c) advanced cirrhosis of the liver
   (d) thyroiditis
   (Clinical Significance of Complement Deficiency)

3. Inadequate complement levels may arise from:
   (a) genetic conditions
   (b) structural defect in the molecule
   (c) hypercatabolism
   (d) none of the above
   (Clinical Significance of Complement Deficiency)

4. C1q deficiency:
   (a) appears to be associated with a sex-linked agammaglobulinemia or a combined immunodeficiency disease
   (b) is frequently associated with loss of B- and T-lymphocytes
   (c) has been found in only one individual
   (d) may be associated with a systemic lupus erythematosus–like syndrome
   (C1q Deficiency)

5. The most common of the human complement deficiencies is:
   (a) C1q deficiency
   (b) C4 deficiency
   (c) C2 deficiency
   (d) C3 deficiency
   (General)

6. In the measurement of complement components, hemolytic assays:
   (a) are highly specific
   (b) have limited usefulness
   (c) provide a crude screening test
   (d) use sheep erythrocytes
   (Hemolytic Assays)

7. Functional assays used for the measurement of individual complement components have the following disadvantages:
   (a) they are complex and time consuming
   (b) they do not require highly purified reagents
   (c) they may not detect the presence of a complement component in certain body fluids
   (d) they are insensitive
   (Measurement of Individual Complement Components)

ANSWER "TRUE" OR "FALSE"

8. The majority of patients with complement deficiencies present with one or another manifestation of autoimmune disease.
   (Clinical Significance of Complement Deficiency)

9. C1s INH deficiency is not known to be associated with any disease state.
   (C1s and C1s INH Deficiency)

10. C4 deficiency has been recognized as an autosomal recessive characteristic in guinea pigs.
    (C4 Deficiency)

11. C2 deficiency has been associated with the HLA haplotype A10, B18.
    (C2 Deficiency)

12. C6 deficiency appears to be associated with increased susceptibility to *Neisseria* infections.
    (C6 and C7 Deficiency)

General References

Bellanti, J. A.: Immunology III. Philadelphia, W. B. Saunders Company, 1985.

Barrett, J. T.: Textbook of Immunology, 4th ed. St. Louis, The C. V. Mosby Co., 1983.

Henry, J. B. (Ed.): Clinical Diagnosis and Management by Laboratory Methods, 17th ed. Philadelphia, W. B. Saunders Company, 1984.

Rapp, J. H., and Borsos, T.: Molecular Basis of Complement Action. Norwalk, CT, Appleton-Century-Crofts, 1970.

SIXTEEN

MISCELLANEOUS SEROLOGY

OBJECTIVES

The student shall have a general understanding of:

1. Opsonocytophagic tests
2. Bacteriolysin test
3. The Moan hemagglutination test
4. The hemagglutination-inhibition test for rubella
5. Skin tests, specifically:
   a. A description of allergic conditions
   b. The performance of skin tests
   c. The *Trichinella spiralis* skin test
   d. The tuberculin skin test
   e. The brucellergin skin test
   f. The coccidioidin skin test
   g. The Frei test
   h. The histoplasmin skin test
   i. The Schick test
   j. The toxoplasmin skin test
   k. The *Trichinella* skin test
   l. Vollmer's patch test
6. The Quellung reaction
7. Lancefield grouping
8. Elek's diffusion test
9. The detection and identification of immunoglobulin and other serum proteins
10. *Toxoplasma gondii*
11. Pregnancy testing
12. The pertussis (whooping cough) agglutination test
13. The leptospiral agglutination test
14. General laboratory techniques, including:
    a. Complement fixation
    b. Complement fixation inhibition
    c. Hemagglutination inhibition
15. The collection and preservation of sheep blood
16. The preparation of sheep red cell hemolysin
17. The preparation and preservation of complement
18. The preparation of red cell concentrations

Many serologic procedures exist that, although not warranting special treatment, are of interest to the student of serology. The purpose of this chapter is to acquaint the student with these procedures and to offer a list of references that might prove useful if any subsection demands further study within a course outline.

Opsonocytophagic Tests

The presence of opsonins in a patient's serum against certain bacteria is demonstrated by mixing the patient's fresh, citrated blood with a saline suspension of the bacteria. The mixture is incubated at 37°C for 20 minutes, and a drop of sedimented cells is then smeared on a glass slide, allowed to dry, and stained with any good stain. Subsequently, the number of bacteria present within a certain number of segmented neutrophil leukocytes (phagocytes) is counted in order to determine the opsonic power of the patient's blood. One to 20 phagocytized bacteria indicate slight phagocytosis; 41 or more indicate marked phagocytosis.

The "opsonic index" is an expression of the opsonic power of the patient's blood in relation to the opsonic power of normal blood. Opsonocytophagic tests are occasionally used in cases of brucellosis (in conjunction with the agglutination test or the skin test); they are, however, of doubtful diagnostic value in this disease.

Bacteriolysin Test

A bacteriolysin is an antibody that causes the dissolution of bacteria. These bacteriolysins are found in the blood serum of animals who are naturally immune to a particular antigen as well as in those who have been artificially immunized against an antigen by injection. Unlike antitoxin, which neutralizes soluble toxin, bacteriolysin destroys the bacterial cell itself. In order for the bacteriolytic reaction to take place, complement is necessary (unlike toxin-antitoxin neutralization).

In 1894, Pfeiffer demonstrated that when cholera vibrios are intraperitoneally injected into a guinea pig previously immunized against cholera, the organisms gradually lose their motility, become swollen, and disintegrate (known as Pfeiffer's phenomenon). Metchnikoff later showed that the same phenomenon can be detected *in vitro* by mixing cholera vibrios in a test tube with peritoneal fluid (or serum) from an immunized guinea pig.

Lysins have been produced for a variety of cells other than bacterial and are highly specific. If red blood cells of an animal or human are injected into an animal of a different species, hemolysins are developed that are specific for that blood. This test is useful in court trials where it is necessary to determine whether blood stains are of human or animal origin.

Serologic Test for Amebiasis

A serologic test for amebiasis, known as the Moan hemagglutination test, is commercially available from Mobac Laboratories, Lansdowne, PA. The Moan antigen is a water-clear aqueous extract of *Entamoeba histolytica*, which, when added to rabbit or human erythrocytes that have been coated with tannic acid according to the Boyden technique, produces agglutination of the cells in the presence of antibodies to *E. histolytica*.

METHOD 1: THE MOAN HEMAGGLUTINATION TEST

Materials

1. Isotonic saline (0.85 gm of C.P. crystal NaCl in 100 ml of distilled water).
2. Tannic acid. Note: This solution is unstable. It should be prepared weekly and kept under refrigeration. A 1 per cent stock solution (distilled water) is sufficient. A 1/5,000 solution (saline) is prepared daily from the 1 per cent stock solution.
3. Erythrocytes—rabbit or human—prepared by washing the cells with isotonic saline until the supernatant is clear. Make a 4 per cent suspension of the cells using isotonic saline as the diluent.
4. Moan antigen (provided commercially)

Method

Preparation of Cell Suspension with Tannic Acid

1. To 5 ml of a 4 per cent suspension of cells, add 5 ml of the 1/5,000 solution of tannic acid. (Note: When the tannic acid is added to cells, flocculation should take place within a few minutes.)
2. Incubate at 37°C for 30 minutes.
3. Wash twice in saline.
4. Restore to 2.5 ml volume in saline.

Preparation of Coated Antigen

1. Place the contents of 1 ampule of antigen in a test tube.
2. Add 2.0 ml of isotonic saline.
3. Add 1.0 ml of tannic cells prepared as just described. Mix to ensure homogeneous suspension, and allow to stand at room temperature for 15 minutes.

4. **Centrifuge and wash twice.**
5. **Restore to 1.5 ml with saline.**

Procedure: Presumptive Tests

1. **Add 1.0 ml of saline to each tube.**
2. **Add 0.3 ml of serum to be tested.**
3. **Add one drop (approximately 0.1 ml) of coated antigen to each tube.**
4. **Gently centrifuge for 1 minute and read as follows.**

Procedure: Quantitative Test

Note: The quantitative test is performed exactly as is the presumptive test, using the serum dilutions as shown in Table 16–1.

Interpretation

Tests should be read macroscopically. Any agglutination denotes a positive test. This agglutination remains intact on gentle shaking of the tube. Negative results show as a resuspension of the cells.

Discussion—The Moan Hemagglutination Test

With respect to the coated antigen, 1 ml is usually sufficient for approximately 15 presumptive tests or 3 quantitative tests. The coated antigen is stable for 24 to 48 hours due to instability of the tannic acid. Coated antigen should be kept refrigerated and should be discarded after use.

Although occasional false-positive results may be encountered in this test with other disease states, they have not been encountered in healthy individuals. A positive test indicates that a patient has clinical symptoms of amebiases. A negative test will appear within a week of remission of clinical symptoms, whether natural or drug induced. The strength of the reaction, as revealed by titration, usually parallels the severity of the infection and will recede with successful treatment. Serial dilutions of all positive tests should be made to determine the efficacy of treatment. A Herxheimer-type reaction takes place during the third to sixth days of treatment, resulting in an increased titer. This is indicative that the amebicide is efficacious.

Glassware for the Moan hemagglutination test must be chemically clean. Lipids, detergents, and other contaminants will cause inaccurate results.

THE HEMAGGLUTINATION-INHIBITION TEST FOR RUBELLA

The most widely used technique for the detection of antibodies to rubella is the hemagglutination-inhibition test. This test, available as Rubindex from Ortho Diagnostics, Raritan, NJ, is as sensitive as the fluorescent antibody or neutralization test. The complement fixation test is unsuitable for this purpose, because the CR antibody disappears after infection.

Hemagglutination-inhibition antibodies rise rapidly, often reaching a peak level within 5 to 7 days of the onset of rash and remaining at a high level for a long period of time. The hemagglutination-inhibition test is based on the ability of the rubella virus to agglutinate the erythrocytes of certain species. Antibodies to the rubella virus inhibit this agglutination and can be quantitated by exposing serially diluted test sera to rubella virus antigen and recording those dilutions in which agglutination does not take place.

Complete inhibition of agglutination represents a positive test and is indicated by the formation of a red cell button at the bottom of the well. The highest dilution at which hemagglutination is still completely inhibited represents the antibody titer. A titer of 8 (dilution 1:8) or greater indicates a positive reaction; a titer of less than 8 indicates a negative reaction. A fourfold or greater increase in titer between two specimens collected at least 1 or 2 weeks apart indicates a recent rubella infection. No increase in titer between two specimens usually indicates a previous rubella infection.

The absence (or low levels) of rubella HI antibody indicates susceptibility to rubella virus. If rubella antibodies appear within a 7-day period following exposure to infection, prior infection with rubella virus can be presumed. If rubella antibodies are absent in a sample at the time of exposure, yet are found to be present in a second sample taken 3 to 4 weeks later, a rubella infection that has resulted from exposure can be presumed. A negative result in this second sample indicates that the infection has not occurred.

Congenital rubella infections can be confirmed serologically through the observation of persisting antibody, above and beyond that which is passively transferred from mother to infant during fetal life, especially if this antibody is present in the infant's blood the first months after birth.

Table 16–1. SERUM DILUTIONS FOR THE MOAN HEMAGGLUTINATION TEST (QUANTITATIVE TEST)

Tube	1	2	3	4	5	6
Serum	0.30	0.00	0.00	0.00	0.00	0.00
Saline	0.30	0.30	0.30	0.30	0.30	0.30

0.30 ml of the serum-saline mixture is transferred serially from tube 1 to tube 6. Then add one drop of coated antigen to each tube and proceed as with the presumptive test (see text)

SKIN TESTS

Skin tests are still in common use, yet *in vitro* allergen tests are now available against a wide variety of allergens using radioimmunoassay techniques. These tests (RAST tests) should be used wherever possible in place of intradermal testing.

Skin tests are usually carried out in allergic or immunological conditions (*e.g.,* diphtheria, scarlet fever).

Allergic Conditions

The term *allergy* refers to hypersensitivity to a certain agent (known as an *allergen*). The process involved is similar to an antigen-antibody reaction, but here the antibody may not be demonstrable. Allergens include foreign proteins (complete antigens), carbohydrates, lipids, and haptens. Certain individuals can also develop sensitivity to drugs and biologicals. Common allergens include pollen, milk, eggs, wheat, dust, mushrooms and other fungi, aspirin, quinine, morphine, barbiturates, animal feathers and hairs, and so on.

There are three types of allergic reactions: The first is known as the immediate (or anaphylactic) reaction. This usually begins within minutes after exposure to the allergen and disappears within 1 hour. Examples of this type of reaction are allergy to pollen and horse serum sensitivity.

The second is known as the delayed reaction, which begins several hours following exposure and may last for several days. Examples of this type of reaction are determined by the tuberculin, coccidioidin, histoplasmin, and Frei tests.

The third is tested by toxin-antitoxin neutralization. Examples of this type are the Schick test, the Dick test, and the Schültz-Charlton phenomenon.

The Performance of Skin Tests

Three types of skin tests can be used, namely:

1. *Intradermal.* These tests are commonly used for tuberculin, histoplasmin, coccidioidin in adults, and so on.
2. *Scratch.* These tests are commonly used in testing for pollen or food allergens.
3. *Patch.* These tests are sometimes used for tuberculin tests in children, but they are not as reliable as the intradermal test. The success of the patch test depends upon the ability of the diagnostic material to diffuse into the skin.

For obvious reasons, only sterile instruments and materials should be used in skin testing. The skin should be cleansed using 70 per cent alcohol. Skin tests are usually carried out on the flexor surface of the forearm, but other areas of the skin are just as reliable.

Skin tests are available for the following conditions: trichinosis, hydatid cyst, schistosomiasis, filariasis, leishmaniasis, mumps, influenza, lymphogranuloma venereum (Frei test), coccidioidomycosis, sporotrichosis, histoplasmosis, certain skin infections by the fungi, primary allergies, serum sickness, tuberculosis (Pirquet's, Vollmer's, Mendel's, Mantoux tests), undulant fever, tularemia, diphtheria (Schick test), scarlet fever (Dick test), glanders (mallein test), brucellosis, chancroid, North American blastomycosis, and others.

Commonly Used Skin Tests

Trichinella spiralis (Pork Trichina) Skin Test

In a typical case of *Trichinella spiralis,* in which uncomplicated trichinosis has run a course of 2 weeks or more, sensitivity to *Trichinella* substance develops and can be detected by injection of *Trichinella* extract. The antigen used for the test is 1:10,000 dilution of a saline extract of larvae of *Trichinella spiralis* freed from the tissues of the host in which the parasites were developed in the laboratory.

Method

1. **A small volume of the antigen (0.1 ml or less) is injected intracutaneously on the forearm some distance from the elbow.**
2. **As a control, a similar injection is made with a saline solution used for extracting the larvae.**

Interpretation

A positive skin reaction (indicating infection at some time, usually within the past 5 years or so, with trichinellae) is of the immediate type. It is characterized by the development, within 20 minutes, of an elevated wheal, or edematous blanched area, from 8 to 15 mm in diameter from which pseudopods may or may not radiate into the surrounding area of pronounced erythema. The contrast between the reaction to the antigen and the control solution constitutes the criterion for reading the results of the test.

The Tuberculin Skin Test

Purified protein derivative (PPD) in first, second, and intermediate strengths is available commercially.

One tenth of a milliliter of PPD is injected intradermally, forming a wheal. The test is read at

48 hours. A positive reaction is characterized by an area of definite palpable induration or edema. Redness can be disregarded. A positive test indicates the presence of a tuberculous focus in the body but does not distinguish between an active and an inactive lesion. A negative test practically rules out the existence of tuberculous infection of any age.

Brucellergin Skin Test

One tenth of a milliliter is injected intradermally and read at 48 hours. Readings are similar to the tuberculin skin test (previously described). A positive reaction occurs as a tender edematous plaque 1 to 6 cm in diameter. Positive tests denote the occurrence of infection without indication as to its activity.

Note: If agglutination tests are to be performed later, the skin test should *not* be performed, because it will stimulate the production of specific agglutinins.

Coccidioidin Skin Test

One tenth of a milliliter of a 1:100 solution is used. The solution is injected intradermally and read at 48 hours. The reading is similar to the tuberculin skin test (previously described).

Note: Previous pulmonary infection must be ruled out if the test is used to diagnose the cutaneous form of the disease, because sensitization persists for a long period of time.

Frei Test (Lymphogranuloma Venereum)

One tenth of a milliliter each of antigen and control are injected intradermally and read after 48 hours. A positive test is characterized by an infiltrated inflammatory area with a small, well-defined papule not smaller than 7 mm in diameter.

Note: This test is not *specific* for lymphogranuloma venereum because of antigenic similarity to other viruses in the group.

Note: The patient should be asked whether he has an allergy to eggs, because the source of the injected material is infected chick embryo.

Histoplasmin Skin Test

For this test, undiluted filtrate is used. One tenth of a milliliter is injected intradermally and read at 48 hours. Readings are similar to the tuberculin skin test (previously described). A high incidence of positive histoplasmin skin tests has been observed in certain areas of the United States, especially the midwest.

Schick Test

This test is used to indicate blood levels of diphtheria antitoxin. Note that 1/250 unit per ml of serum is sufficient to protect against the disease.

Toxoplasmin Skin Test

One tenth of a milliliter each of antigen and control are injected in the flexor part of the arm and read at 48 hours. A positive test reveals induration of 10 mm or more with the control site negative.

Note: Material for the skin test cannot be obtained commercially.

Trichinella Skin Test

One tenth of a milliliter of allergen is injected intradermally. The test reveals an immediate reaction within 20 minutes, characterized by a wheal with an areola of hyperemia. A control should be run in parallel with the test, which must be negative for the result to be considered valid. This test is positive in almost 100 per cent of cases. It becomes positive approximately 2 weeks after contact and remains positive for several years. The positive reactions, however, cannot be considered *conclusive,* particularly if other parasites are present.

Vollmer's Patch Test

This test for tuberculous infection is used mainly for children, because it is painless. The test is made by applying a specially prepared tape, which has three small squares, the middle one being the control and the other two being infiltrated with sensitivity agent. The tape is applied to either the flexor part of the arm or on the sternum and is left in place for 48 hours without wetting, after which time it is removed and read. A positive reaction consists of a red area with tiny vesicles. A negative reaction cannot be regarded as *excluding* tuberculous infection. The test has a further disadvantage in that the redness of a positive reaction can be confused with a simple reaction to the adhesive tape itself.

THE QUELLUNG REACTION

The Quellung (German = swelling) reaction is a diagnostic test for infections caused by various encapsulated bacteria, including *Diplococcus pneumoniae, Klebsiella pneumoniae,* and *Haemophilus influenzae.* When exposed to type-specific antiserum, these bacteria exhibit a marked degree of swelling, which can be observed microscopically and can thus be classified and differentiated. The reaction was first developed by Neufeld in 1902.

Since the advent of antibiotic therapy, it has ceased to be used by most clinical laboratories and is now of more academic than practical value.

LANCEFIELD GROUPING

Lancefield (1933) developed a method of serologic differentiation of human and other groups of hemolytic streptococci by means of precipitin reactions between solutions of the carbohydrate extracted from streptococcal cells and antisera prepared by immunizing rabbits with heat-killed suspensions of streptococci. The separation of hemolytic streptococci into distinct categories by this technique resulted in a classification related to the most characteristic source of the organisms. Thus, group A is composed of strains usually pathogenic for man, group B is composed of strains from bovine mastitis, group C is composed of strains commonly found in streptococcal diseases of lower animals, and so on. The grouping extends to group O.

In serologic testing, the possibility of nonspecificity should not be ignored, particularly when typing rather than grouping *Streptococcus* (Lancefield, 1962). Studies by Edwards and Larson (1973) have shown that counterimmunoelectrophoresis can be used in the serologic grouping of hemolytic streptococci, and this technique appears to offer distinct advantages over the precipitation test for Lancefield classification.

ELEK'S DIFFUSION TEST

Elek (1948) devised a special modification of the double-diffusion method in two dimensions for demonstrating the toxigenicity of a given strain of *Corynebacterium diphtheriae*. In this method, diffusion is achieved in agar, with a special culture medium known as Elek's medium (preparation of Elek's medium follows). A strip of filter paper is soaked in diphtheria antitoxin and embedded in the agar in a Petri plate. The culture (or cultures) under study is then planted perpendicularly to the strips (Fig. 16–1).

At A-B (Fig. 16–1), there is streaked a known toxigenic strain of *C. diphtheriae*. At X-Y is streaked the strain of *C. diphtheriae* under test. With the group of toxin-producing organisms, the toxin diffuses outward from the culture and at right angles to the line of diffusion of the antitoxin from the filter paper. A line of precipitation will form at the sites of cross-diffusion where antigen and antibody are in equal proportions. This precipitation line, which arises when a positive toxigenic organism is placed in the streak X-Y, will give an identical reaction and will so join with the similar line that arises from the reaction between the antitoxin and the known toxigenic strain in the streak A-B.

A simplification of this technique was described by Maniar and Fox (1968). This technique of Elek's method is given below.

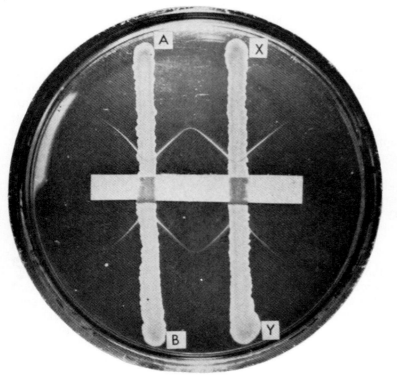

Figure 16–1. Elek's method for demonstrating toxigenicity of an unknown strain of *Corynebacterium diphtheriae*. (From Humphrey, J. H., and White, R. G.: Immunology of Students of Medicine, 3rd ed. Oxford, Blackwell Scientific Publications, 1970.)

METHOD 2: ELEK'S DOUBLE-DIFFUSION TEST

Materials

1. Test culture—a viable *C. diphtheriae* culture
2. Antitoxin—diphtheria antitoxin containing 4000 I.U. per ml
3. Control culture—a toxin-producing strain of *C. diphtheriae*
4. Elek's medium (see preparation that follows)
5. Sterile distilled water
6. Sterile filter-paper strips (0 × 1.0 cm Whatman filter paper No. 1)
7. Sterile Petri dishes

Preparation of Elek's Medium

Preparation A:

Proteose peptone	4 gm
Maltose	0.6 gm
Lactic acid	0.14 ml
Distilled water	100 ml

Dissolve and adjust pH to 7.8

Preparation B:

Agar	3 gm
Sodium chloride	1 gm
Distilled water	100 gm

Dissolve by heat, filter, and adjust pH to 7.8

Preparation C:

Cisamino acid	1 gm
Tween 80	1 ml
Glycerol	1 ml
Distilled water	100 ml

Shake gently, heat to 50°C, dispense in 3.0-ml vials, and autoclave at 115°C for 15 minutes

Store at 4°C

Mix equal parts of preparation A and preparation B, distribute 20-ml portions in screw-capped tubes, and sterilize by flowing steam for 30 minutes on 3 successive days. Store indefinitely at 4°C. For use, melt one tube, cool to below 55°C, and add 3.0 ml of preparation C. Pour plates.

Procedure

1. Aseptically mix 1.9 ml of sterile distilled water and 0.1 ml of antitoxin in a Petri dish.
2. Aseptically dip a filter-paper strip into the mixture until it is completely wet, and transfer it to an empty Petri dish for 30 minutes.
3. Apply a relatively dry strip to the center of a plate of solidified Elek's medium.
4. Inoculate the test culture in streaks perpendicular to the paper strip (see Fig. 16–1).
5. Inoculate at least one similar streak using the control culture.
6. Incubate at 35°C for up to 72 hours.
7. Read every 24 hours. The control culture should demonstrate lines of precipitation. Similar lines of precipitation by test cultures are indicative of toxin production by those cultures.

THE DETECTION AND IDENTIFICATION OF IMMUNOGLOBULIN AND OTHER SERUM PROTEINS

Specific immunoglobulins, as well as a wide range of other serum proteins, may be detected and identified by immunoelectrophoresis and single radial immunodiffusion tests.

The principle of immunoelectrophoresis has been described earlier in this text. Figure 16–2 shows the use of the test in immunoglobulin class differentiation and detection.

Single radial immunodiffusion offers a much more accurate procedure for the identification and measurement of immunoglobulin (Mancini *et al.*, 1965). The test is based on the fact that when antigen diffuses from a well into agar containing

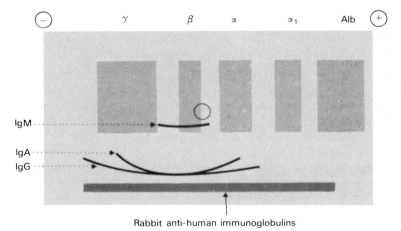

Figure 16–2. Demonstration of major immunoglobulin classes by immunoelectrophoretic analysis. (From Roitt, I.: Essential Immunology, 2nd ed. Oxford, Blackwell Scientific Publications, 1974.)

suitable antiserum, the concentration of antigen continuously falls until the point is reached at which the reactants are in optimal proportions, and a ring of precipitation is formed. The higher the concentration of antigen, the greater the diameter of the ring (Fig. 16–3).

By incorporating standards of known antigen concentration in the plate, a calibration curve can be obtained and used to determine the amount of antigen in the unknown sample.

Absolute values can be determined with the use of plates from commercial companies. These plates can also be used, in most instances, for the detection of several other plasma or serum proteins.

In addition to the immunoglobulins, several proteins (*e.g.*, albumin, haptoglobin, ceruloplasmin, alpha-2-macroglobulin, beta-lipoprotein, transferrin, alpha-1-antitrypsin) can be detected and identified with the use of immunoelectrophoresis and radial immunodiffusion test. Techniques are essentially the same, with the substitution of suitable antibody in each case.

METHOD 3: IMMUNOGLOBULIN QUANTITATION BY IMMUNODIFFUSION

Materials

1. **Radial immunodiffusion plates (R.I.D.) (available from Kallestad Co., Chaska, MN)**
2. **Reference sera (available from Kallestad Co., Chaska, MN)**
3. **5 μL pipettes**
4. **Two-cycle semilog graph paper**
5. **Measuring device (available from Kallestad Co., Chaska, MN)**

Method

1. **Allow the R.I.D. plates and reference sera to reach room temperature.**
2. **Dispense 5 μL each of the three reference sera into wells, and repeat by adding 5 μL of test serum into a well.**
3. **Cover the plate. Place in a ziplock bag (provided), and incubate at room temperature on a level surface for 18 hours (± 1/2 hour).**
4. **Measure the precipitin ring diameter to the nearest 0.1 mm.**
5. **Plot the reference sera concentrations against the zone diameter, and determine the concentration of the test sample from the graph.**

TOXOPLASMA GONDII

The organism *Toxoplasma gondii* is one of the most common infectious agents of humans in the

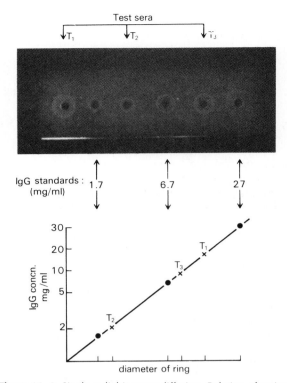

Figure 16–3. Single radial immunodiffusion. Relation of antigen concentration to size of precipitation ring formed. (From Roitt, I.: Essential Immunology, 2nd ed. Oxford, Blackwell Scientific Publications, 1974.)

world. Since its isolation in 1908 in a North African rodent, the gondii, many species of birds, reptiles, and mammals have been found to harbor it.

Humans are infected with *Toxoplasma* from the following sources:

1. Human
   a. Mother to fetus
   b. Immunosuppression (induced or developmental)—organ transplantation, activation of quiescent infections
   c. Transfusion
2. Animal
   a. Ingestion of infected meat, especially mutton or pork
   b. Soil contamination by oocysts from domestic and feral cat feces
3. Unknown (probably most)
   a. Acquisition by vegetarians?
   b. Age, sex, and geographic differences
   c. Other—undefined

Congenital toxoplasmosis is a disease with a very wide range of manifestation—so much so, in fact, that it must be considered in the differential diagnosis of almost all types of obscure illness occurring during early infancy. The symptoms are sometimes nonspecific (including anemia, splenomegaly, jaundice, fever, hepatomegaly, adenopathy, and vomiting), and, because of this, toxoplasmosis is easily misdiagnosed on clinical grounds, even in sick infants who have the generalized form of the disease.

Tests for the Detection of Antibody to *Toxoplasma Gondii*

The Virgo reagent toxoplasma antibody test kit (available from Electronucleonics Lab, Inc., Bethesda, MD) uses the immunofluorescent technique to detect *Toxoplasma* antibody in test serum.

The kit contains fixed *Toxoplasma* organisms that have been dried on each well of each antigen slide. Whenever a human serum sample containing *Toxoplasma* antibody is brought into contact with the organisms on each well, a *Toxoplasma* antibody-antigen complex is formed that can then be detected by staining it with a special dye (FITC), which is visible with a fluorescent microscope. The dye is capable of staining this complex because it is attached to an antibody made against normal human immunoglobulins (of which *Toxoplasma* antibody is a specific example). When this dye (containing antihuman antibody) is brought into contact with the antibody-antigen complex, it reacts with the antibody moiety. A three-member complex, antibody-antigen-antihuman antibody, now exists, which remains on the slide after the nonreacting material has been rinsed away.

If there is no *Toxoplasma* antibody in the test serum, the antibody-antigen complex will not form; therefore, the second (three-member) complex is unable to form. In this case, no detectable fluorescence will be seen microscopically, because it would all be washed away in the rinse cycle.

Note: Clear test serum is essential. If lipids, bacterial contamination, and so on are present, either filtering (0.45 μ) or centrifugation (at 3000 × G for 10 minutes) is required.

Two samples should be submitted, because a single titer is not significant; only a changing titer is meaningful.

The results of the test are interpreted as follows:

Positive Reaction. The reaction observed is positive when yellow-green fluorescence extends around the entire periphery of the organism. This reaction may be intense enough (in lower dilutions of strong positive sera) to mask all internal red counterstain. In higher dilutions, the peripheral staining will become a thin, peripheral halo around an internal red fluorescence.

Negative Reaction. The reaction observed is negative when organisms fluoresce reddish with no yellow-green fluorescence around the periphery; the reaction is also considered negative when only one end of the organism fluoresces bright yellow-green with no extension of yellow-green around the other end. This "polar staining" will occur at lower dilutions and usually disappears at a serum dilution above 1:64.

The clinical significance of the result is measured as follows:

Negative—nondiagnostic

1:16–1:64—usually reflects only some past exposure or may signify early stages of disease with rising titers

1:256—usually indicates relatively recent exposure or present involvement

1:1024—very significant

PREGNANCY TESTING

A number of serologic tests have been used in pregnancy testing, each designed to detect minute amounts of human chorionic gonadotropin (HCG) when it appears in the urine during the first few weeks of pregnancy.

The methods most commonly used now are based on the agglutination-inhibition test developed by Noto and Miale (1964). This test consists of incubation of the patient's urine with anti-HCG, followed by the addition of latex particles coated with HCG. If HCG is present in the urine, it neutralizes the antibody so that no agglutination of the latex particles is seen. If no HCG is present in the urine, agglutination occurs between the anti-HCG and HCG-coated latex particles.

The test gives reliable results about 42 days after the onset of the last normal menstrual period but is not reliable after the first trimester of pregnancy. The first morning urine specimen is required, and it should have a specific gravity of at least 1.015. It should be not more than 12 hours old from the time of collection; fresh urine may be frozen and tested later. Chorioepithelioma, hydatidiform mole, or excessive ingestion of aspirin may give false-positive results.

A number of test kits are available (Warner/Chilcott Laboratories, Morris Plains, NJ; Ortho Diagnostics, Raritan, NJ; and Organon Inc., West Orange, NJ) that give equally satisfactory results.

THE PERTUSSIS (WHOOPING COUGH) AGGLUTINATION TEST

The etiologic agent of pertussis, *Bordetella pertussis* (formerly known as *Haemophilus pertussis*), was isolated by Bordet and Gengou in 1906. It is a small, nonmotile, gram-negative rod. The detection of pertussis agglutinins can be made with suspensions of 10^9 organisms per milliliter of freshly isolated cultures of *B. pertussis* serotype 1,3 in saline, added in 0.4-ml volumes to equal volumes of serum dilutions. After incubation for 18 hours in a 37°C water bath, tests are read with a magnifying glass. The titer is expressed as the highest dilution yielding complete agglutination.

Complement fixation tests are more sensitive for pertussis antibody testing, and, although more complicated, they should probably be considered the method of choice. (See Diagnosis of whooping cough: comparison of serologic tests with isolation of *Bordetella pertussis*. A combined Scottish study. Br. Med. J., *4*:637, 1970.)

THE LEPTOSPIRAL AGGLUTINATION TEST

The leptospiroses are a group of diseases produced by a large number of antigenically distinct members of the genus *Leptospira*. At least 80 different serotypes and subserotypes of the genus have been identified. Several species of *Leptospira* are associated with human infection (Table 16–2). In addition to these pathogenic species, the genus also contains saprophytes, which are collectively designated as *Leptospira biflexa*.

Human leptospirosis can be definitely established either by isolating the disease agent from typical clinical specimens (*e.g.,* blood and cerebrospinal fluid) or by demonstrating a significant rise in leptospiral antibody titer by serologic tests. The leptospiral agglutination test (Cole, 1973) and the hemagglutination test (Sulzer and Jones, 1973) are the most popular. The agglutination test requires microdilution plates available from Falcon Plastics, Oxnard, CA. The hemagglutination test uses a

Table 16–2. *LEPTOSPIRA* SPECIES CAPABLE OF CAUSING HUMAN INFECTION

Species	Disease
L. australis	Canefield fever Field fever Mud fever Pomona fever
L. autumnalis	Akiyami Autumnal fever Fort Bragg fever Seven-day fever
L. bataviae	Ricefield fever Swineherd's disease Weil's disease
L. hebdomadis	Akiyami B Feld-fieber (field fever) B Seven-day fever
L. icterohaemorrhagiae	Infectious or leptospiral jaundice Weil's disease
L. canicola	Canicola fever
L. pyrogenes	Canefield fever Leptospirosis febrilis

soluble antigen coupled to sheep erythrocytes, which are then fixed with glutaraldehyde. The sensitized cells are claimed to be stable for at least 1 year. The test procedure is given in Sulzer and Jones, 1973.

GENERAL LABORATORY TECHNIQUES

Complement Fixation

Methods of complement fixation include manual techniques, test tube techniques, and automated micro methods (slow fixation and rapid fixation). The standard micro method that uses 0.025 ml of all reagents will be described here. The volumes and procedure can easily be adapted from this procedure to suit any specific requirements.

Materials

1. **Hemolysin—This is a serum that contains antibodies to sheep erythrocytes (see preparation of sheep red cell hemolysin, later).**
2. **Sheep erythrocytes (see collection and preservation of sheep blood, later).**
3. **Alsever's solution—This is prepared with 1000 ml distilled water, 0.55 gm citric acid, 8.0 gm sodium citrate, 4.2 gm sodium chloride, and 20.5 gm dextrose.**
4. **Citrate solution—This is prepared with 2.08 gm sodium citrate and 2.5 gm dextrose in 100 ml distilled water.**
5. **Diluent—Veronal-buffered saline is most commonly used. This is prepared with 85.0 gm sodium chloride, 5.75 gm diethylbarbituric acid, and 3.75 gm sodium barbital in 2000 ml distilled water.**
6. **Microtiter plates (available from Canalco, Rockville, MD).**
7. **Complement—Usually from guinea pig serum (see preparation and preservation of complement, later).**
8. **Antigens—A variety are used, available commercially.**
9. **Antigen medium (normal antigen)—This is necessary when testing for viral antibodies and is prepared in the same way as viral antigen except that normal cells (rather than virus-infected cells) are used. The medium serves as a control to test each serum for cellular antibodies, which lead to false-positive results.**
10. **Test serum—Patient's serum, inactivated at 56°C for 30 minutes. Stored sera (*i.e.,* for more than a day) should be reinactivated before use (10 minutes at 60°C). Because antibody titers will decrease on storage and cause the sera to become anticomplementary, they should not be stored for long periods of time**

(see preparation and preservation of complement, later).

Preliminary Tests

Preliminary tests to determine the efficiency of the many reagents used in the complement fixation test should be carried out on each new batch of reagent.

Hemolysin. A titration of hemolysin should be performed whenever a new batch of cells of a new hemolysin is used.

1. Dilute the hemolysin 1:1000.
2. Set up one row of eight test tubes in a test tube rack.
3. Make the following dilutions of hemolysin in buffered saline:

Tube No.	Hemolysin	Buffered Saline	Dilution
1	1.0	0	1000
2	0.66	0.34	1500
3	0.5	0.5	2000
4	0.33	0.67	3000
5	0.25	0.75	4000
6	0.166	0.834	6000
7	0.125	0.875	8000
8	0	1.0	0

4. Using separate pipets for each tube, add 1.0 ml of a 2 per cent suspension of sheep erythrocytes to each tube. Mix.
5. Allow to stand (sensitize) at room temperature.
6. Dilute complement 1:10.
7. Set up one row of eight test tubes in a test tube rack.
8. Make the same dilutions of complement as made for hemolysin (step 3).
9. Deliver 0.025 ml of complement dilutions into the wells of a microplate, as shown:

10. Add 0.05 ml of saline to each well as a substitute for the serum and antigen in the actual tests.
11. Allow plates to stand at 37°C for 90 minutes.
12. After incubation, deliver 0.025 ml of the sensitized cells (step 5) in a checkerboard fashion (as in step 9).
13. Shake gently but firmly. Incubate at 37°C for 30 minutes. Shake again at 15 minutes and on removal from the incubator.
14. Read. (Note: Plates need not be read immediately but may be left for several hours at room temperature if desired.)

Complement. Each new batch of complement should be titrated as follows:

1. Set up test tubes in a test tube rack.
2. Dilute complement 1:10.
3. Make the following dilutions of complement in saline:

Tube No.	Complement	Saline	Dilution
1	1.0	0	1:10
2	0.66	0.34	1:15
3	0.5	0.5	1:20
4	0.33	0.67	1:30
5	0.25	0.75	1:40
6	0.16	0.84	1:60
7	0.12	0.88	1:80
8	0.08	0.92	1:120
9	0.06	0.94	1:160
10	0	1.0	0

4. Mix and deliver 0.025 ml of each dilution into separate wells in a row of wells on a microplate.
5. Incubate plate at 37°C for 90 minutes.
6. After incubation, deliver 0.025 ml of sensitized cells in a checkerboard fashion (see step 12 under titration of hemolysin).
7. Shake gently but firmly and incubate at 37°C for 30 minutes. Shake at 15 minutes and again on removal from the incubator.

Dilutions of Hemolysin	Dilutions of Complement								
	1:10	1:15	1:20	1:30	1:40	1:60	1:80	1:120	0
0	4	4	4	4	4	4	4	4	4
1:8000	2	3	4	4	4	4	4	4	4
1:6000	1	1	1	2	2	3	3	3	4
1:4000	tr.	0	0	0	1	2	3	3	4
1:3000	0	0	0	1	2	3	3	3	4
1:2000	0	0	0	0	0	tr.	2	3	4
1:1500	0	0	0	0	0	0	1	3	4
1:1000	0	0	0	0	0	tr.	1	3	4

Interpretation:
  0 = Complete hemolysis
  tr = 10 per cent cells
  1+ = 25 per cent cells
  2+ = 50 per cent cells
  3+ = 75 per cent cells
  4+ = 100 per cent cells (no hemolysis)

8. **Reading:** The HD_{50} (hemolytic dose, 50 per cent) is taken as the dilution that gives 2+ hemolysis (50 per cent). In the actual test, 2.5 HD_{50} is used. This is derived by dividing the dilution showing 50 per cent hemolysis by 2.5.

Antigen. Each batch of new antigen should be subject to all three of the following titrations:

Anticomplementary Titration

1. Add 0.025 ml of diluent to wells 2 through 9 of a microplate.
2. Add 0.025 ml of antigen to wells 1 and 2. Mix and serially dilute to well 9. Discard 0.025 ml of the final dilution in well 9.
3. Add 0.025 ml of diluent to all wells.
4. Add 0.025 ml of complement (2.5 HD_{50}) to each well and shake gently.
5. Incubate. (Some systems require overnight incubation at 4°C; others, 2 hours at room temperature. Such requirements are usually indicated in the instruction inserts with commercial antigens. As a general rule, bacterial, influenzal, and chlamydial antigens require 2 hours at room temperature; all others give better results if incubated overnight at 4°C.)
6. Add 0.025 ml of sensitized sheep erythrocytes to all wells.
7. Shake gently and place in a 37°C water bath for 30 minutes.
8. Read. No fixation should occur in any well. If, however, a slight degree of fixation is noted in the first or second well, the antigen may be used if the maximal reactivity titer is high.

Hemolytic Titration

1. Repeat steps 1 and 2 under anticomplementary titration.
2. Add 0.05 ml of diluent to each well.
3. Add 0.025 ml of sensitized sheep erythrocytes to all wells.
4. Place immediately in a 37°C water bath for 30 minutes.
5. Read. No hemolysis should occur in any well. If a small degree of hemolysis occurs in a very low titer, however, the antigen may still be used if the maximal specific reactivity is to a higher titer.

Reactivity Titration

1. Set up a block titration by serially diluting a positive serum and the antigen in test tubes and then distributing 0.025 ml of each into the wells of a microplate in a checkerboard fashion.
2. Add 0.025 ml of complement (2.5 HD_{50}) to all wells.
3. Set up controls as described under Test Controls (later).
4. Incubate as for long or short fixation (see step 5 under Anticomplementary Titration).
5. Add 0.025 ml of sensitized sheep erythrocytes to all wells.

6. Shake and place in a 37°C water bath for 30 minutes.
7. Read. A calculation is made to determine two antigenic units per 0.025 ml. The *antigenic unit* is read as the highest dilution of the hyperimmune serum that gives a 4+ reaction in the presence of the highest dilution of antigen.

Procedure

1. Deliver 0.75 ml of diluent to well 1 and 0.025 ml to wells 2 through 7 of one row of wells in a microplate.
2. Add 0.025 ml of test serum to well 1. Mix and transfer 0.025 ml of the mixture to well 2 through to well 6. Wells 7 and 8 serve as serum controls. Discard 0.025 ml of the final 1:128 dilution in well 6.
3. Add 0.025 ml of antigen (two units) to each of wells 1 to 6. Add 0.025 ml of antigen medium to well 8, if necessary (see antigen medium under Materials).
4. Add 0.025 ml of complement (2.5 HD_{50}) to each well.
5. Incubate as required (see step 5 under Anticomplementary Titration).
6. Add 0.025 ml of sensitized sheep erythrocytes to each well.
7. Shake and place in a 37°C water bath for 30 minutes.
8. Read. The titer is expressed as the highest serum dilution that will allow fixation of enough complement to prevent 50 per cent of cell lysis, provided that all controls give the appropriate results (see Test Controls, following).

Test Controls

1. **Antigen hemolytic control:** 0.025 ml of antigen, 0.05 ml of diluent, no complement, 0.025 ml of sensitized erythrocytes. Correct reading, 4+ (no hemolysis)
2. **Antigen anticomplementary control:** 0.025 ml of antigen, 0.025 ml of diluent, 0.025 ml of complement, 0.025 ml of sensitized erythrocytes. Correct reading, 0 (complete hemolysis)
3. **Complement controls:**
   a. 0.05 ml of diluent, 0.025 ml of complement, 0.025 ml of sensitized erythrocytes. Correct reading, 0 (complete hemolysis)
   b. 0.065 ml of diluent, 0.01 ml of complement, 0.025 ml of sensitized erythrocytes. Correct reading, 2+ (50 per cent hemolysis)
4. **Cell control (also diluent control):** 0.075 ml of diluent, 0.025 ml of sensitized erythrocytes. Correct reading, 4+ (no hemolysis)
5. **Known positive and negative serum controls:** Correct readings:

Positive serum—4+ (no hemolysis) up to its titer

Negative serum—0 (complete hemolysis)

6. Test serum—antigen medium control: Well 7 of the actual test. Correct reading, 0 (complete hemolysis)

7. Test serum—anticomplementary control: Well 8 of the actual test. Correct reading, 0 (complete hemolysis)

Complement Fixation Inhibition

Materials

As for complement fixation. In addition, an indicator antibody is used.

1. Indicator antibody—Serum that will fix complement in the presence of the test antigen

2. Test sera—Usually avian serum samples that fail to fix complement in the presence of the test antigen

Preliminary Tests

The same preliminary tests are required as those described under Complement Fixation. In addition, the indicator antibody needs to be titrated prior to use, as follows:

1. Prepare serial twofold dilutions of the indicator serum in 0.025-ml volumes in a row of wells in a microplate.

2. Add to each well 0.025-ml volumes of antigen containing two CF units each.

3. Add 0.025 ml of 2.5 HD_{50} complement to each well.

4. Incubate as required (see step 5 under Anticomplementary Titration).

5. Add 0.025 ml of sensitized erythrocytes to each well.

6. Shake gently and reincubate at 37°C for 30 minutes.

7. Read. The highest serum dilution that will fix 100 per cent of the complement (no hemolysis) is taken as one unit of indicator antibody.

Procedure

1. Proceed with steps 1, 2, and 3 as described under the procedure for complement fixation.

2. Add 0.025 ml of the indicator antibody serum, as determined by titration, to each of wells 1 through 6. Add 0.01 ml of antigen medium to well 7, if necessary.

3. Add 0.025 ml of complement (2.5 HD_{50}) to each well.

4. Incubate as required.

5. Add 0.025 ml of sensitized erythrocytes to each well.

6. Shake gently.

7. Place in a 37°C water bath for 30 minutes.

8. Read. The titer is read as the highest dilution of test serum that will completely inhibit complement fixation. This will be the last well in which complete lysis is demonstrated.

Test Controls

In addition to the controls discussed under Complement Fixation, the following must also be incorporated in each test run:

1. Test serum—antigen control: 0.025 ml of test serum, 0.025 ml of antigen, 0.025 ml of diluent, 0.025 ml of conplement, and 0.025 ml of sensitized erythrocytes. Correct reading, 0 (complete hemolysis)

2. Test serum—indicator antibody control: 0.025 ml of each of the following: diluent, indicator antibody, complement, and sensitized erythrocytes. Correct reading, 0 (complete hemolysis)

3. Antigen—indicator antibody control: 0.025 ml of each of the following: diluent, antigen, indicator antibody, complement, and sensitized erythrocytes. Correct reading, 4+ (no hemolysis)

4. Antigen medium—indicator antibody control (if necessary): 0.025 ml of each of the following: diluent, antigen medium, indicator antibody, complement, and sensitized erythrocytes. Correct reading, 0 (complete hemolysis)

Hemagglutination Inhibition

Materials

1. Test serum—Nonspecific agglutinins present in normal serum must be removed before use (method given later).

2. Antigen—Commercially available from Flow Laboratories Inc., Rockville, MD, and Microbiological Associates, Bethesda, MD. Antigens must be titrated before used (method given later).

3. Red cells—See table below for species recommended with the particular antigen. Make up 50 per cent and 0.05 per cent suspension in appropriate dilution.

4. Diluent—0.85 per cent saline or HEPES-saline-albumin-gelatin (HSAG diluent) (preparation of HSAG diluent given later).

5. Test tubes or microplates—10 × 75 round-bottomed test tubes or V-bottomed microplates (available from Cooke Engineering, Alexandria, VA, and Linbro Chemical Co., New Haven, CT).

CELLS, INCUBATION TIMES, AND TEMPERATURES FOR VARIOUS HEMAGGLUTINATION-INHIBITION SYSTEMS

Virus	Erythrocytes	Time for Ab-Ag Reaction	Time for Agglutination	Temp. of Incubation °C
Influenza Parainfluenza Mumps Sendai Reovirus	Human—Group O	15 min	60	20
Enterovirus	Human— Group O	15 min	60	4
Measles (Rubeola)	Rhesus or vervet monkey	15 min	90	37
Rubella	Baby chick at 4°C	60 min	90	4
Adenovirus	Rhesus monkey	15 min	90	37
Vaccinia Smallpox	Chicken	30 min	90	20

6. **Diluting loops—For microplate technique.**
7. **Positive and negative control sera.**

Preliminary Procedures

The procedure described here uses 0.1-ml volumes of all reagents. Volumes will differ depending upon whether tubes or microplates are used but can be adjusted according to the technique chosen. Temperature and incubation times will also differ depending upon the virus used, as will the erythrocytes used. General instructions given in this procedure can be adjusted to suit the virus under test by the technologist engaged in the testing (see table that follows).

    Preparation of Erythrocytes. See Preparation of Red Cell Concentrations (later).

Preparation of HSAG Diluent (if required)

Solution A

1. **HEPES (N-2-hydroxyethyl-piperazine-N-2-ethanesul-fonic acid)**   **29.8 gm**
2. **Sodim chloride**   **40.95 gm**
3. **Calcium chloride (CaCl$_2$2H$_2$O)**   **0.74 gm**
4. **Distilled water**   **1000 ml**

    Dissolve the chemicals in 900 ml of distilled water. Adjust the pH with approximately 12 ml of 1 N sodium hydroxide to 6.5. Add more distilled water to bring to 1000 ml. Sterilize by filtration and store at 4°C.

Solution B

1. **Bovine albumin powder**   **25 mg**
2. **Distilled water**   **1000 ml**

    Dissolve the albumin in 900 ml of water and adjust the volume to 1000 ml. Sterilize by filtration and store at 4°C.

Solution C

1. **Gelatin**   **25 mg**
2. **Distilled water**   **1000 ml**

    Dissolve the gelatin. Sterilize in an autoclave at 120°C for 15 minutes and store at 4°C.

    HSAG diluent is prepared by mixing 200 ml of solution A, 500 ml of solution B, and 100 ml of solution C in 200 ml of sterile distilled water. Adjust the pH to 6.2 with 1.0 N sodium hydroxide or hydrochloric acid if necessary. Store at 4°C for up to 2 months.

Titration of Antigen

1. **Set out 10 tubes in a test tube rack.**
2. **Add 0.1 ml of diluent to each tube.**
3. **Deliver 0.1 ml of antigen to tube 1, mix, transfer 0.1 ml to tube 2, and so on. Discard 0.1 ml of the final dilution in tube 9.**
4. **Add 0.1 ml of diluent to each tube.**
5. **Add 0.1 ml of 0.5 per cent erythrocytes to each tube. (The same erythrocyte suspension should be used in this preliminary test as that to be used in the actual test.)**
6. **Shake. (Microplates must be shaken on a mechanical vibrator for 1 minute.)**
7. **Incubate.**
8. **Read. The cell control (tube 10) should show no hemagglutination. The antigen titer (one unit) is the reciprocal of the highest dilution yielding complete hemagglutination. In the actual test, four units of antigen must be used. These are obtained simply by dividing the true titer by 4.**

Removal of Nonspecific Agglutinins

1. **To 1.0 ml of test serum add one drop (0.03 ml) of 50 per cent erythrocytes. (These should be of the same species that is required for the test antigen; refer to last table.)**
2. **Shake and leave at room temperature for 15 minutes.**
3. **Centrifuge at 1500 rpm for 10 minutes.**
4. **Aspirate the supernatant fluid.**

Removal of Nonspecific Inhibitors

Absorption with Kaolin

1. **Mix 1.0 ml of test serum (the supernatant fluid collected in the removal of nonspecific agglutinations) with 1.0 ml of a 50 per cent suspension of acid-washed kaolin in saline.**

2. **Leave for 30 minutes at room tempeature, shaking periodically.**
3. **Centrifuge at 1500 rpm for 15 minutes.**
4. **Collect the clear supernatant fluid.**

This method removes all nonspecific inhibitors. It does not, however, lend itself well to the absorption of sera to be tested against some viral antigens, such as rubella.

Absorption with Heparin–Manganese Chloride

1. **Prepare a mixture of equal volumes of 5000 units (U.S.P.) per milliliter of sodium heparin and a filtration-sterilized solution of 19.8 per cent manganese chloride ($MnCl_2 \cdot 4H_2O$). This solution may be stored at 4°C for up to 2 weeks.**
2. **Mix 0.2 ml of test serum (the supernatant fluid removed in the removal of nonspecific agglutinins) with 0.4 ml of HSAG diluent.**
3. **Add 0.2 ml of the heparin–manganese chloride solution.**
4. **Shake, and incubate at 4°C for 15 minutes.**
5. **Centrifuge at 4°C for 15 minutes at 1500 rpm.**
6. **Aspirate the supernatant fluid.**

(Note: When making dilutions in the actual test, the first method given will dilute the test serum 1:2, and the second method, 1:4.)

Procedure

1. **Set up 10 test tubes in a test tube rack. (A microplate may also be used.)**
2. **Deliver 0.1 ml of treated test serum to tubes 1, 2, and 10, and 0.1 ml of diluent to tubes 2 through 10.**
3. **Mix the contents of tube 2, transfer 0.1 ml to tube 3, mix and transfer 0.1 ml to tube 4, and so on up to tube 9. Discard 0.1 ml of the final dilution in tube 9. Tube 10 will serve as the serum-erythrocyte control. Serum treated with kaolin will yield dilutions of 1:2 to 1:512; serum treated with heparin-$MnCl_2$ will yield dilutions of 1:4 to 1:1024.**
4. **Add 0.1 ml of antigen (containing four units) to tubes 1 through 9.**
5. **Shake, and incubate as required (see last table).**
6. **Add 0.1 ml of 0.5 per cent erythrocytes to all tubes.**
7. **Shake and incubate as required (see last table).**
8. **Read. The antibody titer is the reciprocal of the highest serum dilution in which 50 per cent or some of the hemagglutination is inhibited.**

Test Controls

1. **Test serum-erythrocyte control—Tube 10 of each series of test serum dilutions should show no hemagglutination.**
2. **Antigen control—0.1 ml of diluent, antigen, and erythrocytes. Final result, complete hemagglutination.**
3. **Red cell control—0.2 ml of diluent and 0.1 ml of erythrocytes. Final result, no agglutination.**
4. **Positive and negative serum controls—Set up in the same manner as the test sera. These should read their exact, known titers.**

COLLECTION AND PRESERVATION OF SHEEP BLOOD

Blood is collected from the jugular vein of the animal, defibrinated, and stored at 4°C. The sheep red cells may be stored for 1 week provided that no hemolysis becomes visible. If sheep red cells are difficult to obtain, they may be collected in Alsever's solution or citrate in larger volumes and stored at 4°C for approximately 1 month. Cells should not be used until after stabilization, which takes 2 to 3 days' storage at 4°C.

Before use, the cells must be filtered through two layers of cotton gauze and washed three times in buffered saline, with centrifugation of the cells at 2000 rpm each time. After each washing, the buffy coat of white cells should be removed with a pipet. Any red cells that stick to the side of the tube should be removed with a wooden applicator stick. After the final washing, the supernatant fluid must be perfectly clear. This final suspension is centrifuged for 15 to 20 minutes to pack the cells.

To sensitize the cells, a 2 per cent suspension of cells is made up in diluent. An equal volume of hemolysin dilution is prepared, and these two are mixed by pouring the *cells* into the *hemolysin* and then pouring back and forth from one bottle to the other about 10 times. The mixture is then left to sensitize for 30 minutes at 37°C.

PREPARATION OF SHEEP RED CELL HEMOLYSIN

The method of preparing sheep red cell hemolysin is to inject whole sheep blood intracutaneously into rabbits and then to inoculate washed sheep cells intravenously. Sheep red cell hemolysin is readily available commercially, however, and is usually supplied as a 50 per cent glycerinated suspension. A dilution of 1:100 is made by adding 2.0 ml of glycerinated hemolysin to 94.0 ml of buffered saline and then adding 4.0 ml of 5 per cent phenol solution as a preservative. The dilution constitutes the stock solution and is stable for about 3 months at 4°C.

PREPARATION AND PRESERVATION OF COMPLEMENT

Complement, usually from guinea pig serum, is available from many commercial houses. It must be stored in a cold room at 4°C or in an ice bath while tests are being carried out. In a dried state, it can be stored indefinitely in a cold room at 4°C.

Dissolved in distilled water, it should be stored at −20°C. When preparing dilutions of complement, care should be taken to avoid excess shaking or vigorous pipetting, because this can cause inactivation.

PREPARATION OF RED CELL CONCENTRATIONS

Blood collected in anticoagulant from a human, sheep, or other source is washed in three volumes of diluent (saline) by mixing, centrifuging at 1500 rpm for 15 minutes, and aspirating until the supernatant is completely clear. The cells are resuspended to a 50 per cent suspension in diluent and can be stored at 4°C for up to 2 weeks. For most tests, the required suspensions may be made directly from the 50 per cent suspension in diluent. If more exact suspensions are required, a standardization procedure should be performed as follows:

1. Prepare solutions of cyanmethemoglobin (CMG) in CMG diluent reagent containing 80, 60, 40, 20, and 0 mg CMG per 100 ml.
2. Read each solution in a spectrophotometer at the 540-nm wavelength. Plot the readings on regular graph paper against milligrams per 100 ml of the standard CMG. This should produce a straight line.
3. Calculate the factor to be used for determining the target optical density (OD). The factor will be the sum of the concentrations of the standards $(80+60+40+20+0)$ divided by the sum of the OD readings obtained.
4. Calculate the target OD. The target OD is the target number of milligrams of CMG per 100 ml divided by the factor obtained in step 3. Once the targets and factors for a given cell suspension have been established, they can be used for all subsequent standardizations, provided that the spectrophotometer is not moved or jarred.

REVIEW QUESTIONS

MULTIPLE CHOICE

Choose the phrase, sentence, or symbol that completes the statement or answers the question. More than one answer may be correct in each case. Answers are given at the back of this book.

1. The expression of the opsonic power of a patient's blood in relation to the opsonic power of normal blood is known as:
   (a) the opsonic factor
   (b) the opsonic expression
   (c) the opsonic index
   (d) none of the above
   (Opsonocytophagic Tests)

2. Bacteriolysins:
   (a) are antibodies that cause the dissolution of bacteria
   (b) are found in the blood stream of animals who are naturally immune to a particular antigen
   (c) are found in the blood stream of animals who have been artificially immunized against an antigen by injection
   (d) destroy the bacterial cell itself in the presence of complement
   (Bacteriolysin Test)

3. In the Moan hemagglutination test for amebiasis:
   (a) false positives may be encountered in healthy individuals
   (b) false positives may be found in individuals who have other diseases
   (c) the result becomes negative within a week of remission of clinical symptoms

   (d) inaccurate readings may result from the use of glassware containing lipids
   (Discussion—The Moan Hemagglutination Test)

4. The most widely used technique for the detection of antibodies to rubella is:
   (a) the hemagglutination-inhibition test
   (b) the complement fixation test
   (c) radioimmunoassay
   (d) the neutralization test
   (Tests for Rubella)

5. The intradermal skin test is commonly used in cases of:
   (a) tuberculosis
   (b) food allergies
   (c) histoplasmosis
   (d) pollen allergies
   (The Performance of Skin Tests)

6. A positive tuberculin skin test is characterized by:
   (a) an area of definite palpable induration of edema
   (b) redness, indicating recent infection
   (c) an elevated wheal from 8 to 15 mm in diameter from which pseudopods irradiate
   (d) induration of 10 mm or more with the control site also weakly positive
   (Commonly Used Skin Tests)

7. *Toxoplasma gondii:*
   (a) is one of the most common infectious agents of humans in the world
   (b) is an extremely rare infectious agent
   (c) can be passed from mother to fetus
   (d) can infect humans through ingestion of infected meat
   (Toxoplasma Gondii)

ANSWER "TRUE" OR "FALSE"

8. The Moan hemagglutination test is a serologic test for amebiasis.
   (The Moan Hemagglutination Test)

9. Certain carbohydrates may be allergens.
   (Skin Tests)

10. Skin tests are not available for influenza.
    (Skin Tests)

11. The Quellung reaction is a diagnostic test for infections caused by various encapsulated bacteria.
    (The Quellung Reaction)

12. Lancefield grouping is a method of serologic differentiation of human and other groups of hemolytic streptococci by means of counterimmunoelectrophoresis.
    (Lancefield Grouping)

General References

Alba's Medical Technology, 9th ed. Anaheim, CA, Berkeley Scientific Publications, 1980.

Bennington, J. L. (Ed.): Saunders Dictionary and Encyclopedia of Laboratory Medicine and Technology. Philadelphia, W. B. Saunders Company, 1984.

Widman, F. K.: Clinical Interpretation of Laboratory Tests, 9th ed. Philadelphia, F. A. Davis Co., 1983.

BIBLIOGRAPHY

Aach, R. D., Grisham, J. W., and Parker, C. W.: Detection of Australian antigen by radioimmunoassay. Proc. Natl. Acad. Sci. U.S.A., 68:1056, 1971.

Aach, R. D., Hacker, E. J., and Parker, C. W.: Recognition of hepatitis B antigen determinants by a double-label radioimmunoassay: a sensitive means of subtyping hepatitis B antigen. J. Immunol., 111:381, 1973.

Aach, R. D., Szmuness, W., Mosley, J. W., Hollinger, F. B., Kahn, R. A., Stevens, C. E., Edwards, V. M., and Werch, J.: Serum alanine aminotransferase of donors in relation to the risk of non-A, non-B hepatitis in recipients: the transfusion-transmitted viruses study. N. Engl. J. Med., 304:989, 1981.

Abernathy, R. S., and Heiner, D. C.: Precipitation reactions in agar gel in North American blastomycosis. J. Lab. Clin. Med., 57:177, 1966.

Abernethy, T. J., and Francis, T., Jr.: Studies on the somatic C-polysaccharide of pneumococcus. I. Cutaneous and serologic reactions in pneumonia. J. Exp. Med., 69:69, 1937.

Albert, E. D.: The HLA system: serologically defined antigens. Clin. Immunobiol., 3:237, 1977.

Allison, A. S.: Self-tolerance and autoimmunity in the thyroid. N. Engl. J. Med., 295:821, 1976.

Almeida, J. D., Rubinstein, D., and Stott, E. J.: New antigen-antibody system in Australia-antigen-positive hepatitis. Lancet, 2:1225, 1971.

Alper, C. A., Abramson, N., Johnston, R. B., Jandl, J. H., and Rosen, F. S.: Studies in vitro and in vivo on an abnormality in the metabolism of C3 in a patient with increased susceptibility to infection. J. Clin. Invest., 49:1975, 1970.

Alper, C. A., Bloch, K. J., and Rosen, F. S.: Increased susceptibility to infection in a patient with type II essential hypercatabolism of C3. N. Engl. J. Med., 288:601, 1973.

Alper, C. A., and Rosen, F. S.: Complement and clinical medicine. In Vyas, G. N., Stites, D. P., and Brecher, G. (Eds.): Laboratory Diagnosis of Immunologic Disorders. New York, Grune & Stratton, 1975.

Alter, H. J.: The dominant role of non-A, non-B in the pathogenesis of post-transfusion hepatitis: a clinical assessment. Clin. Gastroenterol., 9:155, 1980.

Alter, H. J., Holland, P. V., and Purcell, R. H.: Counterelectrophoresis for detection of hepatitis-associated antigen; methodology and comparison with gel diffusion and complement fixation. J. Lab. Clin. Med., 77:1000, 1971.

Anderson, H. C., and McCarty, M.: Determination of the C-reactive protein in the blood as a measure of the activity of disease process in acute rheumatic fever. Am. J. Med., 8:445, 1950.

Asher, T. M., and Shigekawa, J. M.: Technical evaluation of CR-test. Scientific Report No. 2. Costa Mesa, CA, Hyland Laboratories.

Aubert, E., Pavilanis, V., and Starkey, O. H.: Virus antibody titrations using latex suspensions. Can. J. Public Health, 53:206, 1962.

Audujar, J. J., and Mazurek, R. R.: The plasmacrit (PCT) test on capillary blood. J. Clin. Pathol., 31:197, 1959.

Bach, F. H., and Van Rood, J. J.: The major histocompatibility complex—genetics and biology. N. Engl. J. Med., 295:806, 872, and 927, 1976.

Banatvala, J. E., Best, J. M., and Walker, D. K.: Epstein-Barr virus–specific IgM in infectious mononucleosis, Burkitt's lymphoma, and nasopharyngeal carcinoma. Lancet, 1:1205, 1972.

Barker, L. F., Peterson, M. R., and Murray, R.: Application of the microtiter complement fixation technique to studies of hepatitis-associated antigen in human hepatitis. Vox Sang., 19:211, 1970.

Benacerraf, B.: Role of major histocompatibility complex in genetic regulation of immunologic responsiveness. Transplant. Proc., 9:825, 1977.

Bier, O. G., Leyton, G., Mayer, M. M., and Heidelberger, M.: A comparison of human and guinea-pig complements and their component fractions. J. Exp. Med., 81:445, 1945.

Billingham, R. E., Brent, L., and Medawar, P. B.: "Actively acquired tolerance" of foreign cells. Nature, 172:603, 1953.

Bitter-Suerman, D., Dierich, M., Konig, W., and Hadding, U.: Bypass-activation of the complement system starting with C3. Immunology, 57:267, 1972.

Blount, J. H., and Holmes, K. K.: Epidemiology of syphilis and the non-venereal treponematoses. In Johnson, R. C. (Ed.): The Biology of Parasitic Spirochetes. New York, Academic Press, 1975.

Blum, H. E., and Vyas, G. N.: Non-A, non-B hepatitis: a contemporary assessment. Haematologia, 15:162, 1982.

Blumberg, B. S., Alter, H. J., and Visnich, S.: A new antigen in leukemia sera. JAMA, 191:541, 1965.

Blumberg, B. S., Sutnick, A. I., and London, W. T.: Hepatitis and leukemia: their relation to Australia antigen. Bull N.Y. Acad. Med., 44:1566, 1968.

Borsos, T., Circolo, A., and Ejzemberg, R.: Lack of C4 binding by human IgM during activation of the classical pathway. Key Biscayne, Florida, 9th International Complement Workshop, 1981.

Brown, D. L., and Cooper, A. G.: The in vivo metabolism of radioiodinated cold agglutinins of anti-I specificity. Clin. Sci., 38:175, 1970.

Burnet, F. M., and Fenner, F.: The Production of Antibodies. London, Macmillan, 1941.

Busey, J. F., and Hinton, P. F.: Precipitins in blastomycosis. Am. Rev. Respir. Dis., 95:112, 1967.

Cantor, H., and Boyse, E. A.: Regulation of the immune response by T-cell subclasses. Contemp. Top. Immunobiol., 4:47, 1977.

Capra, J. D., Dowling, P. M., Cook, S., and Kunkel, H. G.: An incomplete cold-reactive γG antibody with i specificity in infectious mononucleosis. Vox Sang., 16:10, 1969.

Caputo, M. J.: Hyland Technical Discussion No. 27. Costa Mesa, CA, Hyland Laboratories.

Carlisle, H. N., and Saslaw, S.: A histoplasmin latex agglutination test. J. Lab. Clin. Med., 51:793, 1958.

Carpenter, K. P., and Lachowicz, K.: The catalase activity of *Sh. flexneri*. J. Pathol. Bact., 77:645, 1959.

Carpenter, P. L.: Immunology and Serology, 3rd ed. Philadelphia, W. B. Saunders Company, 1975.

Cayzer, I., Dane, D. S., Cameron, C. H., and Denning, J. V.: A rapid haemagglutination test for hepatitis B antigen. Lancet, 1:947, 1974.

Chaplin, H. (1980): Personal communication *cited by* Mollison, P. L.: Blood Transfusion in Clinical Medicine. Oxford, Blackwell Scientific Publications, 1983.

Chew, W. H., and Theus, T. L.: Candida precipitins. J. Immunol., 98:220, 1967.

Chrystie, I. L., Islam, M. N., Banatvala, J. E., and Cayzer, I.: Clinical evaluation of the turkey-erythrocyte passive-haemagglutination test for hepatitis B surface antigen. Lancet, 1:1193, 1974.

Cohen, S., and Freeman, T.: Metabolic heterogeneity of human γ-globulin. Biochem. J., 76:475, 1960.

Cole, J. R., Sulzer, C. R., and Pursell, A. R.: Improved microtechnique for the leptospiral microscopic agglutination test. Appl. Microbiol., 25:976, 1973.

Coons, A. H.: Histochemistry with labeled antibody. Int. Rev. Cytol., 5:1, 1956.

Coons, A. H.: Fluorescent antibody methods. *In* Danielli, J. F. (Ed.): General Cytochemical Methods, Vol. 1. New York, Academic Press 1958, pp. 400–422.

Coons, A. H.: The beginnings of immunofluorescence. J. Immunol., 87:499, 1961.

Corbel, M. J., and Cullen, G. A.: Differentiation of the serologic response to *Yersinia enterocolitica* and *Brucella abortus* in cattle. J. Hyg. (Camb.), 68:519, 1970.

Costea, N., Yakulis, V. J., and Heller, P.: Inhibition of cold agglutinins (anti-I) by *M. pneumoniae* antigens. Proc. Soc. Exp. Biol. (N.Y.), 139:476, 1972.

CR Test, Package Insert, Deerfield, IL, Hyland Laboratories, 1979.

Crockson, R. A., Payne, C. J., Ratcliff, A. P., and Soothill, J. F.: Time sequence of acute phase reactive proteins following surgical trauma. Clin. Chim. Acta, 14:435, 1966.

Csonka, G. W.: "Bejel": childhood treponematosis. Med. Illus. (Lond.), 6:401, 1952.

Dacie, J. V.: The Haemolytic Anaemias, 2nd ed. London, J. and A. Churchill Ltd., 1962.

Damp, S. C., Crumrine, M. H., and Lewis, G. E.: Microtiter plate agglutination test for *Brucella canis* antibodies. Appl. Microbiol., 25:489, 1973.

Daniels, J. C., Larson, D. L., Abston, S., and Ritzmann, S. E.: Serum protein profiles in thermal burns. J. Trauma, 14:153, 1974.

Das, P. C., Hopkins, R., Cash, J. D., and Cumming, R. A.: Rapid identification of hepatitis-associated antigen and antibody by counter-immunoelectro-osmophoresis. Br. J. Haematol., 21:673, 1971.

Davidson, I.: Serologic diagnosis of infectious mononucleosis. JAMA, 108:289, 1937.

Dawson, S. F.: The significance of the c-reactive protein estimation in streptococcal and allied diseases. Arch. Dis. Child., 32:454, 1957.

Day, N. K., Geiger, H., McLean, R., Michael, A., and Good, R. A.: C2 deficiency: development of lupus erythematosus. J. Clin. Invest., 52:1601, 1973.

Delaat, A. N. C.: The complement fixation test in virus antibody studies. Can. J. Med. Technol., 26:35, 1964.

Dienhardt, F., Holmes, A. W., Capps, R. B., and Popper, H.: Studies on the transmission of human viral hepatitis to marmoset monkeys. J. Exp. Med., 125:673, 1967.

Dienstag, J. L., Feinstone, S. M., Purcell, R. H., Hoofnagle, J. H., Barker, L. E., London, W. T., Popper, H., Peterson, J. M., and Kapikian, A. Z.: Experimental infection of chimpanzees with hepatitis A virus. J. Infect. Dis., 132:532, 1975.

Dixon, R., Rosse, W., and Ebbert, L.: Quantitative determination of antibody in idiopathic thrombocytopenic purpura. N. Engl. J. Med., 292:230, 1975.

Drake, M. E., Hampil, B., Pennell, R. B., Spizizen, J., Henle, W., and Stokes, J.: Effect of nitrogen mustard on virus on serum hepatitis in whole blood. Proc. Soc. Exp. Biol. (N.Y.), 80:310, 1952.

Dreesman, G. R., Hollinger, F. B., and Melnick, J. L.: Detection of hepatitis B antigen by counter-immunoelectrophoresis: enhancing role of homologous serum diluents. Appl. Microbiol., 24:1001, 1972.

Dubois, E., Drexler, E., and Arteberry, J. D.: A latex nucleoprotein test for diagnosis of systemic lupus erythematosus. JAMA, 117:141, 1961.

Dulbecco, R.: Production of plaques in monolayer tissue culture by particles of an animal virus. Proc. Natl. Acad. Sci. U.S.A., 38:747, 1952.

Edelman, G. M.: Antibody structure and molecular immunology. *In* Kochwa, S., and Kunkel, H. G. (Eds.): Immunoglobulins. Ann. N.Y. Acad. Sci., 190:5, 1971.

Edwards, E. A., and Larson, G. L.: Serologic grouping of hemolytic streptococci by counter-immunoelectrophoresis. Appl. Microbiol., 25:1006, 1973.

Edwards, P. R., and Ewing, W. H.: Identification of Enterobacteriaceae, 2nd ed. Minneapolis, Burgess Publishing Co., 1972.

Elek, S. D.: Recognition of toxicogenic bacterial strains *in vitro*. Br. Med. J., 1:493, 1948.

Ewing, W. H.: Shigella nomenclature. J. Bacteriol., 57:633, 1949.

Ewing, W. H., and Davis, B. R.: The O antigen groups of *Escherichia coli*. Cultures from various sources. Atlanta, GA, Center for Disease Control, U.S. Department of Health Education and Welfare, 1961.

Ewing, W. H., and Johnson, J. G.: Intersubgroup and intrasubgroup antigenic relationships within genus Shigella: subgroup A. Can. J. Microbiol., 7:303, 1961.

Ewing, W. H., Tanner, K. E., and Tatum, H. W.: Investigation of *Escherichia coli* O Group, 18 Serotypes isolated from cases of infantile diarrhea. Public Health Lab., 14:106, 1956.

Feinstone, S. M., Kapikian, A. Z., and Purcell, R. H.: Hepatitis A. Detection by immune electronmicroscopy of a viruslike antigen associated with acute illness. Science, 182:1026, 1973.

Fiedel, B., and Gewurz, H.: Inhibition of platelet aggregation by C-reactive protein. Fed. Proc. (Abstr.), 34:854, 1975.

Fishel, E. E.: Laboratory diagnostic procedures. *In* Cohen, A. S. (ed.): Rheumatic Diseases. Boston, Little, Brown and Co., 1967, pp. 70–83.

Fisher, C. L., Gill, C., Forrester, M. G., and Nakamura, R.: Quantitation of acute phase proteins postoperatively. Am. J. Clin. Pathol., 66:840, 1976.

Forssman, J.: Die Herstellung hochwertiger specifischer Schafhamolysine ohne Verwendung von Schafblut. Ein Beitrag zur Lehre von heterologer Anti-Korperbildung. Biochem. Z., 37:78, 1911.

Franklin, E. C., and Kinkel, H. G.: Comparative levels of high molecular weight (19S) gamma globulin in maternal and umbilical cord sera. J. Lab. Clin. Med., 52:724, 1958.

Fritz, R. B., and Rivers, S. L.: Hepatitis-associated antigen: detection by antibody-sensitized latex particles. J. Immunol., 108:108, 1972.

Fudenberg, H. H., Stites, D. P., Caldwell, J. L., and Wells, J. V.: Basic and Clinical Immunology. Los Altos, CA, Lange Medical Publications, 1976

Gal, K., and Miltenyi, M.: Hemagglutination test for the demonstration of CRP. Acta Microbiol. Acad. Sci. Hung., 3:41, 1955.

Garner, M. F., and Clark, M. E.: The *Treponema pallidum* hemagglutination (TPHA) test. WHO/VDT/RES/,75:332, 1975.

Georg, L. K., Coleman, R. M., and Brown, J. M.: Evaluation of an agar gel precipitin test for the serodiagnosis of actinomycosis. J. Immunol., 100:1288, 1968.

Gershon, R. K.: Immunoregulations by T cells. Miami Winter Symposium, 9:267, 1975.

Gocke, D. J., and Howe, C.: Rapid detection of Australian antigen by counter-immunoelectrophoresis. J. Immunol., 104:1031, 1970.

Goers, J. W. F., and Porter, R. R.: The assembly of early components of complement on antibody-antigen aggregates and on antibody-coated erythrocytes. Biochem. J., 175:675, 1978.

Goldberg, L. S., and Barnett, E. V.: Mixed γG-γM cold agglutinin. J. Immunol., 99:803, 1967.

Goldstein, A. L., Thurman, G. B., Cohen, G. H., and Hooper, J. A.: The role of thymosin and the endocrine thymus on the ontogenesis and function of T cells. Miami Winter Symposium, 9:423, 1975.

Gotschlich, E. C., and Edelman, G. M.: C-reactive protein: a molecule composed of subunits. Proc. Natl. Acad. Sci. U.S.A., 54:558, 1965.

Gotschlich, E. C., and Edelman, G. M.: Binding properties and specificity of C-reactive protein. Proc. Natl. Acad. Sci. U.S.A., 57:706, 1967.

Grady, G. F., and Lee, V. A.: Prevention of hepatitis from accidental exposure among the medical workers. N. Engl. J. Med., 293:1067, 1975.

Gray, D. F.: Immunology. American Elsevier Publishing Co., 1970.

Guerrant, R. L., and Dickens, M. D.: Toxigenic bacterial diarrhea: a nursery outbreak involving multiple strains. Fourteenth Interscience Conference on Antimicrobial Agents and Chemotherapy. Abstr., 130, 1974.

Hanshaw, J. B.: Congenital cytomegalic infection: laboratory methods of detection. J. Pediatr., 75:1179, 1969.

Harrington, W. J., Minnich, V., Hollingsworth, J. W., and Moore, C. V.: Demonstration of a thrombocytopenic factor in the blood of patients with thrombocytopenic purpura. J. Lab. Clin. Med., 38:1, 1951.

Harrison, R. A., and Lachmann, P. J.: The physiologic breakdown of the third component of human complement. Mol. Immunol., 17:9, 1980.

Hayashi, H., and LoGrippo, G. A.: C-reactive protein—potential significance of quantitation in patients with chronic diseases. Henry Ford Hosp. Med. J., 20:91, 1972.

Hazen, E. L., Gordon, M. A., and Reed, F. C.: Laboratory Identification of Pathogenic Fungi Simplified, 2nd ed. Springfield, IL, Charles C Thomas, 1970.

Hedge, U. M., Powell, D. K., Bowes, A., and Gordon-Smith, E. C.: Enzyme-linked immunoassay for the detection of platelet associated IgG. Br. J. Haematol., 48:39, 1981.

Heidelberger, M., and Mayer, M. M.: Quantitative studies on complement. Adv. Enzymol., 8:71, 1948.

Hirata, A. A., Emerick, A. J., and Boley, W. F.: Hepatitis B virus antigen detection by reverse passive haemagglutination. Proc. Soc. Exp. Biol. Med., 143:761, 1973.

Hirst, G. K.: The quantitative determination of influenza virus and antibodies by means of red cell agglutination. J. Exp. Med., 75:49, 1942.

Holland, P. V., Bancroft, W., and Zimmerman, H.: Post-transfusion viral hepatitis and the TTVS. N. Engl. J. Med., 304:1033, 1981.

Hoofnagle, J. H., Seeff, L. B., Bales, Z. B., and Zimmerman, H. J.: Type B hepatitis after transfusion with blood-containing antibody to hepatitis B core antigen. N. Engl. J. Med., 298:1379, 1978.

Hopkins, R., and Das, P. C.: A tanned cell haemagglutination test for the detection of hepatitis-associated-antigen (Au-Ag) and antibody (Anti-Au). Br. J. Haematol., 25:619, 1973.

Hudson, E. H.: Non-Venereal Syphilis. Edinburgh, E and S. Livingstone, 1958, p. 189.

Hudson, E. H.: Treponematosis and anthropology. Ann. Intern. Med., 58:1037, 1963.

Hughes-Jones, N. C.: Nature of the reaction between antigen and antibody. Br. Med. Bull., 19:171, 1963.

Humphrey, J. H., and Dourmashkin, R. R.: Electron microscope studies of immune cell lysis. *In* Wolstenholme, G. E. W., and Knight, J. (Eds.): Ciba Found. Symp. Complement, London, J. & A. Churchill, 1965.

Humphrey, J. H., and Dourmashkin, R. R.: The lesions in cell membranes caused by complement. Adv. Immunol., 11:75, 1969.

Hunder, G. G., McDuffie, F. C., and Mullen, B. J.: Activation of C3 and factor B in synovial fluids. J. Lab. Clin. Med., 89:160, 1977.

Hunter, E. F., Deacon, W. E., and Meyer, P. C.: An improved test for syphilis—the absorption procedure (FTA-ABS). Public Health Rep., 79:5, 1964.

Huppert, M., and Bailey, J. W.: The use of immunodiffusion tests in coccidioidomycosis. Tech. Bull. Reg. Med. Technol., 35:155, 1965.

Hymes, K., Shulman, S., and Karpatkin, S.: A solid-phase radioimmunoassay for bound anti-platelet antibody. Studies on 45 patients with autoimmune platelet disorders. J. Lab. Clin. Med., 94:639, 1979.

Iwakata, S., Rhodes, A. J., and Labzoffsky, N. S.: The significance of specific IgM antibody in the diagnosis of rubella employing the immunofluorescence technique. Can. Med. Assoc. J., 106:327, 1972.

Jambazian, A., and Holper, J. C.: Rheophoresis: a sensitive immunodiffusion method for detection of hepatitis associated antigen. Proc. Soc. Exp. Biol. Med., 140:560, 1972.

Janney, F. A., Lee, L. T., and Howe, C.: Cold hemagglutinin cross-reactivity with *Mycoplasma pneumoniae*. Infect. Immun., 22:29, 1978.

Jawetz, E., Melnick, J., and Adelberg, E. A.: Review of Medical Microbiology. Los Altos, CA, Lange Medical Publications, 1974.

Jenkins, W. J., Koster, H. G., Marsh, W. L., and Carter, R. L.: Infectious mononucleosis: an unsuspected source of anti-i. Br. J. Haematol., 11:480, 1965.

Jerry, L. M., Kunkel, H. G., and Grey, H. M.: Absence of disuseful bonds linking the heavy and light chains: a property of a genetic variant of γA2 globulins. Proc. Natl. Acad. Sci. U.S.A., 65:557, 1970.

Jodal, U., and Hanson, L. A.: Sequential determination of C-reactive protein in acute childhood pyelonephritis. Acta Pediatr. Scand., 65:319, 1976.

Johannson, B. C., Kindermark, C. O., Treil, E. Y., and Wollheim, F. A.: Sequential changes of plasma proteins after myocardial infarction. Scand. J. Clin. Lab. Invest., 124(Suppl. 29):117, 1972.

Joklik, W. K., *et al.* (Ed.): Zinsser Microbiology, 15th ed. Norwalk, CT, Appleton-Century-Crofts, 1972.

Juji, T., and Yokochi, T.: Haemagglutination technique with erythrocytes coated with specific antibody for detection of Australian antigen. Jpn, J. Exp. Med., *39*:615, 1969.

Kaplan, M. H., and Volanakis, J. E.: Interaction of C-reactive protein with the complement system. I. Consumption of human complement associated with the reaction of C-reactive protein with pneumococcal C-polysaccharide and with the choline phosphatides, lecithin and sphingomyelin. J. Immunol., *112*:2135, 1974.

Kauffmann, F.: Enterobacteriaceae, 3rd ed. Baltimore, The Williams & Wilkins Co., 1965.

Kauffmann, L.: The use of immunodiffusion for the detection of histoplasmin antibodies. Public Health Rep., *81*:177, 1966.

Kenyon, R. H., and McManus, A. T.: Rickettsial infectious antibody complexes: detection by antiglobulin plaque reduction technique. Infect. Immun., *9*:966, 1974.

Kindermard, C. O.: Stimulating effect of c-reactive protein on phagocytosis of various species of pathogenic bacteria. Clin. Exp. Immunol., *8*:941, 1971.

Kroop, I. G., and Shackman, N. H.: Levels of c-reactive protein as a measure of acute myocardial infarction. Proc. Soc. Exp. Biol. Med., *86*:96, 1954.

Kunkel, H. G., and Prendegast, R. A.: Subgroups of gamma-A immune globulins. Proc. Soc. Exp. Biol. Med., *122*:910, 1966.

Kushner, I., and Feldmann, G.: Demonstration of c-reactive protein synthesis and secretion by hepatocytes during acute inflammation in the rabbit. J. Exp. Med., *148*:466, 1978.

Lachmann, P. J., and Pangburn, M. K.: The breakdown of C3bi to C3c, C3d, and C3e. IXth International Complement Workshop, Key Biscayne, Florida, 1981.

Lancefield, R. C.: A serologic differentiation of human and other groups of hemolytic streptococci. J. Exp. Med., *57*:571, 1933.

Lancefield, R. C.: Current knowledge of type-specific M antigens of group A streptococci. J. Immunol., *89*:307, 1962.

Landsteiner, K.: Über Beziehungen zwischen dum Blutserum und den Korperzellen. Münch. med. Wschr., *50*:1812, 1903.

Landsteiner, K., and Levine, P.: On the cold agglutinins in human serum. J. Immunol., *12*:441, 1926.

Lawton-Smith, J., David, N. J., Indgin, S., Israel, E. W., Levine, B. M., Justice, J., Jr., McCrary, J. A., III, Mendina, R., Paez, P., Santana, E., Sarkar, M., Schatz, N. J., Spitzer, M. L., Spitzer, W. O., and Walter, E. K.: Neuro-ophthalmologic study of late yaws and pinta. II. The Caracas Project. Br. J. Vener. Dis., *47*:226, 1971.

Leach, J. M., and Ruck, B. J.: Detection of hepatitis-associated antigen by the latex agglutination test. Br. Med. J., *4*:597, 1971.

LeBouvier, G. L.: The heterogeneity of Australia antigen. J. Infect. Dis., *123*:671, 1971.

Lee, C. L., Davidson, I., and Panczyszyn, O.: Horse agglutinins in infectious mononucleosis. Am. J. Clin. Pathol., *49*:3, 1968.

Lennette, E. H., and Schmidt, N. J.: Diagnostic Procedures for Viral and Rickettsial Diseases, 4th ed. New York, American Public Health Association, 1969.

Lofstrom, G.: Comparison between the reactions of acute phase serum with pneumococcus C-polysaccharide and with pneumococcus type 27. Br. J. Exp. Pathol., *25*:21, 1944.

Longbottom, J. L., and Pepys, L.: Pulmonary aspergillosis: diagnostic and immunologic significance of antigens and C-substance in *Aspergillus fumigatus.* J. Pathol. Bacteriol., *84*:141, 1964.

Louria, D. B., Smith, J. K., Brayton, R. G., and Buse, M.: Anti-*Candida* factors in serum and their inhibitors. J. Infect. Dis., *125*:102, 1972.

Luoto, L.: A capillary agglutination test for bovine Q fever. J. Immunol., *71*:222, 1953.

MacLeod, C. M., and Avery, O. T.: The occurrence during acute infections of a protein not normally present in the blood. III. Immunologic properties of the C-reactive protein and its differentiation from normal blood proteins. J. Exp. Med., *73*:191, 1941.

Malin, S. F., and Edwards, J. R.: Detection of hepatitis-associated antigen by latex agglutination. Nature (New Biol)., *235*:182, 1972.

Mancini, G., Carbonara, A. O., and Heremans, J. T.: Immunochemical quantitation of antigens by single radial immunodiffusion. Int. J. Immunochem., *2*:235, 1965.

Maniar, A. C., and Fox, J. G.: Techniques of an *in vitro* method for determining toxigenicity of *Corynebacterium diphtheriae* strains. Can. J. Pub. Health., *59*:297, 1968.

March, R. W., Stiles, G. E., and Forgione, P. S.: *In* Abstracts of Annual Meeting of American Society for Microbiology, 1974, p. 73.

Marrack, J. R.: The Chemistry of Antigens and Antibodies. London, Medical Research Council, Special Report Series. No. 194, 1938.

Martensson, L., and Fudenberg, H. H.: Gm genes and γG-globulin synthesis in the human fetus. J. Immunol., *94*:514, 1965.

Mata, L. J.: The agar cell culture precipitation test: its application to the study of vaccinia virus, adenoviruses, and herpes simplex virus. J. Immunol., *91*:151, 1963.

McCarthy, P. L., Frank, A. L., Ablow, R. C., Masters, S. T., and Dolan, T. F.: Value of C-reactive protein in the differentiation of bacterial and viral pneumonia. J. Pediatr., *92*:454, 1978.

McGrew, B. E., DuCros, M. J. F., Stout, G. W., and Falcone, V. H.: Automation of a flocculation test for syphilis. Am. J. Clin. Pathol., *50*:52, 1968.

Michael, A., and McLean, R.: Evidence for activation of the alternate pathway in glomerulonephritis. Adv. Nephrol., *4*:49, 1974.

Michaelsen, T. E., Frangione, B., and Franklin, E. C.: Primary structure of the "hinge" region of human IgG3. J. Biol. Chem., *252*:883, 1977.

Miller, L. H., Mason, S. J., Clyde, D. F., and McGinniss, M. H.: The resistance factor to *Plasmodium vivax* in blacks. The Duffy blood group geotype *FyFy*. N. Engl. J. Med., *295*:302, 1976.

Miller, L. H., Mason, S. J., Dvorak, J. A., McGinniss, M. H., and Rothman, I. K.: Erythrocyte reception for *(Plasmodium knowlesi)* malaria: The Duffy blood group determinants. Science, *189*:561, 1975.

Miller, M. E., and Nilsson, U. R.: A familial deficiency of the phagocytosis-enhancing activity of serum related to a dysfunction of the fifth component of complement (C5). N. Engl. J. Med., *282*:354, 1970.

Miller, W. J., *et al.:* Specific immune adherence assay for human hepatitis A antibody. Application to diagnostic and epidemiologic investigations. Proc. Soc. Exp. Biol. Med., *149*:254, 1975.

Moore, B. P. L., and Maede, D.: Counter-immunoelectrophoresis for detection of hepatitis by antigen and antibody: a technique for large-scale use. Can. J. Public health, *63*:453, 1972.

Morell, A., Skvaril, F., Van Loghem, E., and Kleemola, M.: Human IgG subclasses in maternal and fetal serum. Vox Sang., *21*:481, 1971.

Mortensen, R. F., Osmand, A. P., and Gerwurz, H.: Effects of C-reactive protein on the lymphoid system. I. Binding to thymus-dependent lymphocytes and alteration of their function. J. Exp. Med., *141*:821, 1975.

Mueller-Eckhardt, C., Kayser, W., Mersh-Baumert, K., Mueller-Eckhardt, G., Breidenbach, M., Kugel, H.-G., and Graubner, M.: The clinical significance of platelet-associated IgG: a study of 298 patients with various disorders. Br. J. Haematol., *46*:123, 1980.

Mueller-Eckhardt, C., Schulz, G., Sauer, K.-H., Dienst, C., and Mahn, I.: Studies on the platelet radioactive anti-immunoglobulin test. J. Immunol., Methods, *91*:1, 1978.

Murray, R.: Viral hepatitis. Bull. N.Y. Acad. Med., *31*:341, 1955.

Nagasawa, S., Ichihara, C., and Stroud, R. M.: Cleavage of C4b and C3b inactivator: production of a nicked form of C4b.C4b′ as an intermediate cleavage product of C4b by C3b inactivator. J. Immunol., *125*:578, 1980.

Nahmias, A., Delbuono, I., Pipkin, J., Hutton, R., and Wickliffe, C.: Rapid identification and typing of *Herpes simplex* virus types 1 and 2 by direct immunofluorescence technique. Appl. Microbiol., *22*:455, 1971.

Nel, J. D., and Stevens, K.: A new method for the simultaneous quantitation of platelet-bound immunoglobulin (IgG) and complement (C₃) employing an enzme-linked immunosorbent assay (ELISA) procedure. Br. J. Haematol., *44*:281, 1980.

Nelson, R. A.: Factors affecting survival of *Treponema pallidum in vitro*. Am. J. Hyg., *48*:120, 1948.

Nelson, R. A., and Mayer, M. M.: Immobilization of *Treponema pallidum in vitro* by antibody produced in syphilitic infection. J. Exp. Med., *89*:369, 1949.

Nisonoff, A., Hopper, J. E., and Spring, S. B.: The Antibody Molecule. New York, Academic Press, 1975.

Noto, T. A., and Miale, J. B.: New immunologic test for pregnancy. Am. J. Clin. Pathol., *41*:273, 1964.

Orskov, F., Orskov, I., Evans, D. J., Jr., Sack, R. B., Sack, D. A., and Wadstrom, T.: Special *Escherichia coli* stereotypes among enteropathogenic strains from diarrhea in adults and children. Med. Microbiol. Immunol., *162*:73, 1976.

Oveinnikov, N. M., and Delektorskij, V. V.: Morphology of *Treponema pallidum*. Bull. WHO, *35*:223, 1966.

Oveinnikov, N. M., and Delektorskij, V. V.: Further study of ultra-thin sections of *Treponema pallidum* under the electron microscope. Br. J. Vener. Dis., *44*:1, 1968.

Overby, L. R., Miller, J. P., Smith, I. D., Decker, R. H., and Ling, C. M.: Radioimmunoassay of hepatitis B virus–associated (Australia) antigen employing ^{125}I-antibody. Vox sang. Suppl., *24*:102, 1973.

Owen, R. D.: Immunogenetic consequences of vascular anastomoses between bovine twins. Science, *102*:400, 1945.

Palmer, D. F., and Woods, R.: Qualitation and quantitation of immunoglobulins. Immunology Series No. 3. Atlanta, GA. Center for Disease Control, U.S. Department of Health, Education, and Welfare, 1972.

Paul, J. R., and Bunnell, W. W.: The presence of heterophile antibodies in infectious mononucleosis. Am. J. Med. Sci., *183*:90, 1932.

Pepys, M. B., Druguet, M., Klass, H. J., *et al.*: Ciba Foundation Symposium 46. Immunology of the Gut, pp 283. Amsterdam, Elsevier, Excerpta Medica, North Holland, 1977.

Perlmann, P.: Cellular immunity: antibody dependent entotoxicity (K-cell activity). Clin. Immunobiol., *3*:107, 1976.

Pirofsky, B.: Autoimmunization and the Autoimmune Hemolytic Anemias. Baltimore, The Williams & Wilkins Company, 1969.

Polley, M. J., Mollison, P. L., and Soothill, J. F.: The role of 19S gamma globulin blood antibodies in the antiglobulin reaction. Br. J. Haematol., *8*:149, 1962.

Portnoy, J.: Modifications of the rapid plasma reagin (RPR) card test for syphilis for use in large scale testing. Am. J. Clin. Pathol., *40*:473, 1963.

Portnoy, J., Carson, W., and Smith, C. A.: Rapid plasma reagin test for syphilis. Public Health Rep., *72*:761, 1957.

Portnoy, J., and Carson, W.: New and improved antigen suspension for rapid reagin test for syphilis. Public Health Rep., *75*:985, 1960.

Prince, A. M.: An antigen detected in blood during the incubation period of serum hepatitis. Proc. Natl. Acad. Sci. U.S.A., *60*:814, 1968.

Purcell, R. H., Holland, P. V., Walsh, J. H., Wong, D. C., Morrow, A. G., and Chanock, R. M.: A complement-fixation test for measuring Australian antigen and antibody. J. Infect. Dis., *120*:383, 1969.

Quevillon, M., and Chagnon, A.: Microtissue culture test for the titration of low concentrations of diphtheria antitoxin in minimal amounts of human sera. Appl. Microbiol., *25*:1, 1973.

Rapp, J. H., and Borsos, T.: Molecular Basis of Complement Action. Norwalk, CT, Appleton-Century-Crofts, 1970.

Rawston, J. R., and Farthing, C. P.: A comparison of tests for thyroglobulin antibody. J. Clin. Pathol., *15*:153, 1962.

Rosenbaum, M. J., Phillips, I. A., Sullivan, E. J., Edwards, E. A., and Miller, L. F.: A simplified method for virus-antigen culture procedures in microtitration plates. Proc. Soc. Exp. Biol. Med., *113*:224, 1963.

Rosenfield, R. E., Schmidt, P. J., Calvo, R. C., and McGinniss, M. H.: Anti-i, a frequent cold agglutinin in infectious mononucleosis. Vox Sang., *10*:631, 1965.

Rosse, W. F., Adams, J. P., and Yount, W. J.: Subclasses of IgG antibodies in immune thrombocytopenic purpura (ITP). Br. J. Haematol., *46*:109, 1980.

Rosse, W. F., and Dacie, J. V.: Immune lysis of normal human and paroxysmal nocturnal hemoglobinuria (PNH) red blood cells. II. The role of complement components in the increased sensitivity of PNH red cells to immune lysis. J. Clin. Invest., *45*:749, 1966.

Rosse, W. F., Dourmashkin, R., and Humphrey, J. H.: Immune lysis of normal human and paroxysmal nocturnal hemoglobinuria (PHN) red blood cells. III. The membrane defects caused by complement lysis. J. Exp. Med., *123*:969, 1966.

Rowe, B., Scotland, S. N., and Gross, R. J.: Enterotoxigenic *Escherichia coli* causing infantile enteritis in Britain. Lancet, *1*:90, 1977.

Sack, R. B.: Serotyping of *E. coli*. Lancet, 1:1132, 1976.

Sack, R. B., Hirschhorn, N., Brownlee, I., Cash, R. A., Woodward, W. E., and Sack, D. A.: Enterotoxigenic *Escherichia coli*–associated diarrheal disease in Apache children. N. Engl. J. Med., *292*:1041, 1975.

Sakazaki, R., Tamura, K., and Saito, M.: Enteropathogenic *Escherichia coli*: associated with diarrhea in children and adults. Jpn. J. Med. Sci. Biol., *20*:387, 1967.

Salk, J. E., Younger, J. S., and Ward, W. N.: Use of color change of phenol red as the indicator in titrating poliomyelitis virus or its antibody in a tissue culture system. Am. J. Hyg., *60*:214, 1954.

Sandoval, O.: Unpublished observations. Cited by Deodhar, S. D., and Valenzuela, R.: C-reactive protein: new findings and specific applications. Lab. Manag. 19(6): 1981.

Scaletter, R., *et al.*: A nucleoprotein complement fixation test in the diagnosis of systemic lupus erythematosus. N. Engl. J. Med., *263*:226, 1960.

Schmidt, N. J., and Lennette, E. H.: Sensitivity of a 1-day complement fixation test for detection of hepatitis-associated antigen. Health Lab. Sci., *8*:238, 1971.

Schubert, J. H., and Hampson, H. C.: An appraisal of serologic tests for coccidioidomycosis. Am. J. Hyg., *76*:144, 1962.

Schultze, H. E., and Heremans, J. F.: Molecular Biology of Human Proteins with Special Reference to Plasma Proteins, Vol. 1, Elsevier, Amsterdam, 1966.

Seeff, L. B., *et al.*: A randomized, double-blind controlled trial of the efficacy of immune serum globulin for the prevention of post-transfusion hepatitis. Gastroenterology, *72*:111, 1977.

Sever, J. L.: Application of a micro-technique to viral serologic investigations. J. Immunol., *88*:320, 1962.

Shiga, K.: Ueber den dysenteriebacillus *(Bacillus dysenteriae)*. Zentralbl. Bakteriol., *24*:817, 913, 1898.

Siegel, J., Rent, R., and Gewurz, H.: Interactions of C-reactive protein with the complement system. I. Protamine-induced consumption of complement in acute phase sera. J. Exp. Med., *140*:631, 1974.

Sim, E., Wood, A. B., Hsiung, L. M., and Sim, R. B.: Pattern of degradation of human complement fragment. C3b. FEBS Letters, *132*:55, 1981.

Smith, S. J., Bos, G., Esseveld, M. R., Van Eijk, H. G., and Gerbrandy, J.: Acute phase proteins from the liver and enzymes from myocardial infarction. Clin. Chim. Acta, *81*:75, 1977.

Soulier, J. P., Patereau, C., and Drouet, J.: Platelet indirect radioactive Coombs' test. Its utilization for P1^A1 grouping. Vox Sang., *29*:253, 1975.

Sternberger, L. A.: *In* Osler, A., and Weiss, L.: Immunocytochemistry. Englewood Cliffs, NJ, Prentice-Hall, Inc., 1974.

Sulzer, C. R., and Jones, W. L.: Evaluation of hemagglutination test for human leptospirosis. Appl. Microbiol., *26*:655, 1973.

Szmuness, W., Stevens, C. E., Harley, E. J., Edith, A., Oleszko, W. R., William, D. C., Sadovsky, R., Morrison, J. M., and Kellner, A.: Hepatitis B vaccine: demonstration of efficacy in a controlled clinical trial in a high-risk population in the United States. N. Engl. J. Med., *303*:833, 1980.

Tabor, E., *et al.*: Experimental transmission and passage of human non-A, non-B hepatitis in chimpanzees. *In* Vyas, G., Cohen, S., and Schmid, R. (Eds.): Viral Hepatitis. Philadelpia, Franklin Institutes Press, 1978, p. 419.

Tanowitz, H. B., Robbins, N., and Leidich, N.: Hemolytic anemia: associated with severe mycoplasma pneumoniae. N.Y. State J. Med., *78*:2231, 1978.

Tenveen, J. H., and Feltkamp, T. E. W.: Formalized chicken red cell nuclei as a simple antigen for standardized antinuclear factor determination. Clin. Exp. Immunol., *5*:673, 1969.

Tillet, W. S., and Francis, T., Jr.: Serologic reactions in pneumonia with a non-protein somatic fraction of pneumococcus. J. Exp. Med., *52*:561, 1930.

Tomasi, T. B., Jr., Tan, E. M., Solomon, A., and Prendergast, R. A.: Characteristics of an immune system common to certain external secretions. J. Exp. Med., *121*:101, 1965.

Troxel, D. B., Innella, F., and Cohren, R. J.: Infectious mononucleosis complicated by hemolytic anemia due to anti-i. Am. J. Clin. Pathol., *46*:625, 1966.

Vaerman, J. P., and Heremans, J. F.: Antigenic heterogenicity of human immunoglobulin A proteins. Science, *153*:647, 1966.

Venezia, R. A., and Robertson, R. G.: Efficacy of the Candida precipitin test. Am. J. Clin. Pathol., *61*:849, 1974.

Volankis, J., Clements, W., and Schohenloher, R.: C-reactive protein physical, chemical characterization. J. Immunol. Methods, *23*:285, 1978.

Von Dem Borne, A. E. G. KR., Verheught, F. W. A., Oosterhof, F., Von Riesz, E., De La Riviere, A. B., and Engelfriet, C. P.: A simple immunofluorescence test for the detection of platelet antibodies. Br. J. Haematol., *39*:195, 1978.

Wallace, A. L., and Harris, A.: Reiter treponema. Bull. WHO, *36*:Suppl. 2, 1967.

Walsh, L., Davies, P., and McConkey, B.: Relationship between erythrocyte sedimentation rate and serum C-reactive protein in rheumatoid arthritis. Ann. Rheumatol. Dis., *38*:362, 1979.

Wara, D. W., Reiter, E. O., and Doyle, N. E.: Persistent Clq deficiency in a patient with a systemic lupus-like syndrome. J. Pediatr., *86*:743, 1975.

Wassermann, A., Neisser, A., and Bruck, C.: Eine serodiagnostische Reaktion bei Syphilis. Deutsch. Med Wschr., *32*:745, 1906.

Weil, E., and Felix, A.: Zür serologischen diagnose des Fleckfiebers. Wien. Klin. Wochenschr., *29*:33, 1916.

Welsh, R. D., and Dolan, C. T.: Sporothrix whole yeast agglutination test: low-titer reactions of sera of subjects not known to have sporotrichosis. Am. J. Clin. Pathol., *59*:82, 1973.

West, C. D., Hong, R., and Holland, N. H.: Immunoglobulin levels from the newborn period to adulthood and in immunoglobulin deficiency states. J. Clin. Invest., *41*:2054, 1962.

WHO: Advances in viral hepatitis. Technical Report Series, *602*, 1977.

Wistreich, G. A., and Lechtman, M. D.: Microbiology and Human Disease. Beverly Hills, CA, Glencoe Press, 1976.

Wollheim, F. A., and Williams, R. C.: Studies on the macroglobulins of human serum. I. Polyclonal immunoglobulin class M (IgM) increase in infectious mononucleosis. N. Engl. J. Med., *274*:61, 1966.

Worlledge, S. M., and Dacie, J. V.: Haemolytic and other anaemias in infectious mononucleosis. *In* Carter, R. L., and Penman, H. G. (Eds.): Infectious Mononucleosis. Oxford, Blackwell Scientific Publications, 1969.

Zak, S. J., and Good, R. A.: Immunochemical studies of human serum gamma globulins. J. Clin. Invest., *38*:579, 1959.

ANSWERS

CHAPTER 1: **INTRODUCTION: NONSPECIFIC (NATURAL, INNATE) IMMUNITY**

1. **b**	6. **b, c, d**	11. **a, b, c, d**	16. **F**
2. **a, b, c, d**	7. **a, c**	12. **a, c**	17. **F**
3. **c**	8. **a, b, c, d**	13. **F**	18. **T**
4. **a, b, c, d**	9. **c**	14. **T**	19. **T**
5. **b**	10. **a, b, c**	15. **T**	20. **F**

CHAPTER 2: **SPECIFIC IMMUNITY**

1. **d**	11. **a**	21. **a, c, d**	31. **F**
2. **a, b, c**	12. **a**	22. **b, c**	32. **T**
3. **a, b, c, d**	13. **c**	23. **d**	33. **F**
4. **a**	14. **b**	24. **a**	34. **F**
5. **c**	15. **b, c**	25. **d**	35. **T**
6. **c**	16. **c**	26. **F**	36. **T**
7. **c**	17. **a, c, d**	27. **T**	37. **T**
8. **c**	18. **c**	28. **T**	
9. **a, b**	19. **b, c**	29. **F**	
10. **a, c, d**	20. **a, b, c**	30. **T**	

CHAPTER 3: **COMPLEMENT**

1. **a, c**	11. **b**	21. **T**
2. **b, c**	12. **a, b, c, d**	22. **F**
3. **a, d**	13. **a, b, c**	23. **F**
4. **c**	14. **c**	24. **T**
5. **a**	15. **a, c, d**	25. **T**
6. **b, d**	16. **T**	26. **T**
7. **c**	17. **F**	27. **T**
8. **a**	18. **T**	28. **F**
9. **a, c**	19. **F**	29. **T**
10. **a**	20. **T**	30. **F**

CHAPTER 4: **THE IMMUNE RESPONSE**

1.	a, b, d	11.	b, d	21.	T
2.	c, d	12.	c, d	22.	T
3.	a, b, c, d	13.	a, c, d	23.	F
4.	a	14.	d	24.	F
5.	c	15.	c	25.	T
6.	a, b, c, d	16.	a, c	26.	T
7.	d	17.	b, d	27.	T
8.	b, c	18.	b, c	28.	F
9.	a, b, c, d	19.	b, c	29.	F
10.	a, b	20.	a, b, c, d	30.	T

CHAPTER 5: **THE ANTIGEN–ANTIBODY REACTION** *IN VITRO*

1.	b, c	5.	a, b, c, d	9.	b, d	13.	F
2.	b	6.	a, b, c	10.	a, d	14.	F
3.	b	7.	a, b, c, d	11.	T	15.	T
4.	a	8.	a, c	12.	T	16.	T

CHAPTER 6: **SYPHILIS**

1.	b	11.	a, b, c, d	21.	a, b, c, d
2.	c	12.	b	22.	a, b, c
3.	a	13.	a, b, c, d	23.	T
4.	d	14.	b	24.	F
5.	a, b, c	15.	a, d	25.	F
6.	d	16.	d	26.	T
7.	b	17.	d	27.	T
8.	a, b, c	18.	b	28.	T
9.	b	19.	a, c	29.	F
10.	a, b, d	20.	a, b, c	30.	F

CHAPTER 7: **HEPATITIS**

1.	a, b, c, d	11.	b, c, d	21.	b
2.	a	12.	a, b, c, d	22.	a
3.	b, c, d	13.	d	23.	T
4.	c, d	14.	a, b, c, d	24.	T
5.	a, b	15.	a, b, c, d	25.	T
6.	a, b, d	16.	a, b, c	26.	F
7.	a, c	17.	b	27.	F
8.	a	18.	a, b, c, d	28.	T
9.	c	19.	b, d	29.	F
10.	b, c	20.	c	30.	T

CHAPTER 8: **C–REACTIVE PROTEIN**

1.	a, c, d	5.	a, b, c, d	9.	d	13.	F
2.	a, b, c, d	6.	b, d	10.	a	14.	F
3.	b	7.	b, c	11.	F	15.	T
4.	b, c	8.	a	12.	T		

CHAPTER 9: **STREPTOLYSIN O**

1.	a, c	5.	a	9.	b, d	13.	F
2.	a, c	6.	b	10.	b	14.	T
3.	b	7.	d	11.	T	15.	F
4.	a, d	8.	c	12.	T		

CHAPTER 10: **COLD AGGLUTININS: STREPTOCOCCUS MG**

1.	a, d	6.	a, b, c	11.	T	16.	T
2.	d	7.	b, d	12.	T	17.	F
3.	a, b	8.	c, d	13.	F	18.	T
4.	a, c	9.	a, c, d	14.	F		
5.	a, c	10.	a	15.	F		

CHAPTER 11: **INFECTIOUS MONONUCLEOSIS**

1.	a, d	5.	a, b, c, d	9.	a, c, d	13.	F
2.	d	6.	a, b, d	10.	a, c	14.	F
3.	a, b	7.	a, b, c, d	11.	T	15.	F
4.	d	8.	a, c	12.	T	16.	T

CHAPTER 12: **AUTOIMMUNE DISEASES**

1.	a, b, d	8.	a, b, c	15.	a	22.	T
2.	b, c	9.	b, c, d	16.	a, c	23.	T
3.	c	10.	a, b	17.	a, b, c, d	24.	T
4.	a, b, c, d	11.	b, c, d	18.	F	25.	F
5.	a, b, d	12.	a, b, c, d	19.	T		
6.	a, b	13.	a, b	20.	F		
7.	a, c, d	14.	a, b	21.	T		

CHAPTER 13: **THE ENTEROBACTERIACEAE**

1.	a, c	5.	c	9.	a	13.	F
2.	b, d	6.	b	10.	c	14.	F
3.	a, b, c	7.	a, b	11.	T	15.	T
4.	a, b, d	8.	a	12.	T	16.	T

CHAPTER 14: **FUNGAL ANTIBODY TESTS, FEBRILE ANTI-BODY TESTS, VIRAL ANTIBODY TESTS**

1. **a**	5. **b**	9. **a**	13. **T**
2. **a, b, c, d**	6. **d**	10. **T**	14. **F**
3. **a**	7. **b**	11. **T**	15. **T**
4. **c**	8. **a, b, c**	12. **F**	

CHAPTER 15: **COMPLEMENT LEVELS**

1. **a, b, c, d**	4. **a, b, d**	7. **a**	10. **T**
2. **b, d**	5. **c**	8. **T**	11. **T**
3. **a, b, c**	6. **b, c, d**	9. **F**	12. **T**

CHAPTER 16: **MISCELLANEOUS SEROLOGY**

1. **c**	4. **a**	7. **a, c, d**	10. **F**
2. **a, b, c, d**	5. **a, c**	8. **T**	11. **T**
3. **b, c, d**	6. **a**	9. **T**	12. **F**

GLOSSARY

ABO Antigens The antigens of the major human blood group system.

Absorption The removal of antibodies from serum by the addition of red cells that possess the corresponding surface antigen.

Accuracy A term used to describe the proximity of the "average" value and the "true" value.

Acquired Antigen An antigen that is not genetically determined and is sometimes transient.

Acquired Immunity Immunity that is developed subsequent to birth. The acquisition of immunity in the form of immunologically competent cells from an immune donor.

Activated Macrophage A macrophage from an antigen-sensitized or otherwise stimulated animal.

Active Immunity Immunity that is generated by the actual production of antibody by the host in response to foreign antigen.

Adjuvant A substance that can increase the specific antibody production to, or the degree of sensitization against, an antigen by increasing its size or length of survival in the circulation. A substance (usually injected with an antigen) that improves the immune response, either humoral or cellular, to the antigen.

Adsorption The attachment of one substance to the surface of another; in particular, the attachment of antibody to specific receptors on a cell surface.

Agammaglobulinemia A condition in which all the immunoglobulins are missing (absent) from a serum.

Agglutination The aggregation or clumping of cellular or particulate antigens by an antiserum containing antibodies to one or more of the surface antigens.

Agglutinin An antibody that is capable of causing agglutination with surface antigens.

Agglutinogen Another term for red cell antigen.

Alexin An old term for "complement."

Allele The alternative form(s) of a gene at a particular locus.

Allergen A substance that causes an allergy (i.e., that stimulates IgE synthesis or causes a delayed hypersensitivity).

Allergy An altered state of reactivity to an allergen (i.e., usually antigen or hapten). The term is used synonymously with *hypersensitivity*.

Alloantibody An antibody that reacts with an antigen from another animal of the *same* species.

Alloantigen An antigen that is present in other members of one's own species.

Allogeneic Being of different genetic (and therefore antigenic) type within one species.

Allograft A tissue graft in which the donor and the recipient are the same individual (or are genetically identical).

Alloimmunization The immunization of an individual with antigens from within the same species.

Alternative Complement Pathway A system for activating complement beginning at C3 and not involving a serologic reaction.

Amino Acid Any one of a class of organic compounds containing the amino (NH_2) group and the carboxyl (COOH) group. Amino acids form the chief structure of proteins.

Anamnestic Response A rapid rise in immunoglobulin concentration following a second or subsequent exposure to antigen. Also known as "secondary" or "booster" response.

Anaphylactic Allergy An allergy that is caused by IgE.

Anaphylatoxin Specific peptides from complement fractions 3 and 5, which release histamine from mast cells and basophils. (Note: originally believed to be a substance that caused histamine release.)

Anaphylatoxin Inhibitor The anaphylatoxin inhibitor is an enzyme that destroys the biologic activity of C3a and C5a (complement components).

Anaphylaxis An unexpected, detrimental reaction to a second exposure to antigen in which histamine, serotonin, etc. are released by reaction of the antigen with IgE on the surface of mast cells.

Anergy The inability to respond to an antigen (especially in the allergic sense).

Antibody A globulin formed in response to exposure to an antigen; an immunoglobulin.

Antigen A macromolecule that, when introduced into a foreign circulation, will induce the formation of immunoglobulins or sensitized cells that react specifically with that antigen.

Antigen Competition The failure of a mixture of antigens to stimulate as high a titered antiserum to one or more of the antigens, compared with when the antigens are administered independently.

Antigen Determinant Sites Unique portions of the structure of an antigen that are responsible for its activity.

Antiglobulin Test A test used to determine the presence of a globulin using an antibody to that globulin.

Antiserum A serum containing antibodies.

Antitoxin An antibody (or antiserum) prepared in response to a toxin or toxoid.

Arthus Reaction A necrotic, dermal reaction caused by antigen-antibody precipitation, complement fixation, and neutrophilic inflammation in tissues of an animal inoculated intracutaneously with antigen.

Attenuation Weakening the virulence of a pathogenic organism while retaining its viability.

Autoantigen A molecule that behaves as a "self" antigen.

Autocoupling Hapten A hapten that can combine spontaneously with a carrier.

Bacteria Large groups of unicellular microorganisms, existing morphologically as oval or spherical cells (cocci), rods (bacilli), spirals (spirilla), or comma-shaped organisms (vibrios).

Bacteriortropin An immune opsonin that stimulates phagocytosis of a bacterium, other cell type, or particle.

Basophil A blood granulocyte whose granules release histamine during anaphylactic reactions.

B Cell A lymphocyte from the bursa of Fabricius or that is of the immunoglobulin-forming type.

Bence Jones Protein An immunoglobulin L chain that is found in the urine or blood of patients with a myeloma.

Blastogenic Factor A lymphokine that stimulates T cell growth.

Blocking Antibody An antibody that prevents (blocks) the action of another antibody.

Blood Group Antigen Antigens that are genetically determined and present on the surface of erythrocytes.

Boivin Antigen A heat-stable antigen that is extractable from gram-negative bacteria. It can, for the most part, be considered synonymous with *endotoxin*.

Booster Response See *Anamnestic response*.

Buffer Any substance(s) in solution that resist changes in pH.

Bursa of Fabricius A cloacal organ in fowl from which the immunoglobulin-synthesizing B lymphocytes originate.

C1 Esterase An esterase that is formed subsequent to the activation of the C1s component of complement.

Capping Phenomenon The movement of antigens on the surface of B lymphocytes to a single position (or locus).

Cell-Mediated Immunity Immunity that is dependent on T lymphocytes and phagocytic cells.

Central Lymphoid Tissue Bone marrow, thymus, and bursa of Fabricius.

Chemotaxis Attraction of leukocytes or other cells by chemicals; with respect to white blood cells, the term can be used synonymously with *leukotaxin*.

Classic Complement Pathway The major system of complement activation that involves all nine components of complement and is initiated by a serologic reaction.

Cold Agglutinin An agglutinin or hemagglutinin that is active at 4°C but not at 37°C.

Complement Fixation The fixation (or binding) of complement in a reaction with antigen and antibody.

Complementoid An "altered" type of complement (usually partly damaged, for example, by heating) that is capable of combining with sensitized cells without producing the usual lysis and that is also capable of blocking the normal action of complement.

Con A (Abbr) Concanavalin A

Concanavalin A A mitogen highly specific for T lymphocytes.

Conglutinin A protein that is normally present in bovine serum that reacts with the C3 component of complement.

Constant Domain The region in an immunoglobulin whose amino acid sequence is identical to the sequence in another region.

Counterimmunoelectrophoresis The electrophoresis of antigen and antibody toward one another through a gel medium.

Cross-reactive Antigen An antigen so structurally similar to a second antigen that it will react with antibody to the second antigen.

Cryoglobulin Globulin that precipitates from serum at 0 to 4°C.

Disulfide Bonds The links between antibody molecule chains.

Domain A section or region in the peptide chain of an immunoglobulin.

Electrophoresis (of serum) The separation of serum proteins according to their rate of travel when an electric current is passed through a buffer solution. The supporting medium can be Whatman paper, starch, or agar gels.

Enzyme-linked Immunosorbent Assay A serologic test in which one of the reagents is labeled with an enzyme (ELISA).

Eosinophil A white blood cell that contains cytoplasmic granules with an affinity for acid dyes (also referred to as an *acidophil*).

Epitope An antigenic determinant.

Equivalence Point The point of dilution in a serologic reaction in which all the antigen and all the antibody are mutually involved in complexes.

Fab Fragment The fragment of an antibody molecule that is capable of antigen binding. It consists of a light chain and part of a heavy chain of the molecule.

Fc Fragment The fragment of the antibody molecule that in certain species can be crystallized. It consists of two pieces of heavy chain.

Flocculation A specific type of precipitation that occurs over a narrow range of antigen concentration, aggregation of colloidal particles in a serologic reaction (as in syphilis serology).

Fluorescent Antibody An antibody (immunoglobulin) that is conjugated to a fluorescent dye for use in ultraviolet microscopy.

Gammopathy An imbalance in immunoglobulin concentration.

Globulin A class of proteins to which antibodies belong. They can be separated by electrophoresis into alpha, beta, and gamma fractions.

Gm Group An allotypic group based on antigenic changes in H chain antigens of IgG.

Graft-Versus-Host Reaction A reaction resulting from the attack of immunocompetent tissue in a graft against an immunologically compromised host.

Granulocyte A collective term for white blood cells with pronounced cytoplasmic granulation.

H-2 The major histocompatibility antigen system of mice.

Half-life The time taken to decrease to half the original value.

H Antigen The flagella antigens of bacteria.

Haplotype One half of the histocompatibility genes that are present on one chromosome and are inherited from one parent.

Hapten A nonantigenic material that, when combined with an antigen, conveys a new antigenic specificity on the antigen.

H Chain (Abbr) The heavy chain of an immunoglobulin. Two such heavy chains exist in the basic four-peptide structure of an immunoglobulin.

HDN (Abbr) See *Hemolytic disease of the newborn*.

Heavy Chain See H chain.

Helper Cell A subclass of T cells that assists B cells in antibody formation.

Hemagglutination The agglutination (or clumping) of red blood cells, especially by antiserum.

Hemolysin An antibody that, in cooperation with serum complement, will cause the hemolysis of erythrocytes.

Hemolysis The lysis of red blood cells by specific antibody and serum complement.

Hemolytic Disease of the Newborn (HDN) A disease of the newborn in which maternal antibodies cross the placenta and contribute to the destruction of fetal red cells.

Heteroimmunization The immunization of an individual with antigens from another species.

Heterophil Antigen An antigen that is broadly distributed in nature.

Hinge Region The region of the H chain of an immunoglobulin near where the L chain joins it and near the sites of papain and pepsin cleavage. It allows the immunoglobulin to have flexibility.

Histamine A specific chemical compound that is released from mast cells and produces vasodilation, smooth muscle contraction, and edema during anaphylaxis.

Histocompatibility Antigen The antigen on a cell surface that, upon transplantation into a different host, induces a response that leads to graft rejection. Also known as *transplant antigen*.

HLA (Abbr) Human leukocyte antigen. The major histocompatibility antigen system in humans.

Horror Autotoxicus A term used to describe the inability of an antigen to serve as an autoantigen.

H Substance An antigen on human red cells that acts as a precursor for the A and B antigens.

Humoral Immunity Immunity that results from the formation of antibody.

Hypersensitivity An unexpected, exaggerated reaction to an antigen. The term is used synonymously with *allergy*.

Hypogammaglobulinemia Decreased levels of gamma globulin in plasma.

IFN (Abbr) See *Interferon*.

IL-1 (Abbr) See *Interleukin 1*.

IL-2 (Abbr) See *Interleukin 2*.

Immune Adherence A term referring to the "adhesive" nature of antigen-antibidy complexes to inert substances when complement is fixed.

Immune-associated Antigen An antigen present on B lymphocytes and macrophages and inherited with Ir genes (short form is Ia antigen).

Immediate Hypersensitivities Allergy that is related to IgE or to similar immunoglobulins in lower species such as hay fever, food allergies, certain drug allergies, and other allergies of the intermediate type.

Immune Complex A complex of antigen with antibody (which may involve complement) that can be soluble or can deposit on tissues.

Immune Response Any reaction demonstrating specific antibody response to antigenic stimulus.

Immune Response Gene A structural gene in the major histocompatibility complex that exerts a regulatory role on the immune response.

Immune Suppression The suppression of an immunologic response by chemical, physical, or biologic means.

Immunity The condition of resistance to infection.

Immunization The process by which an antibody is produced in response to antigenic stimulus.

Immunoblast A cell intermediate between the lymphocyte and plasma cell.

Immunoconglutinin An antibody directed against the antigenic sites of the C3 component of complement that is revealed or created by antigen-antibody fixing of complement.

Immunocyte A cell that is capable of synthesizing immunoglobulin.

Immunodominant Region The most potent epitope (antigenic determinant) in an antigen.

Immunogen Antigen.

Immunologic Tolerance A failure (or depression) in the immune response on proper exposure to antigen (especially massive doses). Also sometimes known as *immune paralysis*.

Inherited Immunity Immunity resulting from genetic factors (*i.e.,* genetic constitution) that is not the result of exposure to infectious agents.

Inhibition The prevention of a normal reaction between an antigen and its corresponding antibody, usually because an antigen of the same specificity but from another source is present in the serum.

Interferon Protein(s) released from a cell that is infected with an intracellular parasite, which protects neighboring cells from invasion by the same or other intracellular parasites.

Interleukin (IL) A monokine that acts on other leukocytes.

Interleukin 1 (IL-1) A monokine that activates T cells and possibly B cells.

Interleukin 2 (IL-2) A monokine that serves as a growth factor for T cells.

In Vitro Outside the body.

In Vivo Inside the body.

Ir Gene An immune response gene.

Isoantigen An antigen present in another member of one's own species (also known as alloantigen).

Isohemagglutinin An antibody of an animal that will agglutinate the red cells of another animal of the same species. Also referred to as *isoagglutinin*.

Isoimmunization Immunization of an individual with antigens of another individual of the same species.

Isotype A synonym of class (when referring to immunoglobulins).

J Chain A polypeptide chain found attached to secretory IgA and IgM that may function as a joining chain.

Kupffer's Cell A macrophage of the liver.

Laked Hemolyzed.

Langerhans' Cells Macrophages found in the skin.

LC (Abbr) See *Langerhans' cells*.

L Chain (Abbr) The light chain of an immunoglobulin: two such chains exist in the four-peptide unit of an immunoglobulin.

Lectin An extract from seeds that possesses the ability to agglutinate red cells (usually directed against a specific antigen).

Leukocyte A white cell.

Light Chain See *L chain*.

Locus The position on a chromosome occupied by a gene.

LPS (Abbr) Lipopolysaccharide, the endotoxic portion of the cell wall of most gram-negative bacteria; mitogenic for B lymphocytes.

Lymphocyte The agranular leukocyte with sparse cytoplasm and round nucleus derived from the thymus (T type) or bone marrow or bursa (B type) found in lymph, lymph nodes, blood, spleen, etc.

Lymphocyte Transformation The active nucleic acid metabolism and nuclear enlargement of a lymphocyte on contact with antigen.

Lymphotoxins A family of lymphokines that are cytolytic for target cells.

Lyt Marker An antigen marker on T lymphocytes.

Macrophage A tissue or blood phagocyte, 20 to 80 μm in diameter, containing lysosomes, vacuoles, and partially digested debris in its cytoplasm.

Major Histocompatibility Complex A collection of structural genes associated with transplantation antigens and the immune response.

M Component The serum protein produced in excessive concentration in cases of myeloma or macroglobulinemia.

Memory Cell A cell that responds more quickly to the second exposure to antigen than to the primary exposure and is responsible for the anamnestic response.

MHC (Abbr) See *Major histocompatibility complex*.

Mitogen A substance that stimulates mitosis.

Monocyte A white blood cell, 12 to 30 μm in diameter, with rounded nucleus. A precursor to macrophages.

Monokine A protein elaborated by a monocyte or macrophage that acts on other host cells.

Multiple Myeloma See *Myeloma.*

Myeloma A plasma cell neoplasm resulting in excessive production of one or more immunoglobulins.

Myeloperoxidase An enzyme in lysosomes that aids intraphagocyte killing.

Natural Resistance See *Inherited immunity.*

Neoantigen A "new" antigen, formed by modification of an "old" antigen by haptenic addition or other means.

Neutrophil A leukocyte with granules that are not predominant in their affinity for acid or basic dyes.

O Antigen The surface somatic antigens of bacteria, *or* one of the antigens of the ABO blood group system.

Opsonin An antibody that attaches to a cellular or particulate antigen and that "prepares" it for phagocytosis.

Optimal Proportions The point of dilution in a serologic reaction that gives a positive reaction.

Paraproteinemia The presence of protein molecules in plasma that are antigenically similar to, but lack the biologic activity of, normal molecules, especially regarding immunoglobulins.

Passive Hemagglutination Hemagglutination resulting from antibodies that are directed against antigens adsorbed to the erythrocyte surface.

Passive Immunity Immunity that results from contribution of protection (*e.g.,* antibody) from one individual to another.

Passive Immunization The acquisition of immunity through the injection of antibodies or antiserum produced by another animal.

Peripheral Lymphoid Tissue Lymphoid tissues other than bone marrow, thymus, and bursa.

Phagocytosis The engulfment of cells or particulate matter by leukocytes, macrophages, or other cells.

Phlebotomy The removal (withdrawal) of blood from a vein.

Phytohemagglutinin An extract of plants, usually legumes, that will agglutinate red cells.

Plasma Cell A cell 10 to 20 μm in diameter that can actively synthesize immunoglobulins and can be distinguished morphologically from similar cells.

PMN (Abbr) See *Polymorphonuclear neutrophilic leukocyte.*

Polymorphonuclear Neutrophilic Leukocyte A white blood cell with a granular cytoplasm and a multi-lobed nucleus that is very active in phagocytosis.

Postzone The failure of a serologic reaction to occur in extreme dilutions of the antibody.

Precipitation The formation of an insoluble complex of antibody with soluble antigen.

Precursor Substance A substance in a stage of a process that precedes a later development.

Primary Response The initial response to a foreign antigen.

Protein A A protein on the surface of *Staphylococcus aureus* that binds IgG.

Prozone The failure of a serologic reaction to occur in high concentration of the antibody.

Pseudoagglutination The clumping of cells caused by agents other than antibodies.

Radioimmunoassay An immunologic test using radio-labeled antigen, antibody, complement, or other reactants.

Reagin IgE, with specificity for allergens; *or* syphilitic reagin, with specificity for cardiolipin antigens.

RES (Abbr) See *Reticuloendothelial system.*

Reticulocyte A type of immature erythrocyte.

Reticuloendothelial Blockade Malfunction of phagocytic cells by prior exposure to phagocytosable particles.

Reticuloendothelial System A collective term for cells of varying morphology and tissue residence, with the common feature of being actively phagocytic.

Rheumatoid Factor An IgM with specificity toward IgG, which is associated with arthritis.

RIA (Abbr) See *Radioimmunoassay.*

SC (Abbr) See *Secretory component.*

Secondary Response See *Anamnestic response.*

Secretory Component A portion of secretory IgA and secretory IgM not present in serum IgA or IgM and not produced in plasma cells.

Secretory Immunoglobulin An immunoglobulin found in colostrum, saliva, mucous secretions, etc., as secretory IgA or secretory IgM.

Sequestered Antigen An antigen not found in the circulatory system.

Serum Sickness A reaction caused by the presence of antigen at the time antibody is being formed.

Shared Antigen A cross-reactive antigen (*i.e.,* one that will react with an antibody induced by some other antigen).

Solid Phase Radioimmunoassay A radioimmunoassay in which one of the reactants is bound to a surface.

Soluble Immune Response Suppressor A lymphokine that suppresses B cells.

Specificity The special affinity between an antigen and its corresponding antibody.

Suppressor Cell A subclass of T cells that suppresses the capacity of B cells to become immunoglobulin producers.

T Cell–Dependent Antigen An antigen that requires the cooperation of T and B cells to induce specific antibody production.

T Cell Growth Factor See *Interleukin 2.*

T Cell–Independent Antigen An antigen that does not require the cooperation of B and T cells in the production of specific antibody.

TGGF (Abbr) T cell growth factor. See *Interleukin 2*.

Th Cell A T helper cell.

THY 1 Antigen An antigen found on T cells.

Thymoroirtin A thymic hormone.

Thymosin A hormone-like substance from thymus believed to be the active component of T lymphocytes.

Thymus A gland located near the parathyroid and thyroid whose lymphocytes (T type) regulate cell-mediated hypersensitivity and interact with B cells for immunoglobulin formation.

Titer The greatest dilution of a substance used in a serologic reaction that will produce the desired result.

T Lymphocyte (T Cell) A thymus-derived lymphocyte responsible for cell-mediated hypersensitivity.

Tolerance A state of specific nonreactivity to an antigen due to prior exposure to the same antigen under special circumstances. In short, the failure to respond to antigenic stimulus.

Toxoid A toxin treated to preserve its native antigenicity but to eliminate its toxicity.

Ts Cell A T suppressor cell.

Vaccination The inoculation or ingestion of organisms or antigens to produce immunity to those organisms in the recipient.

Vaccine A suspension of living or dead organisms used as an antigen and injected into individuals as protection against disease.

Variable Domain A region in an immunoglobulin whose amino acid sequence is not constant from one molecular species to another.

Waldenström's Macroglobulinemia A myeloma involving IgM or IgM-like molecules.

Warm Agglutinin An antibody (agglutinin) or hemagglutinin that is active at 37°C but not at 4°C.

Witebsky's Postulates A set of conditions that must be met before a disease can be considered to be an autoimmune disease.

Xenoantigen An antigen present in another species.

Xenoimmunization The immunization of an individual with antigens from another species (also known as *heteroimmunization*).

INDEX

Page numbers followed by (t) refer to tables.

213